T0259209

Approach to Consultations for Patients with Liver Disease

Guest Editor

STEVEN L. FLAMM, MD

CLINICS IN LIVER DISEASE

www.liver.theclinics.com

Consulting Editor
NORMAN GITLIN, MD

May 2012 • Volume 16 • Number 2

SAUNDERS an imprint of ELSEVIER, Inc.

W.B. SAUNDERS COMPANY

A Division of Elsevier Inc.

1600 John F. Kennedy Boulevard, Suite 1800 • Philadelphia, PA 19103-2899

http://www.theclinics.com

CLINICS IN LIVER DISEASE Volume 16, Number 2
May 2012 ISSN 1089-3261, ISBN-13: 978-1-4557-3886-1

Editor: Kerry Holland
Developmental Editor: Donald Mumford

Clinics in Liver Disease (ISSN 1089-3261) is published quarterly by Elsevier Inc., 360 Park Avenue South, New York, NY 10010-1710. Months of issue are February, May, August, and November. Business and Editorial Offices: 1600 John F. Kennedy Blvd., Ste. 1800, Philadelphia, PA 19103-2899. Customer Service Office: 3251 Riverport Lane, Maryland Heights, MO 63043. Periodicals postage paid at New York, NY and additional mailing offices. Subscription prices are $271.00 per year (U.S. individuals), $134.00 per year (U.S. student/resident), $365.00 per year (U.S. institutions), $360.00 per year (foreign individuals), $185.00 per year (foreign student/ resident), $440.00 per year (foreign instituitions), $313.00 per year (Canadian individuals), $185.00 per year (Canadian student/resident), and $440.00 per year (Canadian institutions). Foreign air speed delivery is included in all *Clinics* subscription prices. All prices are subject to change without notice. **POSTMASTER:** Send address changes to *Clinics in Liver Disease*, Elsevier Health Sciences Division, Subscription Customer Service, 3251 Riverport Lane, Maryland Heights, MO 63043. **Customer Service: Telephone: 1-800-654-2452 (U.S. and Canada); 314-447-8871 (outside U.S. and Canada). Fax: 314-447-8029. E-mail: journalscustomerservice-usa@elsevier.com (for print support); journalsonlinesupport-usa@elsevier.com (for online support).**

Reprints. For copies of 100 or more of articles in this publication, please contact the Commercial Reprints Department, Elsevier Inc., 360 Park Avenue South, New York, NY 10010-1710. Tel.: 212-633-3812; Fax: 212-462-1935; E-mail: reprints@elsevier.com.

Clinics in Liver Disease is covered in *MEDLINE/PubMed (Index Medicus)*, Science Citation Index Expanded, Journal Citation Reports/Science Edition, and Current Contents/Clinical Medicine.

Printed and bound by CPI Group (UK) Ltd, Croydon, CR0 4YY
Transferred to Digital Print 2012

Contributors

CONSULTING EDITOR

NORMAN GITLIN, MD, FRCP (LONDON), FRCPE (EDINBURGH), FACG, FACP
Formerly, Professor of Medicine, Chief of Hepatology, Emory University; Currently, Consultant, Atlanta Gastroenterology Associates, Atlanta, Georgia

GUEST EDITOR

STEVEN L. FLAMM, MD
Professor of Medicine and Surgery, Medical Director, Liver Transplantation, Department of Medicine, Division of Gastroenterology and Hepatology, Northwestern University Feinberg School of Medicine, Chicago, Illinois

AUTHORS

NEZAM AFDHAL, MD
Department of Medicine, Liver Center, Beth Israel Deaconess Medical Center, Harvard Medical School, Boston, Massachusetts

ALAN BONDER, MD
Department of Medicine, Liver Center, Beth Israel Deaconess Medical Center, Harvard Medical School, Boston, Massachusetts

ROBERT S. BROWN Jr, MD, MPH
Frank Cardile Professor of Medicine, Center for Liver Disease and Transplantation, New York Presbyterian Hospital; Columbia University College of Physicians and Surgeons, New York, New York

CHALERMRAT BUNCHORNTAVAKUL, MD
Division of Gastroenterology and Hepatology, Department of Medicine, University of Pennsylvania, Philadelphia, Pennsylvania; Department of Medicine, Rajavithi Hospital, College of Medicine, Rangsit University, Rajthewi, Bangkok, Thailand

GINA CHOI, MD
Department of Medicine, David Geffen School of Medicine, University of California, Los Angeles, Los Angeles, California

TIMOTHY J. DAVERN, MD
Director, Acute Liver Failure Program, Department of Transplantation, California Pacific Medical Center, San Francisco, California

STEVEN L. FLAMM, MD
Professor of Medicine and Surgery, Medical Director, Liver Transplantation, Department of Medicine, Division of Gastroenterology and Hepatology, Northwestern University Feinberg School of Medicine, Chicago, Illinois

ALYSON N. FOX, MD, MSCE
Assistant Professor of Medicine, Center for Liver Disease and Transplantation, New York Presbyterian Hospital; Weill Cornell Medical Center, New York, New York

ROBERT GISH, MD
Professor of Clinical Medicine, Division of Gastroenterology, University of California, San Diego, San Diego, California

FREDRIC D. GORDON, MD
Associate Professor of Medicine, Tufts Medical School, Boston, Massachusetts; Director of Hepatology, Lahey Clinic Medical Center, Burlington, Massachusetts

STEPHEN A. HARRISON, MD
Division of Gastroenterology and Hepatology, Department of Medicine, Brooke Army Medical Center, San Antonio Military Medical Center, Fort Sam Houston, Texas

VANDANA KHUNGAR, MD, MSc
Gastroenterology Fellow, Department of Medicine, Cedars-Sinai Medical Center; Department of Medicine, David Geffen School of Medicine, University of California, Los Angeles, Los Angeles, California

W. RAY KIM, MD
Division of Gastroenterology and Hepatology (PL 6), Mayo Clinic College of Medicine, Rochester, Minnesota

KRIS V. KOWDLEY, MD, FACP
Director, Liver Center of Excellence, Digestive Disease Institute, Virginia Mason Medical Center, Benaroya Research Institute, Seattle, Washington

ALEXANDER KUO, MD
Associate Professor of Clinical Medicine, Division of Gastroenterology, University of California, San Diego, San Diego, California

PAUL Y. KWO, MD
Professor of Medicine, Medical Director, Liver Transplantation, Gastroenterology/Hepatology Division, Indiana University School of Medicine, Indianapolis, Indiana

TAE HOON LEE, MD
Clinical Associate Professor, Department of Internal Medicine, Marshall University, Huntington, West Virginia

ARJMAND R. MUFTI, MD, MRCP
Fellow, Department of Medicine, Section of Gastroenterology, Hepatology and Nutrition, University of Chicago Medical Center, Chicago, Illinois

ANDREW J. MUIR, MD, MHS
Director, Gastroenterology/Hepatology Research, Division of Gastroenterology, Duke Clinical Research Institute, Duke University School of Medicine, Durham, North Carolina

ANGELO H. PAREDES, MD
Division of Gastroenterology, Department of Medicine, Walter Reed National Military Medical Center, Bethesda, Maryland

FRED POORDAD, MD
Professor, Department of Medicine; Department of Surgery, Cedars-Sinai Medical Center, Los Angeles, California

JOHN J. POTERUCHA, MD
Division of Gastroenterology and Hepatology, Mayo Clinic College of Medicine, Rochester, Minnesota

NANCY REAU, MD
Associate Professor of Medicine, Department of Medicine, Section of Gastroenterology, Hepatology and Nutrition, University of Chicago Medical Center, Chicago, Illinois

K. RAJENDER REDDY, MD
Professor of Medicine, Division of Gastroenterology and Hepatology, Department of Medicine, University of Pennsylvania, Philadelphia, Pennsylvania

BRUCE ALLEN RUNYON, MD
Clinical Professor of Medicine, Director of Hepatology, Department of Medicine, University of California, Santa Monica, Santa Monica, California

ASMA SIDDIQUE, MD
Fellow in Hepatology, Department of Gastroenterology, Center for Liver Disease, Digestive Disease Institute, Seattle, Washington

DAWN M. TORRES, MD
Division of Gastroenterology, Department of Medicine, Walter Reed National Military Medical Center, Bethesda, Maryland

Contents

is important that liver disease during pregnancy is recognized because early diagnosis may improve maternal and fetal outcomes, with resultant decreased morbidity and mortality. Liver diseases that occur in pregnancy can be divided into 3 different groups: liver diseases that are unique to pregnancy, liver diseases that are not unique to pregnancy but can be revealed or exacerbated by pregnancy, and liver diseases that are unrelated to but occur coincidentally during pregnancy.

Evaluation of Liver Lesions **271**

Alan Bonder and Nezam Afdhal

The differential diagnosis of a liver mass is large and requires understanding of the clinical and imaging features of liver lesions. A detailed history, physical examination, hepatic biochemical tests, and imaging studies are all essential in making the diagnosis. Decisions regarding specific imaging modalities for diagnoses, the use of liver biopsy, therapeutic options, and appropriate follow-up are all determined by the presentation of the lesion and associated patient characteristics.

Ascites **285**

Fredric D. Gordon

Ascites is the pathologic accumulation of fluid in the peritoneum. It is the most common complication of cirrhosis, with a prevalence of approximately 10%. Over a 10-year period, 50% of patients with previously compensated cirrhosis are expected to develop ascites. As a marker of hepatic decompensation, ascites is associated with a poor prognosis, with only a 56% survival 3 years after onset. In addition, morbidity is increased because of the risk of additional complications, such as spontaneous bacterial peritonitis and hepatorenal syndrome. Understanding the pathophysiology of ascites is essential for its proper management.

Hepatic Encephalopathy **301**

Vandana Khungar and Fred Poordad

Hepatic encephalopathy (HE) represents a continuum of transient and reversible neurologic and psychiatric dysfunction. It is a reversible state of impaired cognitive function or altered consciousness in patients with liver disease or portosystemic shunting. Over the last several years, high-quality studies have been conducted on various pharmacologic therapies for HE; as more data emerge, it is hoped that HE will become a more easily treated complication of decompensated liver disease. In the interim, it is important that physicians continue to screen for minimal HE and treat patients early in addition to continuing to provide current treatments of overt HE.

Shortness of Breath in the Patient with Chronic Liver Disease **321**

Paul Y. Kwo

Shortness of breath is a common complaint in those with chronic liver disease. The differential diagnosis for this complaint includes primary pulmonary disorders, systemic disorders that affect the liver and lungs, and extrahepatic manifestations of portal hypertension. Orthotopic liver transplant, when appropriate, is the most effective therapy for many patients

with dyspnea and chronic liver disease, although therapies to treat the underlying complications of cirrhosis may provide relief. Shortness of breath in patients with cirrhosis often portends a poor prognosis, and these patients should be evaluated for orthotopic liver transplant because this therapy is most likely to provide long-lasting benefit.

Pruritus in Chronic Cholestatic Liver Disease 331

Chalermrat Bunchorntavakul and K. Rajender Reddy

Pruritus is a troublesome complication in patients with cholestatic liver disease. Several links to its pathogenesis have been proposed, including the role of bile acids, endogenous opioid and serotonins, and lysophosphatidic acid. The management of pruritus in cholestasis is challenging. Medical treatment of the underlying cholestatic condition may provide benefit. Extracorporeal albumin dialysis can be pursued for those who have a poor quality of life and failed the various therapeutic interventions, while awaiting liver transplantation. Experimental interventions, and the management of pruritus in certain conditions such as intrahepatic cholestasis of pregnancy and benign recurrent intrahepatic cholestasis, are also briefly reviewed.

Chronic Hepatitis B Infection 347

Alexander Kuo and Robert Gish

The management of chronic hepatitis B virus (HBV) infection requires understanding the natural history of the disease as well as the risks, benefits, and limitations of the therapeutic options. This article covers the principles governing when to start antiviral therapy, discusses recent advances using hepatitis B surface antigen quantification to better define various phases of infection, describes the use of HBV core, precore, and viral genotyping as well as host IL28B genotyping to predict response to interferon therapy, and reports on the management of HBV in 3 special populations (pregnancy, postliver transplantation, and in the setting of chemotherapy or immunosuppression).

Alcoholic Hepatitis: A Clinician's Guide 371

Gina Choi and Bruce Allen Runyon

Alcoholic hepatitis is a frequent reason for admission and a common consultation request for hepatologists and gastroenterologists. Although it seems to occur acutely, it is usually subacute and often superimposed on underlying alcoholic cirrhosis. Typically patients have a background of drinking on a daily basis, but, in response to a life crisis, patients have started drinking massively.

Granulomatous Liver Disease 387

Steven L. Flamm

Hepatic granulomata are not infrequently encountered in liver biopsy and often are associated with systemic disease. The clinical presentation varies with the particular systemic process. From a biochemical standpoint, the most common abnormalities are elevated serum alkaline phosphatase and γ-glutamyltransferase. The observation of granulomata in a liver biopsy specimen warrants workup to identify a possible cause.

Clues may be obtained in the medical history, on physical examination, or with specialized blood testing or radiologic studies. Treatment involves therapy of the underlying cause of the disease associated with the development of the granulomatous hepatitis.

Nonalcoholic Fatty Liver Disease **397**

Angelo H. Paredes, Dawn M. Torres, and Stephen A. Harrison

As the hepatic manifestation of the metabolic syndrome, nonalcoholic fatty liver disease (NAFLD) has become the most common cause of asymptomatic liver enzyme elevations in Western nations. Although it is easy to diagnose NAFLD, a liver biopsy is currently required to diagnose nonalcoholic steatohepatitis (NASH). Patients with NASH are those at greatest risk of progression to cirrhosis and, thus, treatment efforts are targeted to these individuals. Although currently there are no FDA-approved treatments for NASH, a multidisciplinary approach that addresses comorbid conditions and promotes modest weight loss comprises the backbone of therapy.

Surgical Clearance for the Patient with Chronic Liver Disease **421**

Andrew J. Muir

Patients with chronic liver disease face greater risk of perioperative morbidity and mortality, with the greatest risk among patients with cirrhosis. Both the Child-Pugh score and the Model for End-Stage Liver Disease have been evaluated as predictors of postoperative mortality. Other comorbidities, age, and American Society of Anesthesiologists physical status classification are also important predictors of these outcomes. In patients with liver disease, elective surgeries should be delayed to allow complete evaluation of the severity of liver disease, including the role of transplantation in the event of hepatic decompensation postoperatively.

Is the Patient a Candidate for Liver Transplantation? **435**

Alyson N. Fox and Robert S. Brown Jr

Identifying whether someone is a good candidate for liver transplantation is a complex process that requires a team approach. There are several medical and psychosocial considerations involved, each of which is thoroughly explored during the evaluation process. Both the indications and contraindications to transplantation can change over time, reflecting advances in understanding of, and ability to treat, certain disease processes. Ultimately, the goal of liver transplantation remains to provide a survival benefit to those with acute or chronic liver diseases.

Index **449**

CLINICS IN LIVER DISEASE

FORTHCOMING ISSUES

August 2012
NASH
Arun Sanyal, MD, *Guest Editor*

November 2012
Alcoholic Liver Disease
David Bernstein, MD, *Guest Editor*

February 2013
Novel and Combination Therapies for HCV
Paul J. Pockros, MD, *Guest Editor*

RECENT ISSUES

February 2012
Hepatic Encephalopathy: An Update
Kevin D. Mullen, MD, FRCPI and
Ravi K. Prakash, MBBS, MD, MRCP (UK),
Guest Editors

November 2011
Liver Transplant: Reaching the Half Century
Cynthia Levy, MD, and Paul Martin, MD,
Guest Editors

August 2011
Hepatitis C Direct Acting Antivirals:
The New Standard of Care
Fred Poordad, MD, *Guest Editor*

RELATED INTEREST

Neurologic Clinics, February 2010, (Vol. 28, No. 1)
Neurology and Systemic Disease
Alireza Minagar, *Guest Editor*

Preface

Consultations for Liver Disease Patients

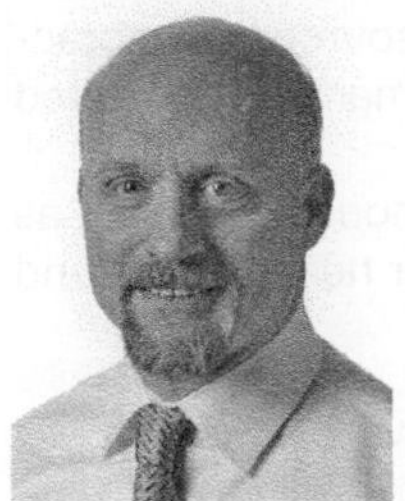

Steven L. Flamm, MD
Guest Editor

Inpatient and outpatient consultation for patients with liver disease is commonly encountered in clinical gastroenterology practice. Many issues are complicated and infrequently seen. Some of the disease states have potential life-threatening consequences, causing anxiety for the practitioner. Further, there have been diagnostic and therapeutic advances for many of the problems, making the gastroenterologist somewhat uncomfortable when consultation is sought. This issue of *Clinics in Liver Disease* is entitled "Approach to Consultations to Patients with Liver Disease" and is intended to provide a framework for dealing with many of the vexing issues that face the clinical gastroenterologist on a daily basis. The articles are not exhaustive literature reviews: rather, they are clinical discussions that guide the practitioner on how to handle common consultations.

The first article is entitled "Evaluation of Elevated Liver Enzymes" by Dr Kim. The next discussion is a clinical approach to the complicated topic of drug-induced liver disease by Dr Davern. The next article is a clinical approach to the patient with elevated alkaline phosphatase and hepatic cholestasis by Dr Kowdley.

The following series of articles deal with troubling symptoms and complications observed in patients with chronic liver disease. Dr Gordon discusses the evaluation and management of ascites and hepatorenal syndrome, and Dr Poordad provides a description of the state-of-the-art assessment and management of hepatic encephalopathy. A presentation of shortness of breath in the cirrhotic patient involves a unique set of problems that is described by Dr Kwo. Dr Reddy outlines the management of the particularly troublesome issue of pruritus in patients with chronic liver disease.

Several difficult disease entities are presented thereafter. Alcoholic hepatitis is discussed by Dr Runyon, and hepatitis B virus infection is presented by Dr Gish. I have written an article on the common problem of granulomatous liver disease. The frequently encountered issue of evaluation and management of liver lesions is outlined

Clin Liver Dis 16 (2012) xiii–xiv
doi:10.1016/j.cld.2012.04.001

by Dr Afdhal, and a clinical approach to the assessment and management of nonalcoholic liver disease is presented by Dr Harrison.

The last section involves general enigmatic issues that are frequent reasons for consultation for the gastroenterologist. Dr Brown discusses liver transplantation candidacy and Dr Muir presents an approach to surgical clearance in patients with chronic liver disease. Finally, Dr Reau outlines an approach to the unsettling problem of liver disease in pregnancy.

This issue of *Clinics in Liver Disease* should be an invaluable resource to the practicing gastroenterologist and allow for appropriate handling of many complicated problems in liver disease.

I would like to thank Dr Norman Gitlin for bestowing on me the honor of serving as editor of this issue of *Clinics in Liver Disease* and Kerry Holland for her patience and assistance in preparing the articles for publication.

Steven L. Flamm, MD
Liver Transplantation, Department of Medicine
Division of Gastroenterology and Hepatology
Northwestern University Feinberg School of Medicine
Chicago, IL 60611, USA

E-mail address:
s-flamm@northwestern.edu

Evaluation of Elevated Liver Enzymes

Tae Hoon Lee, MD[a], W. Ray Kim, MD[b,*], John J. Poterucha, MD[c]

KEYWORDS

- Aminotransferase • Alkaline phosphatase
- Gamma glutamyl transferase • Liver enzymes
- Diagnostic algorithm

Activities of certain enzymes detectable in the serum, commonly called the liver enzymes, are one of the most frequently used panel of blood tests in a physician's practice. These enzymes include aspartate aminotransferase (AST), alanine aminotransferase (ALT), alkaline phosphatase (AP), and γ-glutamyltransferase (GGT). Their uses are broad, ranging from screening for liver disease, to monitoring side effects of medications, and to determining responses to treatment for a given liver disease. Because of the widespread use of the tests, abnormal liver enzymes are encountered commonly.

When a liver enzyme is found to be abnormal, mild elevations (eg, <2–3 times of the upper limit of normal) without a symptom may be considered benign.[1] It is also well accepted that abnormal liver enzymes correlate with "hard end points" in liver disease, such as mortality and need for liver transplantation, as well as progression of fibrosis and development of hepatocellular carcinoma. Most recently, several observations have been reported that question the conventional definitions of normal and abnormal liver enzymes. These findings include data suggesting that normal ranges of liver enzymes may need to be redefined, and those showing that even a mild increase in liver enzymes correlates with an increased risk of future mortality.[2,3]

Regardless of how the normal range is defined, liver enzymes may remain normal in patients with well-established liver disease such as chronic hepatitis C, autoimmune hepatitis, and nonalcoholic steatohepatitis.[4,5] The converse may also be true in that abnormal liver enzymes may be seen in otherwise healthy subjects. Thus, it is important that liver enzymes should be interpreted within the clinical context of an individual patient.

No conflict of interest exists.

[a] Department of Internal Medicine, Marshall University, 1249 15th Street, Huntington, WV 25701, USA; [b] Division of Gastroenterology and Hepatology (PL 6), Mayo Clinic College of Medicine, 200 1st Street Southwest, Rochester, MN 55905, USA; [c] Division of Gastroenterology and Hepatology, Mayo Clinic College of Medicine, 200 1st Street Southwest, Rochester, MN 55905, USA
* Corresponding author.
E-mail address: kim.ray@mayo.edu

Clin Liver Dis 16 (2012) 183–198
doi:10.1016/j.cld.2012.03.006
liver.theclinics.com
1089-3261/12/$ – see front matter

AMINOTRANSFERASES

AST and ALT catalyze the transfer of the α-amino group from alanine and aspartic acid to α-ketoglutaric acid, respectively.[6] AST is found in liver, cardiac and skeletal muscle, kidney, brain, pancreas, lung, leukocyte, and erythrocyte.[6] ALT exists mainly in liver and exists in low concentrations in other tissue.[7] Recently, an isoform of ALT2 has been cloned in a separate chromosome (chr. 16) from the classic ALT (chr. 8). There is a high homology (69% identical at the protein level) between the 2 isoenzymes. ALT2 has a wider organ distribution, including skeletal muscles and adipose tissue. To date, however, the clinical significance of ALT2 in the diagnosis of liver disease remains to be defined.[8]

Aminotransferase activities may be measured by several methods such as chromatography, spectrophotometry, fluorimetry, and colorimetry.[9] Although the assay results may differ slightly according to the method used, there is a high degree of correlation between the 2 most common methods, namely colorimetry and spectrophotometry, particularly near the normal range.[9]

Recently, there has been renewed attention about what constitutes the normal range for serum activities of aminotransferase, particularly ALT. Traditionally a level around 40 has been considered the upper limit of normal based on the mean and standard deviation calculated in apparently healthy reference subjects.[9] There is an increasing consensus that the conventional normal range may have been set too high, because the reference subjects presumed to be healthy may have included individuals with asymptomatic liver disease, such as nonalcoholic fatty liver disease and chronic hepatitis C. When more stringent criteria are applied to exclude subjects with a high probability of liver disease, the upper limit of the normal range becomes considerably lower. Prati and colleagues[10] analyzed samples of blood donors carefully selected to exclude those at risk of liver disease by using criteria such as normal body mass index (BMI), normal cholesterol, triglyceride, and glucose levels, and no potentially hepatotoxic medications. The upper limit of normal ALT in that study was determined to be 30 U/L for men and 19 U/L for women. Although these updated normal values are frequently cited, one may note that they way the upper limit of normal was set in that particular study was different from the usual convention. Whereas most laboratory normal ranges are taken from the middle 95%, ie, 2.5th to 97.5th percentiles of the population, Prati and colleagues[10] chose to take the lower 95th percentile as normal. The authors believe that the normal ranges proposed in that study are set too low.

Others have taken a different approach and have hypothesized that normal ALT defined in a cross section of a population may not equate with absence of disease. In other words, normal ALT is not necessarily healthy ALT. In a large population-based study from South Korea, serum ALT activity measured at baseline was correlated with subsequent mortality. In particular, compared with men with ALT less than 20 IU/L, those with ALT of 20 to 29 IU/L had a 2.9-fold increase in liver mortality and those with ALT of 30 to 39 IU/L had a 9.5-fold increase in mortality.[2] The authors also have evaluated ALT and AST activities as a predictor of future mortality. Using population-based data in Olmsted County, AST and ALT results in a given year were correlated with subsequent all-cause mortality. Similar to the data by Kim and colleagues,[3] there was a positive correlation between the standardized mortality ratio and the aminotransferase results. Further, the increase in mortality could be discerned with aminotransferase values less than the upper limit of normal set by the laboratory at that time.

Another aspect of serum aminotransferase activities that the clinician must be aware of is the variability between, as well as within, individual subjects. Several factors such as age, sex, and BMI influence its activities in subjects without known liver disease.[11] In addition, an early study by Friedman showed that ALT elevation was intermittent in 36% and persistent in 28% during up to 7 months of observation.[12] One limitation of the study is that it included a large proportion (63%) of patients who were consuming alcohol regularly, making it possible that not all of the fluctuation of ALT was simply a result of its variability. A subsequent study by Lazo and colleagues[13] investigated variability of liver enzymes using the samples of the National Health and Nutrition Examination Survey. Out of nearly 20,000 survey respondents, 1864 had 2 biochemical assessments separated by a mean of 18 days. In the initial testing, 6.2% and 5.9% had abnormal AST and ALT, respectively, using normal ranges defined by the laboratory. Of those with initially elevated results, more than 30% (35.6% for AST and 31.2% for ALT) were reclassified as normal in the follow-up tests. As expected, mildly elevated of AST and ALT were more likely to normalize on repeat testing; most people who transitioned from abnormal to normal had initial elevation within 1.1 to 2.0 times the normal range. Another element of intraindividual variability in aminotransferases is diurnal variation. According to Cordoba and colleagues,[14] ALT level is lowest at night and highest in the afternoon.

CAUSES OF ELEVATED AMINOTRANSFERASES

Serum aminotransferase activities may be elevated as a result of a variety of causes. Although they are most commonly derived from hepatobiliary disorders, increased aminotransferase levels may be seen in extrahepatic conditions.[15] **Table 1** summarizes potential causes of abnormal aminotransferases.

Nonalcoholic Fatty Liver Disease

Nonalcoholic fatty liver disease (NAFLD) is thought to be the most common cause of abnormal liver enzymes. In a study where magnetic resonance spectroscopy was used to measure liver triglyceride contents, the prevalence of NAFLD in the United States was estimated to be about 30%.[16] NAFLD may or may not increase the aminotransferase level, and mild elevation of aminotransferase level may be the only finding in NAFLD patients. In early NAFLD, ALT is usually higher than AST (AST/ALT < 1).[17] As NAFLD advances and causes liver fibrosis, the AST/ALT ratio reverses to the degree that ALT in patients with cirrhosis from NAFLD may be normal.[18] This trend is reflected in the NAFLD fibrosis score ($-1.675 + 0.037 \times$ age [years] $+ 0.094 \times$ BMI [kg/m^2] $+ 1.13 \times$ impaired fasting glucose/diabetes [yes = 1, no = 0] $+ 0.99 \times$ AST/ALT ratio $- 0.013 \times$ platelet [$\times 10^9$/L] $- 0.66 \times$ albumin [g/dL]), which may be used to estimate liver fibrosis.[19]

Alcoholic Liver Disease

Alcoholic liver disease (ALD) has been the most common cause of both liver-related mortality and alcohol-related mortality in the United States. There is a large degree of variability in the pattern and amount of alcohol consumption seen in patients with ALD. ALD is probably underdiagnosed because the most common form, alcoholic fatty liver, is asymptomatic. More severe forms of ALD include alcoholic hepatitis and alcoholic cirrhosis.

Depending on the severity of ongoing liver damage, aminotransferase levels can range from normal to more than 10 times the upper limit of normal.[15] A high AST/ALT ratio is thought to be an the indicator of ALD. If the ratio is more than 3, ALD is highly likely, whereas a ratio greater than 2 is strongly suggestive.[20] On the other hand, an AST/ALT ratio of less than 2 does not necessarily exclude ALD; even a ratio

Table 1
Potential causes of abnormal aminotransferases

			Initial Test	Secondary Test
Hepatobiliary cause	Metabolic cause	Wilson disease	Serum ceruloplasmin, 24-h urinary copper, Kayser-Fleischer ring	Liver biopsy
		Hemochromatosis	Fasting morning transferrin saturation, ferritin	Genetic test, liver biopsy
		α1-Antitrypsin deficiency	Clinical suspicion	α1-Antitrypsin phenotype
		Other liver metabolic disorder (pophyrias, cystic fibrosis)		
	Infectious	Viral hepatitis (A, B, C, D, E)	See text	See text
		Other virus (CMV, EBV, HSV, VZV, SARS)		
		EBV	Mono spot	EBV IgM Ab
		CMV	CMV IgM Ab (in acute primary infection), PCR	CMV culture, liver biopsy
		HSV	Clinical suspicion/Mucocutaneous lesion	Liver biopsy
		Bacterial, parasitic, and fungal infection	Culture	
	Medication/ toxin/alcohol	Alcohol	History	Liver biopsy
		Hepatotoxic medication/toxin	History	
		Allergic reaction	History	Liver biopsy
	NAFLD		US	Liver biopsy
	Immunology	Autoimmune hepatitis	SPEP	ANA, anti–smooth muscle Ab, LKMA, liver biopsy
		HELLP syndrome	Clinical situation	
		Acute fatty liver of pregnancy	Clinical situation	
	Biliary tract disease	Primary biliary cirrhosis	AMA	Anti-Sp100, Anti-gp210
		Primary sclerosing cholangitis	pANCA, ANA, SMA	ERCP, MRCP, cholangiography
		Secondary cholangitis	US abdomen, CT abdomen	ERCP, MRCP, cholangiography

	Vascular disease	Budd-Chiari syndrome	Doppler ultrasound	MRI
		Sinusoidal obstruction syndrome	Clinical feature	Liver biopsy
		Ischemic hepatitis	ALT/LDH ratio	
	Infiltrative liver disease	Sarcoidosis, amyloidosis	ACE level, gastrointestinal biopsy	
Nonhepatic		Cardiac disease	Echocardiogram, cardiac enzymes	Cardiology referral
		Thyroid disease	Thyroid function test	Endocrinology referral
		Myopathy	CPK, aldolase	
		Macro AST	Polyethyleneglycol precipitation assay	Electrophoresis of AST
		Strenuous exercise	CPK, history	
		Celiac disease	IgA EMA or tTG serology	EMA, tTG
		Adrenal insufficiency	Early-morning serum cortisol	Endocrinology referral
		Anorexia nervosa	History and physical examination	

Abbreviations: Ab, antibody; ACE, angiotensin-converting enzyme; ALT, alanine aminotransferase; AMA, antimitochondrial antibody; ANA, antinuclear antibody; AST, aspartate aminotransferase; CMV, cytomegalovirus; CPK, creatine phosphokinase; CT, computed tomography; EBV, Epstein-Barr virus; EMA, endomysial antibody; ERCP, endoscopic retrograde cholangiopancreatography; HELLP, hemolysis, elevated liver enzymes, low platelet count; HSV, herpes simplex virus; IgM, immunoglobulin M; LDH, lactate dehydrogenase; LKMA, liver/kidney microsomal antibody; MRCP, magnetic resonance cholangiopancreatography; MRI, magnetic resonance imaging; pANCA, perinuclear antineutrophil cytoplasmic antibodies; PCR, polymerase chain reaction; SARS, severe acute respiratory syndrome; SMA, anti-smooth muscle antibodies; SPEP, serum protein electrophoresis; tTG, tissue transglutaminase; US, ultrasonography; VZV, varicella zoster virus.

less than 1 may be seen in patients with significant intake of alcohol, which may suggest alcoholic steatosis rather than more serious forms of ALD.[21]

It is important for the clinician to keep in mind the possibility of a concomitant cause of liver disease in a patient with alcohol abuse or ALD. In patients with polysubstance abuse, hepatitis C virus infection commonly coexists with ALD. Alcohol may also potentiate hepatotoxicity of other drugs.[22] Although rarely necessary just to establish the diagnosis, a liver biopsy may show the characteristic features including ballooning degeneration of hepatocyte, Mallory bodies, and infiltrate of polymorphonuclear leukocytes.[23]

Drug-Induced Hepatotoxicity

A wide range of prescription drugs may cause elevation in liver enzymes. Although almost all medications can potentially cause elevation of serum aminotransferase, certain antibiotics, antivirals, statins, hormonal agents, anesthetics, and antiseizure medications are well-known examples of hepatotoxic drugs. Clinical presentation of drug-induced liver injury (DILI) is variable, ranging from asymptomatic enzyme elevation to acute hepatic failure.

DILI can be dose dependent or idiosyncratic (dose independent).[24] The prototypical example of the former is acetaminophen. Although acetaminophen overdose is recognized as a common cause of acute liver failure, a recent randomized trial showed that its use within the maximum allowed dose was also associated with a high incidence of ALT elevations. Further, the clinician must be aware that hepatotoxicity of a dose-dependent hepatotoxin may develop within the recommended maximum daily doses, depending on genetic predisposition, other medications, and sometimes food intake, which may affect the patient's ability to metabolize the drug (eg, cytochrome P450 enzymes). Idiosyncratic reaction is not very common and, by definition, unpredictable. Essentially any medication can cause idiosyncratic reaction, including over-the-counter medications such as ranitidine. The latent period can be up to several months before the onset of idiosyncratic features.[25,26] Occasionally DILI may be accompanied by a hypersensitivity reaction (ie, fever, rash, eosinophilia).[24]

These characteristics of DILI make its diagnosis sometimes difficult - careful history taking with a high index of suspicion is needed for the diagnosis. Liver biopsies have a limited role in the diagnosis and differential diagnosis of DILI, because histologic features of DILI are often nonspecific and not distinguishable from those of viral or immune-mediated injury.[27] Careful exclusion of other diagnoses and assessing response to withdrawal of the suspected drug constitute an important diagnostic and therapeutic step. Rechallenge of the offending drug is reserved for selected situations whereby the benefit of the drug outweighs the risk of potentially severe hepatotoxicity.

Besides medications, herbal preparations, chemicals, pesticides, and metals can cause hepatotoxicity. Illicit drugs such as cocaine, 3,4-methylenedioxymethamphetamine (Ecstasy), phencyclidine (PCP, Angel Dust), glue/solvents, and anabolic steroids are also known for their hepatotoxicity.[7] Detailed history clearly is crucial, because the patient using these drugs may be reluctant to reveal the exposure history, whereas in other circumstances exposure to hepatotoxic materials may be inadvertent. The clinician must be aware that excessive alcohol use and drug abuse often coexist.[22] Thus in a patient with a history of heavy drinking or ALD, the clinician must inquire after exposure to other hepatotoxic drugs and be aware of their potential interaction with alcohol.

Viral Hepatitis

Hepatitis A, B, C, D, and E viruses may cause elevation of aminotransferase. Among these, hepatitis A and E viruses cause acute infection, whereas hepatitis B, C, and

D are commonly chronic. Aminotransferases are almost always abnormal with acute hepatitis, whereas some chronic hepatitis patients may have normal values.

Hepatitis A can be diagnosed with the detection of immunoglobulin M (IgM) anti–hepatitis A virus (HAV) in serum.[28] The diagnosis of hepatitis B virus (HBV) infection is usually made by the detection of hepatitis B surface antigen (HBsAg), although sometimes anti–hepatitis B core antibodies may be the only clue to the diagnosis.[23] Hepatitis D virus (HDV) can replicate only in a host with HBV infection. HDV RNA by reverse transcriptase polymerase chain reaction (RT-PCR) is the most reliable test. IgM or immunoglobulin G (IgG) anti-HDV can be used, whose sensitivity is less than that of the HDV RNA RT-PCR method.[29,30] Hepatitis C virus (HCV) infection can be screened by anti-HCV antibodies and confirmed with HCV RNA detection.[31] For the diagnosis of hepatitis E virus (HEV), anti-HEV antibodies (IgM/IgG) may be used. However, the availability of tests for HEV has been limited in the United States.[32]

Systemic infections with viruses such as Epstein-Barr virus (EBV), cytomegalovirus (CMV), herpes simplex virus (HSV), varicella zoster virus (VZV), and severe acute respiratory syndrome (SARS) virus, may cause elevated aminotransferase. Aminotransferase elevation caused by EBV is usually seen in conjunction with acute mononucleosis. It is usually self-limited, even though chronic infection is possible.[33] Similarly, in immune-competent hosts, CMV infection presents as subclinical or mild symptomatic cases and resolves by itself. CMV infection is more serious in immune-compromised hosts, including patients with AIDS and solid organ recipients, in whom disseminated infection may cause major organ damage or mortality.[34] HSV hepatitis is most commonly seen in neonatal, pregnant, or immune-compromised patients. Many cases present with fulminant hepatitis with high mortality.[35]

Metabolic Disorders

Hemochromatosis is the most common genetic disease in Caucasians.[36] All subjects with persistently elevated aminotransferase must be evaluated for hemochromatosis.[37] The initial diagnostic test should start with serum ferritin transferrin saturation, followed by the HFE genotyping.[37] Wilson disease can present as acute liver failure as well as chronic liver disease. Patients with unexplained liver disease, especially if it is accompanied by neurologic or psychiatric manifestations, or those with atypical autoimmune or nonalcoholic fatty liver disease must be considered for Wilson disease.[38] Serum ceruloplasmin level, 24-hour urine copper level, and ophthalmologic examination for a Kayser-Fleischer ring are the initial tests for the diagnosis.[38] α1-Antitrypsin (A1AT) deficiency may present as mildly abnormal liver enzymes to liver cirrhosis. The prevalence of genetic phenotypes for A1AT deficiency is estimated to be 1 in 11.3 in the United States.[39] The preferred screening test for A1AT deficiency is phenotyping rather than the serum level.[23] Several rare metabolic/genetic liver diseases may cause elevated liver enzymes, which include glycogen storage disease, porphyrias, tyrosinemia, urea cycle defects, cystic fibrosis, and mitochondrial liver disease.[23]

Autoimmune and Cholestatic Liver Disease

The prevalence of autoimmune hepatitis is about 5 to 200 per 1 million Caucasian population of Northern Europe and North America.[40] Presence of autoantibodies (antinuclear, anti–smooth muscle, or anti-LKM1 antibodies) is suggestive of the diagnosis, especially when elevated serum levels of γ-globulins are present. A scoring system proposed by the International Autoimmune Hepatitis Group may be used for diagnosis.[41]

Primary biliary cirrhosis (PBC) and primary sclerosing cholangitis (PSC) represent the most commonly encountered forms of cholestatic liver disease, which is characterized by elevated alkaline phosphatase rather than aminotransferases. Both are uncommon, with a prevalence of 40 per 100,000 persons for PBC and 14 per 100,000 persons for PSC in the United States.[42,43] A liver biopsy may not be necessary for diagnosis in a patients who present with a clinical picture consistent with PBC and positive antimitochondrial antibodies (AMA).[44] The diagnosis of PSC is usually made by cholangiography. Inflammatory bowel disease coexists in up to 80% of PSC patients.[44] Autoantibodies such as perinuclear antineutrophil cytoplasmic antibodies may be found in PSC patients, but their diagnostic utility is limited. In patients with features of cholestatic liver disease who have significantly increased aminotransferase (>5 × upper limit of normal), an overlap syndrome with autoimmune hepatitis should be considered.[45] Secondary sclerosing cholangitis shares the same cholangiographic features as PSC and must be considered in the differential diagnosis.[44]

Vascular Disease of the Liver

Budd-Chiari syndrome is caused by obstruction of either the hepatic vein or inferior vena cava, and results in acute to chronic diseases. Although liver enzymes may not be strikingly abnormal, jaundice and ascites are commonly seen. Doppler ultrasound is a sensitive (88%) screening test. Sinusodial obstruction syndrome (SOS, also known as veno-occlusive disease) is caused by the endothelial injury in hepatic sinusoid and hepatic venule. It is typically associated with bone marrow transplantation, certain chemotherapeutic agents, or abdominal radiation.[46] SOS is suspected with clinical features consisting of jaundice, portal vein hypertension, and abnormal liver enzymes. A transjugular liver biopsy is a common method of diagnosis.[46] Ischemic hepatitis is caused by hypoperfusion to liver and presents with an extremely high aminotransferase level (usually >3000 U/L). The ALT/lactate dehydrogenase ratio may also be useful, as it stays below 1.5 in most cases.[47] The diagnosis is relatively straightforward based on the clinical setting.

Aminotransferase Elevation from Nonhepatobiliary Causes

Aminotransferase can be elevated in certain nonhepatic conditions. Obviously, AST is one of the cardiac enzymes whose elevation can be seen in cardiac conditions such as ischemic heart disease and congestive heart failure. Systemic diseases such as celiac disease, adrenal insufficiency, hyperthyroidism, and hypothyroidism may be associated with aminotransferase elevation, even when there is no demonstrable concomitant liver disease.[48] Both AST and ALT are expressed in skeletal muscles and conditions associated with myocyte damage including primary muscle diseases, and strenuous exercise may increase the aminotransferase. Some patients with anorexia nervosa may have increased liver enzymes, although the mechanism for this is not clear.[49] Isolated AST elevation may be seen in macro AST. Macro AST and other macroenzymes are high molecular mass complexes of plasma enzymes with immunoglubulins or other proteins, which lead to reduced plasma clearance and prolonged half-life. At the Mayo Clinic, a polyethyleneglycol precipitation assay has been developed to assay macro AST.[50]

ALKALINE PHOSPHATASE AND γ-GLUTAMYLTRANSFERASE

Alkaline phosphatase is a group of enzymes that is present in the bone, liver, small intestine, kidney, placenta, and white blood cells. In adults, the most common clinical situations for elevated serum alkaline phosphatase activities are hepatobiliary and bone diseases, and pregnancy.[6] In isolated elevation of alkaline phosphatase, electrophoresis can be used to fractionate the isoenzymes to suggest the source.

GGT is present in the kidney, pancreas, liver, spleen, heart, brain, and seminal vesicles.[6] One of the clinical uses of serum levels of GGT is to identify the source of elevated alkaline phosphatase. Because it is not increased in bone disease, a concomitant elevation of alkaline phosphatase and GGT would suggest a hepatobiliary source rather than a skeletal source. The other common use of GGT is in patients with suspected ALD, as GGT can be induced by alcohol ingestion. Medications such as barbiturates and phenytoin may also increase GGT, presumably by the same mechanism. Recently, several reports correlated elevated GGT with increased mortality. Compared with reference populations with normal GGT, those with increased GGT had higher mortality from liver disease, cancer, and diabetes, as well as cardiac disease.[51,52]

Because of the nonspecific nature of serum alkaline phosphatase and GGT results, greater than 1.5 times that of upper limit of alkaline phosphatase and greater than 3 times that of GGT have been suggested as thresholds for a diagnostic workup in asymptomatic patients.[44] Careful history and physical examination is the first step in evaluation, together with abdominal ultrasonography. Magnetic resonance cholangiopancreatography (MRCP), endoscopic retrograde cholangiopancreatography (ERCP), and endoscopic ultrasonography (EUS) as well as serum markers such as antimitochondrial antibody can be used for the evaluation of the hepatobiliary system. Liver biopsy can be used, although the diagnostic yield may vary significantly depending on the clinical setting.

EVALUATION OF ABNORMAL LIVER ENZYMES

The decision to evaluate a patient for abnormal liver enzymes should be individualized according to the patient's history and other clinical data.[7] Even though it is frequently the abnormal enzymes that motivate the clinician to initiate an evaluation for liver disease, it is important to remember that normal liver enzymes do not necessarily rule out hepatobiliary disease. On the other hand, mild elevation of liver enzymes can be nonspecific. As shown in the study by Lazo and colleagues,[13] more than 30% of cases with abnormal liver enzymes ended up being reclassified as normal on follow-up.

The initial consultation should include detailed history taking and a full physical examination. For the essential components of this evaluation, the reader is referred to available textbooks on liver disease. Based on clinical data available, patients with abnormal liver enzymes may be categorized into hepatocellular versus cholestatic. The former is characterized by elevated aminotransferases whereas the latter is characterized by alkaline phosphatase. Obviously there are conditions in which both patterns coexist. An algorithm that may help guide a clinician to evaluate a patient with abnormal liver enzymes is shown in **Fig. 1**.

A common clinical scenario for a hepatologist is that of an asymptomatic patient in whom elevated liver enzymes are detected incidentally for the first time. A patient who is initially seen with elevated aminotransferase can be monitored if (1) there is no clear risk factor for liver disease, (2) liver enzyme levels are less than 3 times normal, (3) liver function (as gauged by serum bilirubin and albumin and prothrombin time) is preserved, and (4) the patient feels well. If these conditions are not met or a repeated testing shows persistent abnormalities, the patient has acute or chronic hepatitis. Based on various causes of acute and chronic hepatitis, subsequent testing is outlined in the algorithm. Often, a liver biopsy is considered the ultimate diagnostic test for abnormal liver enzymes. However, given the risk of bleeding and other complications, discomfort/pain, and expenses associated with a liver biopsy, a clear risk-benefit calculation is needed before one is performed. In general, the clinician must be

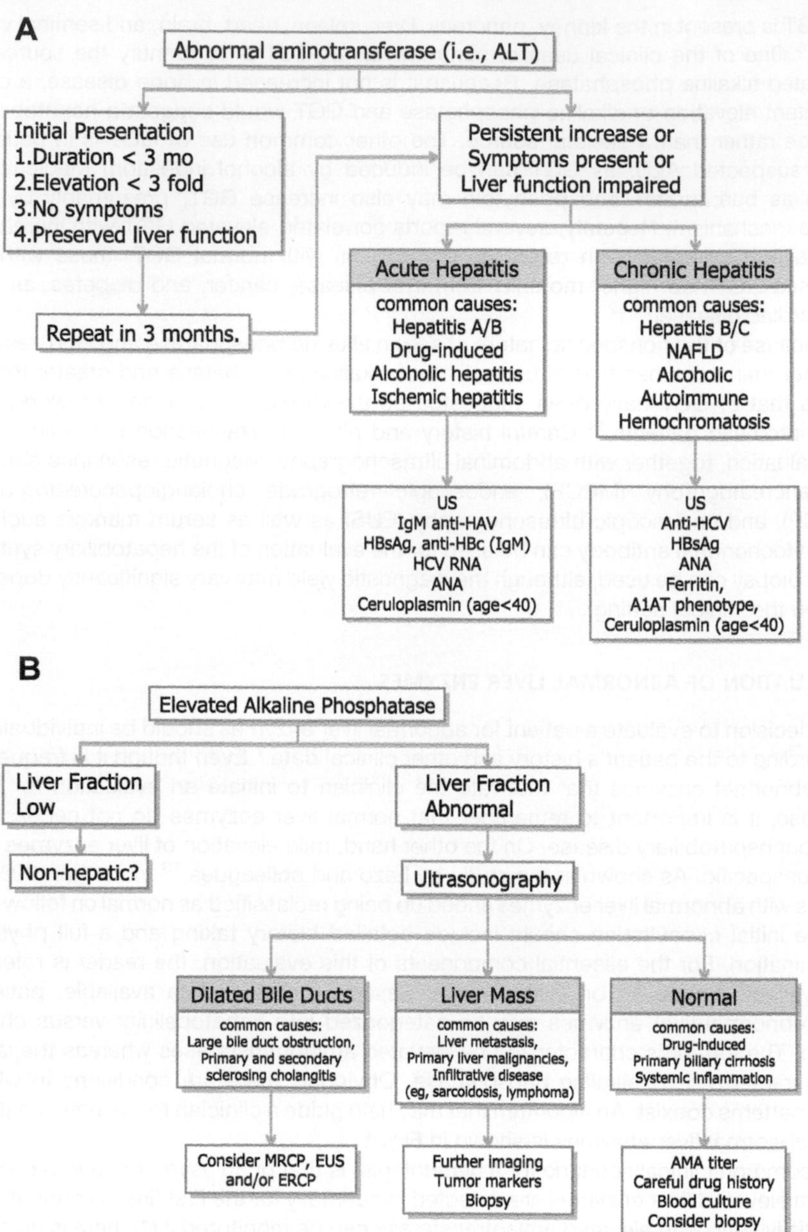

Fig. 1. (*A–B*) Algorithm for the evaluation of abnormal liver enzymes. A1AT, α1-antitrypsin; Ab, antibody; ALT, alanine aminotransferase; AMA, antimitochondrial antibody; ANA, antinuclear antibody; CMV, cytomegalovirus; ERCP, endoscopic retrograde cholangiopancreatography; EUS, endoscopic ultrasound; GGT, γ-glutamyltransferase; HAV, hepatitis A virus; HBsAg, hepatitis B surface antigen; HBc, hepatitis B core; HCV, hepatitis C virus; IgM, immunoglobulin M; MRCP, magnetic resonance cholangiopancreatography; NAFLD, nonalcoholic fatty liver disease; pANCA, perinuclear antineutrophil cytoplasmic antibodies; SMA, anti-smooth muscle antibodies; SPEP, serum protein electrophoresis; US, ultrasonography.

convinced that the histologic information gained by the biopsy will lead to a key therapeutic decision that is not possible otherwise.

For patients who present with cholestatic pattern of enzyme abnormalities, ultrasonography represents a key diagnostic step, which may detect dilated intrahepatic and/or extrahepatic bile ducts, mass lesions, and vascular abnormalities. Further evaluation of a mass lesion or vascular abnormalities is relatively straightforward. If a biliary disease is suspected, further diagnostic modalities such as MRCP, EUS, and ERCP may be used to locate and characterize the biliary abnormalities.[53] In light of the appreciable risk of complication after ERCP with and without sphincterotomy,[54] MRCP and EUS have increasingly been used to enhance the pretest diagnostic probabilities before initiating ERCP. If the cholangiography is unrevealing, biliary obstruction may be at the level of small bile ducts (eg, PBC) or canalicular (eg, sepsis or DILI).

ABNORMAL LIVER ENZYMES IN POSTOPERATIVE SETTING

The interpretation of abnormal liver enzymes in the postoperative setting is unique because of the concentration of many procedures and medications in the short time period. In addition to the presence of liver disease at baseline, the type of surgery, choice of anesthetic agent, administration of blood products and postsurgical analgesic agents can affect the liver, potentially resulting in abnormal liver enzymes. Preexisting liver disease can affect the risk of surgery and anesthesia. In patients with diminished liver function, additional insult to the liver such as ischemia or drug-induced hepatotoxicity may precipitate serious hepatic insufficiency. However, liver abnormality to that degree in asymptomatic patients undergoing elective surgery is not encountered frequently and routine screening by liver biochemistry is deemed not to be cost-effective.[55] The following discussion addresses potential causes of postoperative liver enzyme abnormalities other than underlying primary liver disease the patient may have had at baseline.

Ischemia

Ischemic liver injury is one of the most common causes of elevated liver enzymes after surgery. Hepatic blood flow in general is decreased by general anesthetic agents.[56] Blood loss during the surgery obviously contributes to hypoperfusion and ischemic injury to the liver. The type of surgery and anesthesia affects blood flow to the liver and may determine ischemic injury. For example, increased intra-abdominal pressure from carbon dioxide inflation during a laparoscopic procedure can cause the compression of the inferior vena cava, leading to a decreased cardiac output and systemic hypotension.[57] Transient decrease of cardiac output from any cardiopulmonary procedure can cause liver enzyme elevation from ischemia. Spinal anesthesia is not necessarily safer than general anesthesia. In most cases, ischemic liver injury is transient and does not require specific therapy. It is important, however, to ensure adequate blood flow to the liver in the postoperative period, especially in cardiopulmonary surgical patients in whom systemic perfusion may be compromised.

Anesthetic Agent Induced Hepatotoxicity

Volatile anesthetics can be a possible cause of elevated liver enzymes. Halothane may cause liver damage in 2 different ways. First, it causes asymptomatic elevation of liver enzymes, which may occur in as many as 20% of all patients undergoing halothane anesthesia. The elevation of liver enzyme is mild and usually improves spontaneously.[58] Second, a much more serious form of liver damage is severe acute hepatitis, which may progress to fulminant hepatic failure. This syndrome includes systemic symptoms such as high fever, chills, nausea and vomiting, and eosinophilia, which occur typically a week after the anesthesia. This immune-mediated idiosyncratic reaction has an incidence of fatal cases of about 1 in 35,000.[59] More modern anesthetics such as enflurane, isoflurane, desflurane, and sevoflurane may also be associated with idiosyncratic reactions, but at a much lower frequency than halothane.[60]

Propofol is used for sedation and induction of anesthesia. Propofol infusion syndrome is a rare fatal occurrence, which can present as acute fatty liver together with acute bradycardia and metabolic acidosis.[61] Inappropriate use of multidose propofol vials has recently been implicated in a point-source epidemic of hepatitis B and C virus transmission.[62]

Transfusion/Transplantation-Mediated Viral Hepatitis

Transfusion-mediated viral hepatitis from hepatitis A, B, and C has become extremely rare. The rare residual cases of posttransfusion hepatitis may occur as a result of false-negative results on screening tests and, at least in theory, a blood donor in the so-called window period with negative serologic tests may escape detection of the hepatitis virus infection.[63] In organ transplantation settings, nonhepatitis viruses such as EBV, CMV, and human herpes virus may cause hepatitis from reactivation or de novo infection because of immunosuppression.[64] For patients in whom these viral infections are considered, incubation and latent periods are a useful clue to gauge the probability that they are responsible for the given clinical presentation. In recipients of an organ transplant, hepatotoxicity from the multitude of drugs used in the setting should also be considered.[65]

Postoperative Jaundice

If hyperbilirubinemia and jaundice complicate increased liver enzymes, it may indicate that the extent of the liver damage is severe enough to decrease the liver function to a critical level. These cases, particularly if coagulopathy is also present, must be monitored carefully. For the purpose of differential diagnosis, other causes of postoperative jaundice are mentioned briefly.

A common cause of postoperative jaundice is indirect hyperbilirubinemia as a result of pigment overload (eg, hematoma), which in conjunction with mild liver dysfunction, or underlying Gilbert syndrome may lead to pronounced hyperbilirubinemia. Severe postoperative jaundice may follow a prolonged and difficult surgery and postoperative course complicated by hypotension, hypoxemia, and sepsis, or the systemic inflammatory response syndrome. An important differential diagnosis, particularly if the jaundice follows biliary tract surgery, is obstructive jaundice. Such cases clearly require anatomic diagnosis followed by endoscopic, surgical, or percutaneous relief of the obstruction.

SUMMARY

Liver enzymes represent some of the most commonly used blood tests in a physician's office. Although there are still some uncertainties about exactly how to define normal cutoffs for the aminotransferases, they remain inexpensive and sensitive tests for the screening, diagnosis, and monitoring of patients with a variety of liver diseases. This article outlines the authors' approach in evaluating patients with abnormal liver enzymes at the Mayo Clinic. In most patients with the aminotransferase-predominant picture, careful history and examination and a small number of laboratory tests can guide subsequent management. In patients with elevated alkaline phosphatase, imaging evaluation becomes more essential, as outlined in the presented algorithm (see **Fig. 1**).

Postoperative patients can sometimes present a management challenge, so a judicious and expeditious evaluation must be performed about whether an invasive intervention is necessary. In other patients, monitoring and careful supportive care allow resolution of the postoperative liver abnormalities.

REFERENCES

1. Pratt DS, Kaplan MM. Evaluation of abnormal liver-enzyme results in asymptomatic patients. N Engl J Med 2000;342:1266–71.
2. Kim HC, Nam CM, Jee SH, et al. Normal serum aminotransferase concentration and risk of mortality from liver diseases: prospective cohort study. BMJ 2004;328:983.
3. Lee TH, Kim WR, Benson JT, et al. Serum aminotransferase activity and mortality risk in a United States community. Hepatology 2008;47:880–7.
4. Haber MM, West AB, Haber AD, et al. Relationship of aminotransferases to liver histological status in chronic hepatitis C. Am J Gastroenterol 1995;90:1250–7.
5. Sanyal AJ. AGA technical review on nonalcoholic fatty liver disease. Gastroenterology 2002;123:1705–25.
6. Schiff ER, Sorrell MF, Maddrey WC, editors. Schiff's diseases of the liver. 10th edition. Philadelphia: Lippincott Williams & Wilkins; 2007.
7. Green R, Flamm S. AGA technical review on the evaluation of liver chemistry tests. Gastroenterology 2002;123:1367–84.
8. Yang RZ, Blaileanu G, Hansen BC, et al. cDNA cloning, genomic structure, chromosomal mapping, and functional expression of a novel human alanine aminotransferase. Genomics 2002;79:445–50.
9. Wroblewski F. The clinical significance of transaminase activities of serum. Am J Med 1959;27:911–23.
10. Prati D, Taioli E, Zanella A, et al. Updated definitions of healthy ranges for serum alanine aminotransferase levels. Ann Intern Med 2002;137:1–10.
11. Piton A, Poynard T, Imbert-Bismut F, et al. Factors associated with serum alanine transaminase activity in healthy subjects: consequences for the definition of normal values, for selection of blood donors, and for patients with chronic hepatitis C. MULTIVIRC Group. Hepatology 1998;27:1213–9.
12. Friedman LS, Dienstag JL, Watkins E, et al. Evaluation of blood donors with elevated serum alanine aminotransferase levels. Ann Intern Med 1987;107:137–44.
13. Lazo M, Selvin E, Clark JM. Brief communication: clinical implications of short-term variability in liver function test results. Ann Intern Med 2008;148:348–52.
14. Cordoba J, O'Riordan K, Dupuis J, et al. Diurnal variation of serum alanine transaminase activity in chronic liver disease. Hepatology 1998;28:1724–5.
15. Ellis G, Goldberg DM, Spooner RJ, et al. Serum enzyme tests in diseases of the liver and biliary tree. Am J Clin Pathol 1978;70:248–58.
16. Browning JD, Szczepaniak LS, Dobbins R, et al. Prevalence of hepatic steatosis in an urban population in the United States: impact of ethnicity. Hepatology 2004;40:1387–95.
17. Bacon BR, Farahvash MJ, Janney CG, et al. Nonalcoholic steatohepatitis: an expanded clinical entity. Gastroenterology 1994;107:1103–9.
18. Wong VW, Vergniol J, Wong GL, et al. Diagnosis of fibrosis and cirrhosis using liver stiffness measurement in nonalcoholic fatty liver disease. Hepatology 2010;51:454–62.

19. Angulo P, Hui JM, Marchesini G, et al. The NAFLD fibrosis score: a noninvasive system that identifies liver fibrosis in patients with NAFLD. Hepatology 2007;45: 846–54.
20. Cohen JA, Kaplan MM. The SGOT/SGPT ratio—an indicator of alcoholic liver disease. Dig Dis Sci 1979;24:835–8.
21. Nyblom H, Berggren U, Balldin J, et al. High AST/ALT ratio may indicate advanced alcoholic liver disease rather than heavy drinking. Alcohol Alcohol 2004;39:336–9.
22. Regier DA, Farmer ME, Rae DS, et al. Comorbidity of mental disorders with alcohol and other drug abuse. Results from the Epidemiologic Catchment Area (ECA) Study. JAMA 1990;264:2511–8.
23. Feldman M, Friedman LS, Brandt LJ, editors. Sleisenger and Fordtran's gastrointestinal and liver disease. 8th edition. Philadelphia: Saunders; 2006.
24. Verma S, Kaplowitz N. Diagnosis, management and prevention of drug-induced liver injury. Gut 2009;58:1555–64.
25. Ramrakhiani S, Brunt EM, Bacon BR. Possible cholestatic injury from ranitidine with a review of the literature. Am J Gastroenterol 1998;93:822–6.
26. Yokoyama M, Yokoyama A, Mori S, et al. Inducible histamine protects mice from P. acnes-primed and LPS-induced hepatitis through H2-receptor stimulation. Gastroenterology 2004;127:892–902.
27. Ramachandran R, Kakar S. Histological patterns in drug-induced liver disease. J Clin Pathol 2009;62:481–92.
28. Kao HW, Ashcavai M, Redeker AG. The persistence of hepatitis A IgM antibody after acute clinical hepatitis A. Hepatology 1984;4:933–6.
29. Zignego AL, Deny P, Feray C, et al. Amplification of hepatitis delta virus RNA sequences by polymerase chain reaction: a tool for viral detection and cloning. Mol Cell Probes 1990;4:43–51.
30. Madejon A, Castillo I, Bartolome J, et al. Detection of HDV-RNA by PCR in serum of patients with chronic HDV infection. J Hepatol 1990;11:381–4.
31. Pawlotsky JM. Use and interpretation of virological tests for hepatitis C. Hepatology 2002;36:S65–73.
32. Mast EE, Alter MJ, Holland PV, et al. Evaluation of assays for antibody to hepatitis E virus by a serum panel. Hepatitis E Virus Antibody Serum Panel Evaluation Group. Hepatology 1998;27:857–61.
33. Markin RS. Manifestations of Epstein-Barr virus-associated disorders in liver. Liver 1994;14:1–13.
34. Goodgame RW. Gastrointestinal cytomegalovirus disease. Ann Intern Med 1993; 119:924–35.
35. Sharma S, Mosunjac M. Herpes simplex hepatitis in adults: a search for mucocutaneous clues. J Clin Gastroenterol 2004;38:697–704.
36. Adams PC, Reboussin DM, Barton JC, et al. Hemochromatosis and iron-overload screening in a racially diverse population. N Engl J Med 2005;352:1769–78.
37. Bacon BR, Adams PC, Kowdley KV, et al. Diagnosis and management of hemochromatosis: 2011 practice guideline by the American Association for the Study of Liver Diseases. Hepatology 2011;54:328–43.
38. Roberts EA, Schilsky ML. Diagnosis and treatment of Wilson disease: an update. Hepatology 2008;47:2089–111.
39. de Serres FJ, Blanco I, Fernandez-Bustillo E. Genetic epidemiology of alpha-1 antitrypsin deficiency in North America and Australia/New Zealand: Australia, Canada, New Zealand and the United States of America. Clin Genet 2003;64: 382–97.

40. Manns MP, Vogel A. Autoimmune hepatitis, from mechanisms to therapy. Hepatology 2006;43:S132–44.
41. Alvarez F, Berg PA, Bianchi FB, et al. International Autoimmune Hepatitis Group Report: review of criteria for diagnosis of autoimmune hepatitis. J Hepatol 1999;31:929–38.
42. Kim WR, Lindor KD, Locke GR 3rd, et al. Epidemiology and natural history of primary biliary cirrhosis in a US community. Gastroenterology 2000;119: 1631–6.
43. Bambha K, Kim WR, Talwalkar J, et al. Incidence, clinical spectrum, and outcomes of primary sclerosing cholangitis in a United States community. Gastroenterology 2003;125:1364–9.
44. European Association for the Study of the Liver. EASL Clinical Practice Guidelines: management of cholestatic liver diseases. J Hepatol 2009;51:237–67.
45. Czaja AJ. The variant forms of autoimmune hepatitis. Ann Intern Med 1996;125: 588–98.
46. Kumar S, DeLeve LD, Kamath PS, et al. Hepatic veno-occlusive disease (sinusoidal obstruction syndrome) after hematopoietic stem cell transplantation. Mayo Clin Proc 2003;78:589–98.
47. Cassidy WM, Reynolds TB. Serum lactic dehydrogenase in the differential diagnosis of acute hepatocellular injury. J Clin Gastroenterol 1994;19:118–21.
48. Olsson RG, Lindgren A, Zettergren L. Liver involvement in Addison's disease. Am J Gastroenterol 1990;85:435–8.
49. Miller KK, Grinspoon SK, Ciampa J, et al. Medical findings in outpatients with anorexia nervosa. Arch Intern Med 2005;165:561–6.
50. Litin SC, O'Brien JF, Pruett S, et al. Macroenzyme as a cause of unexplained elevation of aspartate aminotransferase. Mayo Clin Proc 1987;62:681–7.
51. Ruhl CE, Everhart JE. Elevated serum alanine aminotransferase and gamma-glutamyltransferase and mortality in the United States population. Gastroenterology 2009;136:477–485.e11.
52. Schindhelm RK, Dekker JM, Nijpels G, et al. Alanine aminotransferase predicts coronary heart disease events: a 10-year follow-up of the Hoorn Study. Atherosclerosis 2007;191:391–6.
53. Rosch T, Meining A, Fruhmorgen S, et al. A prospective comparison of the diagnostic accuracy of ERCP, MRCP, CT, and EUS in biliary strictures. Gastrointest Endosc 2002;55:870–6.
54. Freeman ML, Nelson DB, Sherman S, et al. Complications of endoscopic biliary sphincterotomy. N Engl J Med 1996;335:909–18.
55. Hanje AJ, Patel T. Preoperative evaluation of patients with liver disease. Nat Clin Pract Gastroenterol Hepatol 2007;4:266–76.
56. Gelman S. General anesthesia and hepatic circulation. Can J Physiol Pharmacol 1987;65:1762–79.
57. Cunningham AJ, Brull SJ. Laparoscopic cholecystectomy: anesthetic implications. Anesth Analg 1993;76:1120–33.
58. Kharasch ED. Adverse drug reactions with halogenated anesthetics. Clin Pharmacol Ther 2008;84:158–62.
59. Summary of the national Halothane Study. Possible association between halothane anesthesia and postoperative hepatic necrosis. JAMA 1966;197:775–88.
60. Mikatti NE, Healy TE. Hepatic injury associated with halogenated anaesthetics: cross-sensitization and its clinical implications. Eur J Anaesthesiol 1997;14:7–14.
61. Fudickar A, Bein B. Propofol infusion syndrome: update of clinical manifestation and pathophysiology. Minerva Anestesiol 2009;75:339–44.

62. Gutelius B, Perz JF, Parker MM, et al. Multiple clusters of hepatitis virus infections associated with anesthesia for outpatient endoscopy procedures. Gastroenterology 2010;139:163–70.
63. Dwyre DM, Fernando LP, Holland PV. Hepatitis B, hepatitis C and HIV transfusion-transmitted infections in the 21st century. Vox Sang 2011;100:92–8.
64. Eid AJ, Razonable RR. New developments in the management of cytomegalovirus infection after solid organ transplantation. Drugs 2010;70:965–81.
65. Kowdley KV, Keeffe EB. Hepatotoxicity of transplant immunosuppressive agents. Gastroenterol Clin North Am 1995;24:991–1001.

Approach to a Patient with Elevated Serum Alkaline Phosphatase

Asma Siddique, MD[a], Kris V. Kowdley, MD[b,*]

KEYWORDS

• Cholestasis • Bile • Cirrhosis • Liver

The term *cholestasis* is derived from the Greek word "chole," which means bile, and "stasis," meaning standing still. Cholestasis develops either from a defect in bile synthesis, impairment in bile secretion, or obstruction to bile flow. Cholestasis may occur as a result of an acute or chronic process involving either the extrahepatic or intrahepatic biliary tree. This syndrome is characterized by an elevated serum alkaline phosphatase (AP) and gamma-glutamyltransferase (GGT) out of proportion to elevation of aminotransferase enzymes. Clinically, pruritus and fatigue are the most common presenting symptoms of chronic cholestatic disorders. Key elements to the diagnostic workup include visualization of the biliary tree by cholangiography and evaluation of liver histology. The hope is that recent advances in understanding the genetic factors and immune mechanisms involved in the pathogenesis of cholestasis will lead to newer therapeutic interventions in the treatment of these diseases.

REPRESENTATIVE CASE

A 68-year-old man presented with history of right upper quadrant pain. He described the pain as a dull aching sensation present intermittently for the past 2 years. He also reported a 20-lb weight loss and intermittent episodes of dark-colored urine and pale stools. He denied taking any medications or excessive alcohol consumption. He had no other significant past medical history. The physical examination revealed jaundice and mild tenderness in the right upper quadrant but was otherwise normal. Laboratory tests revealed an elevated serum total bilirubin of 2.7 mg/dL, AP of 437 U/L, alanine aminotransferase (ALT) of 85 U/L, and aspartate aminotransferase (AST) 54 U/L. CT of the abdomen revealed mild prominence of extrahepatic bile ducts in the porta hepatis, and intrahepatic biliary ductal dilation in both lobes with a patchy distribution.

This work was supported in part by NIH grant DK02957 to Kris V. Kowdley.

[a] Department of Gastroenterology, Center for Liver Disease, Digestive Disease Institute, 1100 Ninth Avenue, PO Box 900, Seattle, WA 98111, USA; [b] Liver Center of Excellence, Digestive Disease Institute, Virginia Mason Medical Center, Benaroya Research Institute, 1201 Ninth Avenue, Seattle, WA 98101, USA

* Corresponding author.

E-mail address: kris.kowdley@vmmc.org

Clin Liver Dis 16 (2012) 199–229

doi:10.1016/j.cld.2012.03.012 liver.theclinics.com

Endoscopic retrograde cholangiography (ERCP) confirmed multifocal intrahepatic biliary ductal strictures with beading and focal dilatation, which was reported to be consistent with sclerosing cholangitis. Cytology from the brushings was negative for malignancy. A liver biopsy revealed hepatic parenchyma with moderate to marked mixed portal inflammation, consisting of lymphocytes and plasma cells. Immunostain for IgG4 revealed numerous scattered IgG4-positive plasma cells in portal tracts up to 20 per high-powered field. The serum IgG4 level was 320 mg/dL.[1] A diagnosis of IgG4-related autoimmune cholangitis was established and corticosteroid therapy was initiated.

PHYSIOLOGY OF BILE FORMATION

Bile acids are the predominant organic solutes in the bile and the driving force for the generation of bile flow. Conjugated bile acids, which represent the major fraction of bile acids in the blood, are transported across the basolateral membrane of hepatocytes by two distinct basolateral transporters: Na+-dependent transport represented by sodium taurocholate cotransporting polypeptide (NTCP; *SLC10A1*) and Na+-independent transport mediated by organic anion transporting proteins (OATPs; OATP2, *SLC21A6*).[2] NTCP is exclusively expressed in hepatocytes and is involved in the transport of both conjugated and unconjugated bile acids.[3] OATP on the other hand facilitates uptake of both conjugated and unconjugated bile salts, and also other organic anions and xenobiotics.[4] Therefore, these uptake and export transporters are essential for not only bile synthesis but also hepatic elimination of various xenobiotics, including bile salts, bilirubin, cholesterol, and drugs. Bile acids are actively transported across the hepatocyte canalicular membrane into the bile by these transporters. Bile acid efflux is mediated by a superfamily of ATP-binding cassette (ABC) transporters. The predominant ABC transporter has been identified as bile salt export pump (BSEP; *ABCB 11*), which mediates export of bile acids.[5]

Some of the other ABC transporters identified include multidrug resistance–associated protein MRP2 (efflux of multiple organic anions, including bilirubin; *ABCC2*) and multidrug-resistance proteins MDR1 (exports organic cation; *ABCB1*) and MDR2 (phospholipid export pump; *ABCB4*).[6] MRP2 also plays an important role in detoxification via its role in transport of drugs, including chemotherapeutic agents, antibiotics, and toxins.[7] MDR3 (multidrug-resistance P-glycoprotein 3; *ABCB4*) is a special ABC transporter that flips phosphatidylcholine, a major lipid constituent, from the inner to the outer leaflet of the canalicular membrane into bile.[8] The expression of these transporters is tightly controlled to prevent accumulation of toxic bile acids in hepatocytes. The primary hepatic bile excreted by the hepatocytes into the bile canaliculus undergoes modifications during its passage through the biliary tree. Cholangiocytes take up bile salts via the apical sodium-dependent bile salt transporter (ASBT; *SLC10A2*), allowing intrahepatic cycling of bile salts.[9] Furthermore, the cholangiocyte transporters, chloride-bicarbonate anion exchanger 2 (AE2; *SLC10A2*) and cystic fibrosis transmembrane conductance regulator (CFTR; *ABCC7*), add cholangiocellular bile to hepatocellular bile.

However, the most critical step in bile acid homeostasis, and a major determinant of bile acid pool size, is the intestinal reabsorption of bile salts.[10] Bile acids are reabsorbed into ileal columnar epithelium (via ASBT) and effluxed into the portal circulation (via MRP3) from where the hepatocytes then extract the bile salts, completing the enterohepatic circulation.[11] The bile acid transporters are subject to extensive regulation at both the transcriptional and posttranscriptional levels.[12] Nuclear receptors play an important role in bile acid metabolism and are activated by different compounds to promote transcription. The known nuclear receptors include farnesoid X receptor (FXR), pregnane X receptor (PXR), vitamin D receptor (VDR), and constitutive androstane (CAR) receptor. During cholestasis both FXR and PXR are activated, resulting in downregulation of *CYP7A1* and thereby decreased conversion of cholesterol to bile acid and decreased bile acid synthesis.[13] FXR is involved in upregulation of BSEP and downregulation of hepatic transporters NTCP. PXR activates OATP2, whereas CAR regulates MRP2 and MPR3.[14] Taken together, activation of nuclear receptors results in decreased bile acid synthesis and uptake and increased bile acid efflux, thereby preventing further accumulation of toxic bile salts in the hepatocytes.

PATTERN OF LIVER TEST ABNORMALITIES IN CHOLESTASIS

Liver disease is often reflected by elevation in liver enzymes and/or liver function. The term *liver function test* is a misnomer, because these tests do not reflect liver function and may be abnormal in conditions unrelated to liver diseases. Liver function tests are often used to describe both serum liver enzymes (aminotransferases, AP) and true function tests, such as prothrombin time, bilirubin, and albumin. The pattern of liver enzyme abnormalities may help characterize the disease as hepatocellular, cholestatic, mixed, or infiltrative (**Table 1**).

Persistent elevation of serum AP is frequently encountered and can pose a diagnostic dilemma. The highest concentration of AP is present in liver and bone; an elevated AP concentration is therefore generally attributed to either liver or bone disease. However, AP is also present in other organs, including intestine, kidney, placenta, and leukocytes. Serum AP levels vary with age, gender, and blood type.[15] Mild elevation of AP is seen in the first 3 months of life and puberty, and a gradual increase is also noted between ages 40 and 65 years, especially in women. AP in adolescent boys may be two to five times greater than in normal adults and correlates with bone growth.[16] Likewise, African Americans have a 10% to 15% higher serum AP, and smokers may have up to 10% higher AP compared with nonsmokers. Finally, individuals with blood type O and B may have elevated AP after a fatty meal because of influx of intestinal AP. Some of the hepatic and extrahepatic causes of elevated and low AP are shown in **Box 1** and **Tables 2** and **3**.

EVALUATION OF CHOLESTASIS

The first step in evaluating a patient with an elevated AP level is to try and identify the source of the AP. This evaluation can be performed through either fractionation of isoenzymes by electrophoresis or obtaining 5′-nucleotidase and GGT levels, both of which are elevated in hepatobiliary disease.[17] The next step is to determine whether cholestasis is secondary to intrahepatic or extrahepatic disease process. Cholestasis is considered intrahepatic when impairment in bile excretion occurs at the

Table 1
Categories based on liver tests

	Liver Disease Category			
Test	**Hepatocellular**	**Cholestatic**	**Infiltrative**	**Mixed**
ALT/AST	++	N/+	N/+	++
AP	N/+	++	+/++	++
TB	N/+ to ++	N/+ to ++	N/+	N/+ to ++

Abbreviations: ALT, alanine aminotransferase; AP, alkaline phosphatase; AST, aspartate aminotransferase; N, normal; TB, total bilirubin; + to ++, degree of elevation.

Box 1 Low alkaline phosphatase
Malnutrition
Wilsons disease
Hypothyroidism
Zinc deficiency
Vitamin C deficiency
Low phosphorus level
Pernicious anemia

hepatocellular level and extrahepatic cholestasis refers to large bile duct involvement, either from an intrinsic process or secondary to extrinsic compression.[18] However, certain conditions such as primary sclerosing cholangitis (PSC) may involve both intrahepatic and extrahepatic bile ducts.[19]

HISTORY AND PHYSICAL

A comprehensive history and physical examination is essential and may provide important clues that help with diagnosis. A history of painless jaundice, with or without a palpable mass, strongly favors malignant biliary obstruction.[20] Choledocholithiasis, however, frequently presents with abdominal pain and jaundice.[21] Life-threatening complications, such as acute ascending cholangitis, may occur in patients with common bile duct stones, mandating urgent intervention. Cholangitis may occur due to partial or complete biliary obstruction and may present with the classic triad of fever with chills, right upper quadrant pain, and jaundice.[21] A history of previous biliary surgery and biliary manipulations increases the possibility of cholangitis in a patient with jaundice.[22] History should also include details regarding alcohol consumption, recreational drug use, and medications, including recently discontinued

Table 2
Nonhepatic cause of elevated alkaline phosphatase

Physiologic	Pregnancy Adolescence After a fatty meal in subjects with blood group O or B
Bone disease	Healing fracture Paget disease Osteomalacia Vitamin D insufficiency Rickets Malignancy: osteogenic sarcoma, metastatic
Renal	Renal failure
Heart	Heart failure
Endocrine	Hyperthyroid Hyperparathyroid
Malignancy	Lymphoma Leukemia Renal cell carcinoma Multiple endocrine neoplasia II

Table 3
Causes of cholestatic liver disease

Intrahepatic Cholestasis	Extrahepatic Cholestasis
Hepatitis: viral (B,C), alcoholic	Extrinsic obstruction
Genetic	stones
Benign recurrent intrahepatic cholestasis	Malignancy
	Pancreas
Progressive familial intrahepatic cholestasis	Gallbladder
	Metastatic
Dubin-Johnson, Rotor syndrome	Cholangiocarcinoma
Drugs and herbal remedies	Ampullary cancer
Pregnancy	Pancreatitis
PBC	Pancreatic pseudocyst
PSC	Parasitic infection
Granulomatous liver disease	Secondary sclerosis (surgery, chemotherapy)
Infections	
Sarcoidosis	
Infiltrative	
Amyloidosis	
Lymphoma	
Idiopathic adult ductopenia	
Autoimmune cholangitis (PSC-like)	
Autoimmune cholangiopathy (PBC-like)	
Prolonged TPN	
Postoperative state	
Sepsis	
Malignancy	
Hepatocellular	
Metastatic	

Abbreviations: PBC, primary biliary cirrhosis; PSC, primary sclerosing cholangitis; TPN, total parenteral nutrition.

medications, herbal remedies, and over-the-counter medications. The clinical setting in which cholestasis occurs should be considered. For example, cholestasis in a severely ill patient is likely secondary to sepsis.[23] Finally, a family history of cholestatic liver disease may suggest a hereditary disorder.[24]

The two most common symptoms suggestive of intrahepatic cholestasis are pruritus and fatigue. These symptoms, however, are nonspecific and may be observed in extrahepatic cholestasis and other liver diseases, such as viral and alcoholic hepatitis.[25] Pruritus can be severe, leading to impaired quality of life. Scratching can result in skin mutilation, and severe refractory itching may be an indication for liver transplant.[26] Pruritus in infants usually manifests as irritability and failure to thrive, whereas older children may experience poor school performance, sleep impairment, and attention deficits.[27] The mechanism of pruritus in liver disease is not entirely understood, and may be related to retention of bile salts or endogenous opioids.[28] Fatigue is an intriguing but poorly recognized symptom in patients with chronic cholestatic liver disease. Fatigue can be very disabling, particularly in patients with primary biliary cirrhosis (PBC).[29,30]

Hypercholesterolemia is a common feature of intrahepatic cholestasis.[28] The abnormal lipoprotein observed in patients with cholestasis is lipoprotein X, which has low atherogenic potential.[31] Clinically, lipid abnormalities may present with xanthomas (cholesterol deposition in tendon sheaths; bony prominences such as elbow and knee; buttocks; and peripheral nerves) and/or xanthelasmas (cholesterol deposits in the periorbital skin folds).[32] Occasionally, xanthomas may develop in acute extrahepatic biliary obstruction, and are usually the eruptive type. Surgical removal of xanthelasmas is usually not effective and recurrence is typical. Malabsorption of fat-soluble vitamins E, D, K, and A is common. Careful attention to prevent and treat these vitamin deficiencies plays an important role in the treatment of chronic cholestatic diseases.[33] Osteopenia and osteoporosis are seen in 10% to 50% of patients with chronic cholestatic liver disease.[34]

INVESTIGATION

Laboratory investigation should include complete blood count with differential, liver enzymes (aminotransferase enzymes and AP), GGT, liver synthetic function (albumin, bilirubin, prothrombin time), viral serologies, autoantibodies antinuclear antibody (ANA), smooth muscle antibody (SMA), antimitochondrial antibody (AMA), pronuclear antineutrophil cytoplasmic antibody (p-ANCA), and immunoglobulin levels.

Transcutaneous abdominal ultrasound (TUS) is usually the first imaging modality to evaluate for intrahepatic and extrahepatic biliary dilatation.[35] TUS is a noninvasive and relatively inexpensive test with a high degree of specificity to identify bile duct obstruction.[36] However, TUS may be technically difficult in obese patients and the pancreas is often difficult to image with the technique; furthermore, approximately 60% of common bile duct (CBD) stones may be missed on TUS. A CT scan is comparable to TUS in detection of stones and provides additional information regarding the liver parenchyma and may help identify mass lesions, such as a pancreatic tumor. CT scan, however, is not very helpful in delineating the biliary tree.[37] A negative TUS and CT in a patient strongly suspected to have extrahepatic obstruction should be followed by further imaging. Magnetic resonance cholangiopancreatography (MRCP) and endoscopic ultrasound are safe and accurate options for detecting lesions causing extrahepatic obstruction.[38] The gold standard for visualizing the biliary tract is endoscopic cholangiopancreatography (ERCP). ERCP can identify the cause and level of obstruction; in addition, brushings and biopsy may be obtained and therapeutic interventions can be undertaken, such as stone extraction, dilatation of biliary strictures and stent placement, if required.[39] Percutaneous transhepatic cholangiography may be required in patients with altered anatomy, such as a history of prior surgery such as gastrectomy or a choledochojejunostomy.

Once extrahepatic cholestasis is excluded, further workup of intrahepatic cholestasis is warranted. Certain autoantibodies are highly specific; a positive AMA is highly suggestive of PBC.[40] The diagnostic criteria for PBC include an elevated AP, positive AMA, and characteristic liver biopsy features, although liver biopsy is no longer considered essential for the diagnosis of PBC.[41] Liver histology consistent with PBC in a patient with biochemical tests suggestive of PBC but a serologic pattern suggestive of autoimmune hepatitis (positive ANA or ASMA) is classified as autoimmune cholangiopathy.[42] However, low titers of ANA and SMA may be seen in several include conditions, including PBC, PSC, and other cholestatic diseases.[43] In the absence of a positive AMA, MRCP is indicated to exclude PSC. The characteristic features of PSC include diffuse multifocal stricturing and dilatation involving the intrahepatic and/or extrahepatic ducts.[44] In an appropriate clinical setting, an abnormal cholangiogram similar to PSC may indicate AIDS cholangiopathy or other secondary cholangitis.[45] When diagnosis is unclear or for staging purpose, a percutaneous liver biopsy is indicated. The liver biopsy specimen should contain at least 10 portal tracts for accurate diagnosis. An algorithm for evaluating the adult patient with cholestasis is presented in **Fig. 1**.

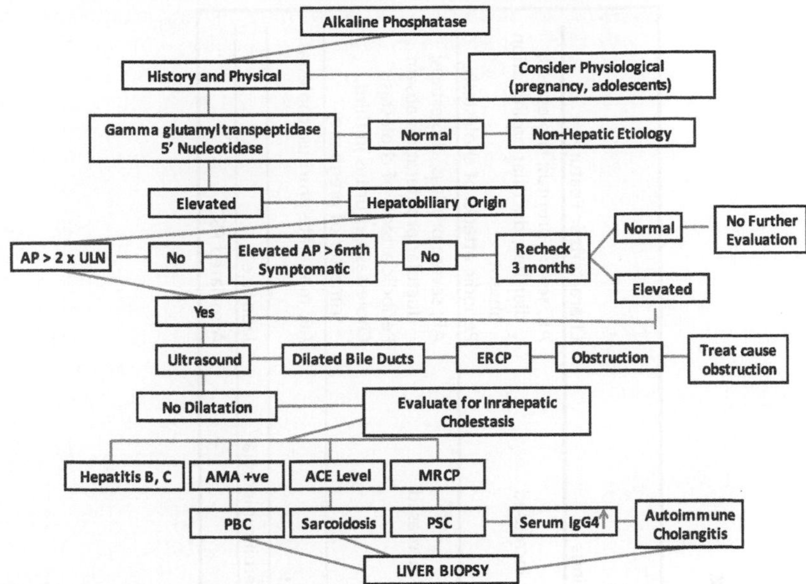

Fig. 1. Proposed algorithm for workup of elevated AP.

GENETIC DISORDERS OF CHOLESTASIS

Several genetic disorders characterized by defects in the hepatocellular transport system have been described, including progressive familial intrahepatic cholestasis (PFIC), benign recurrent intrahepatic cholestasis (BRIC), cystic fibrosis, and Dubin-Johnson syndrome (**Table 4**).

PFIC refers to a heterogeneous group of autosomal recessive cholestatic liver diseases that often present in the neonatal period or first year of life. Without a liver transplant, death from liver failure may occur in the first decade.[24] Three types of PFIC have been described, and the inheritance pattern of all three forms is autosomal recessive. The phenotypic findings of PFIC1 (Byler disease) and PFIC2 (Byler syndrome) are similar. PFIC1 is caused by a mutation in *FIC1* (familial intrahepatic cholestasis 1) located on chromosome 18q21–22, whereas PFIC2 is caused by a mutation in the *BSEP* gene located on chromosome 2q24.[46,47] These children present with severe cholestasis, pruritus, elevated bile acids, and a normal serum GGT level.[48] Patients with PFIC2 usually have higher serum aminotransferase levels and are at an increased risk for developing hepatocellular carcinoma, which may occur in the first or second decade of life.[49] Patients with PFIC1 may show extrahepatic features, such as watery diarrhea, bile acid malabsorption, pancreatitis, and nephrolithiasis. PFIC3 involves mutations in the *ABCB4* gene, the gene that encodes multidrug resistance protein 3 (MDR3)[50]; is characterized by markedly elevated serum GGT; and usually presents in later infancy or early childhood.[48] Liver failure can occur in childhood or adulthood in people with PFIC3.[50] Women who are obligate carriers of heterozygous *MDR3* have an increased risk for developing cholestasis during the third trimester of pregnancy.[51]

BRIC is a rare autosomal recessive or sporadic liver disease characterized by intermittent episodes of cholestasis. Two types of BRIC have been described: BRIC1 is caused by mutations in *FIC1* and BRIC2 by a *BSEP* mutation. This condition follows

Table 4
Hereditary cholestatic syndromes

Protein/Gene	Chromosome	Clinical Disease State	Laboratory Findings	Characteristic Features
FIC1/ATP8B1	18q21	PFIC1	GGT low Serum bile acids increased	AR; severe pruritus; cholestasis; diarrhea; ductular proliferation absent
		BRIC1	GGT low	Periodic attacks of cholestasis
BSEP/ABCB11	2q24	PFIC2	GGT low Serum bile acids increased	AR; severe pruritus; cholestasis; ductular proliferation absent
		BRIC2	GGT low	Periodic attacks of cholestasis
		ICP	GGT low or high	Cholestasis, pruritus in third trimester of pregnancy
MDR3/ABCB4	7q21	PFIC3 ICP	GGT increased Bile acids normal	AR; moderate pruritus; cholestasis
MRP2/ABCC2	10q24	Dubin-Johnson	Conjugated hyperbilirubinemia	Jaundice
CFTR/ABCC7	7q31	Cystic fibrosis		Associated PSC

Abbreviation: ICP, intrahepatic cholestasis of pregnancy.

a benign course, with no progression to chronic liver disease.[52,53] During a cholestatic episode, both the serum bilirubin and AP are elevated, whereas GGT remains normal. Symptom-free periods may last several weeks to months.

Other rare genetic cholestatic conditions include Dubin-Johnson syndrome, a rare benign autosomal recessive, relapsing disorder caused by a *MRP2* mutation.[54] This condition is characterized by conjugated hyperbilirubinemia and an elevated GGT level. Cystic transmembrane regulator (*CFTR*) mutations results in impairment in chloride secretion and cholestasis.[55] Finally, Alagille syndrome (caused by a mutation in *JAG1*) is a rare condition characterized by hypoplasia of the intrahepatic bile ducts and other developmental defects.[56]

PRIMARY BILIARY CIRRHOSIS OR CHRONIC NONSUPPURATIVE DESTRUCTIVE CHOLANGITIS

The exact origin of PBC is not known; however, PBC is believed to develop when a genetically susceptible individual is exposed to an environmental trigger.[57] Evidence that genetic factors play a major role is based on a high concordance rate of 63% in monozygotic twins versus 0% in dizygotic twins, and 5% to 6% of patients have a first-degree relative with PBC.[58] A link between PBC and HLA-DR8 and HLA-DPB1 and other genetic variants of HLA class II suggest an inherited immune system abnormality resulting in inability to suppress the inflammatory injury contributing to biliary cell lysis observed in PBC.[59] Xenobiotics (drugs, pesticides, cosmetics) and certain infections (*Chlamydia pneumoniae*, *Escherichia coli*, retrovirus, *Novosphingobium aromaticivorans*, lactobacilli) are thought to play a role in the pathogenesis of PBC through possibly either triggering an autoimmune reaction or causing a direct toxic effect.[60,61] Smoking is a possible risk factor for the development of PBC, and possibly accelerates progression.[62]

Clinical Features

PBC is more common among women, with a female:male ratio of 10:1.[62] Nearly 60% are asymptomatic at diagnosis and are incidentally detected to have an elevated serum AP level.[63] Fatigue and pruritus are common symptoms and may be present in 40% to 80% of patients, although these symptoms do not correlate with the severity of liver disease.[29,64] Fat-soluble vitamin deficiencies (vitamins A, D, E, and K) and osteoporosis, however, are usually seen in patients with advanced PBC.[34,65]

Diagnosis

PBC is characterized by a cholestatic pattern of liver enzyme abnormalities, with a predominant elevation of serum AP and GGT. An elevated serum bilirubin is an independent predictor of survival.[66] However, the hallmark of PBC is the presence of AMA, which is positive in 90% to 95% of patients, with a sensitivity of 98% and specificity 96%.[40,67] ANA may be present in 20% to 50% of patients with PBC.[68] The role of imaging in PBC is mainly to exclude possible biliary obstruction and cirrhosis, and screen for hepatocellular carcinoma in patients with advanced PBC and cirrhosis. The characteristic histology in PBC is the "florid duct lesion," with involvement of interlobular bile ducts, inflammation, and bile duct injury. The infiltrate comprises plasma cells, macrophages, and eosinophils. Noncaseating granulomas may be present.[69] Occasionally the only finding on histology may be ductopenia, defined as absence of bile ducts in greater than 50% of portal tracts (**Fig. 2**).

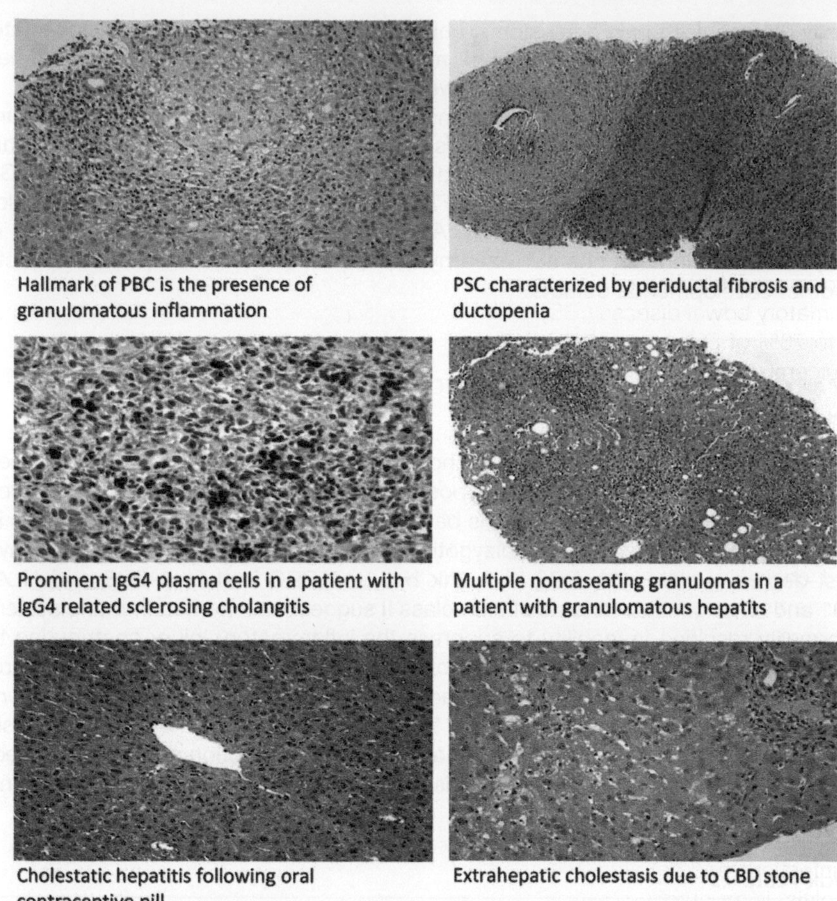

Hallmark of PBC is the presence of granulomatous inflammation
PSC characterized by periductal fibrosis and ductopenia
Prominent IgG4 plasma cells in a patient with IgG4 related sclerosing cholangitis
Multiple noncaseating granulomas in a patient with granulomatous hepatits
Cholestatic hepatitis following oral contraceptive pill
Extrahepatic cholestasis due to CBD stone

Fig. 2. Histologic features in cholestatic liver disease.

Treatment

Ursodeoxycholic acid (UDCA) is the only drug approved by the U.S. Food and Drug Administration for PBC, and is used at a dose 13 to 15 mg/kg/d. UDCA improves liver tests, including serum bilirubin and other serum biochemical markers, and liver histology.[70] When used in the early stages of PBC, UDCA halts progression of disease. Patients with a favorable biochemical response have a significantly reduced likelihood of needing a liver transplant and reduced mortality from decompensated liver disease.[71] Liver transplantation is reserved for patients with decompensated PBC. Liver transplant does not change the AMA-positive status, even though only 20% have recurrence of PBC at 5 years posttransplant.[72]

AUTOIMMUNE CHOLANGIOPATHY

Autoimmune cholangiopathy (AIC) describes the 5% to 8% of patients with AMA-negative PBC. AIC is characterized by a cholestatic liver enzymes pattern, liver histology consistent with PBC, and a negative AMA.[73] Hypergammaglobulinemia and positive ANA and SMA results may be present. AIC is treated similarly to PBC and may represent a single disease with a variable autoantibody profile. The autoantibodies found in autoimmune cholestatic conditions are shown in **Table 5**.

PSC

PSC is a chronic cholestatic liver disease characterized by concentric and obliterative fibrosis of the intrahepatic or extrahepatic bile ducts, which may progress to biliary cirrhosis.[74] Although the first case of PSC was most likely described in 1929 in a patient with ulcerative colitis who developed cirrhosis, it was only in 1960 that the term *primary sclerosing cholangitis* was coined.[75] PSC is frequently associated with inflammatory bowel disease (IBD), most commonly ulcerative colitis.[76] Approximately 62% to 73% of patients with PSC have ulcerative colitis, and 3% to 4% of patients with ulcerative colitis develop PSC. Even though IBD is more frequent in women, PSC has a 2:1 male predominance.[77] The median age of onset is approximately 40 years and it is more common among nonsmokers.[78]

PSC is a multifactorial disease. Environmental factors and genetic predisposition likely play a role, because siblings of patients with PSC have a prevalence of 1.5%; approximately a 100-fold increased risk.[79] The major histocompatibility complex (MHC) encodes human leukocyte antigen (HLA) class I and II molecules and MHC class I chain-like alpha-molecules (MICA). MICA has a role in the innate immune response as ligands for natural killer cells. Polymorphisms in MICA*008 have been associated with PSC.[80] Furthermore an increased prevalence of HLA-B8, HLA-DR3, and HLA-DRw52a is seen in patients with PSC, with HLA-B8 in up to 60% to 80% of patients with PSC.[81] More recently, several genome-wide association studies (GWAS) have shown that, outside of the HLA complex, at least three non-HLA susceptibility loci (chromosome 13q31, chromosome 2q35, and chromosome 3p21), all three of which are also implicated in ulcerative colitis, may contribute toward the risk of PSC development.[82]

The association between PSC and ulcerative colitis has led to considerations of both infectious and autoimmune contributions to the pathogenesis. PSC, like ulcerative colitis, is an autoimmune disease, and bacterial or viral antigens may enter the portal circulation through an inflamed colonic wall, triggering an immune reaction.[83–85] The autoimmune hypothesis is further supported by the presence of autoantibodies, such as p-ANCA or ANA in patients with PSC.[86] However, unlike other autoimmune conditions, PSC has a male predominance and does not respond to corticosteroids.[87]

Clinical Features

PSC should be suspected in any patient with IBD presenting with cholestatic liver enzyme abnormalities. Similar to PBC, most patients are asymptomatic at presentation.[88] The most common symptoms at presentation include intermittent episodes

Table 5
Autoimmune antibodies in cholestatic liver disease

	PBC	AIC	PSC	IgG4-SC
ANA	20%–50%	79%–100%	7%–77%	43%–80%
SMA	20%	50%	15%–20%	<5%
AMA	95%	0	0	0
p-ANCA	3%–33%	unknown	80%	<5%
Ig	IgM	IgG	IgG, IgM	IgG

Abbreviations: Ig, immunoglobulin; IgG4-SC, IgG4-related sclerosing cholangitis.

of fatigue, pruritus, or abdominal discomfort. During the initial course of the disease, most symptoms resolve spontaneously.[89] The serum AP and bilirubin may also fluctuate, indicating transient biliary obstruction from biliary sludge or stones. Episodes of fever, chills, and jaundice may reflect bacterial cholangitis from biliary obstruction rather than advanced disease. Persistent jaundice suggests advanced PSC and should raise the suspicion of cholangiocarcinoma.

Diagnosis

ERCP has traditionally been the gold standard for diagnosing PSC; however, MRCP is increasingly being used as a noninvasive alternative to ERCP.[90] ERCP should currently be reserved for when an intervention such as dilatation and stenting of biliary stricture is anticipated or if MRCP is suboptimal for diagnosis. ERCP is also indicated if a dominant stricture is present to obtain cytologic brushings to rule out cholangiocarcinoma.[91] On cholangiography, the strictures are short and alternate with dilated segments, producing the characteristic "beaded" appearance.[92] The characteristic histologic finding in PSC is the "onion skin" fibrosis pattern present in 7% to 50% (see **Fig. 2**).[93] This feature describes the periductal concentric fibrosis that occurs around the interlobular and septal bile ducts, resulting in ductopenia and bile duct proliferation. The classical PSC finding of obliterative fibrous cholangitis, which represents concentric fibrosis with obliterative cholangitis, is present in less than 10% patients with PSC.[93]

Conditions that result in secondary sclerosing cholangitis should be ruled out before making a diagnosis of PSC, including intraductal stones, ischemic cholangiopathy, bile duct injury from intraarterial chemotherapy, AIDS cholangiopathy, recurrent pyogenic cholangitis, and bile duct injury during surgery.[94]

Patients with PSC are at risk for development of several malignancies. Patients with PSC have a 5% to 10% lifetime risk for developing cholangiocarcinoma.[95] Risk factors for cholangiocarcinoma include older age at diagnosis of PSC, longer duration of IBD, smoking, and alcohol use, and patients who have undergone proctocolectomy.[95] An annual MRI/MRCP or ultrasound along with CA19-9 is recommended for screening for cholangiocarcinoma.[96] Patients with PSC also have increased prevalence of gallbladder cancer, colorectal cancer or dysplasia, and hepatocellular cancer.[97] Therefore, an annual colonoscopy with multiple biopsies is recommended for screening purposes.[98]

Treatment

UDCA has been evaluated for the treatment of PSC.[99] Results from studies using low-dose UDCA were inconclusive and a high-dose (28–30 mg/kg/d) trial was discontinued early because of development of serious adverse events, including cirrhosis, death, and liver transplant.[100] UDCA at a dose up to 13 to 15 mg/kg/d, may show improvement in some features of cholestasis but does not have survival benefit or delay the need for transplant.[101] Therefore, UDCA is not recommended for the treatment of PSC.[102]

IGG4-RELATED SCLEROSING CHOLANGITIS

IgG4-related sclerosing disease is a systemic inflammatory condition characterized by IgG4-positive plasma cells and T-lymphocyte infiltration frequently involving multiple organs.[103] The tissues commonly involved include the pancreas, bile duct, gallbladder, kidney, retroperitoneum, and salivary glands.[104] IgG4-related sclerosing cholangitis (IgG4-SC) is a variant of this condition, characterized by bile duct involvement.[105] IgG4-SC is associated with autoimmune pancreatitis (AIP) in 80% to 90% of patients.[105]

Clinical Features

IgG4-SC clinically and cholangiographically resembles PSC. It is, however, important to differentiate the conditions, because IgG4-SC is responsive to steroid therapy.[106] **Table 6** outlines some of the differences between the conditions.

Diagnosis

IgG4-SC is easy to diagnose when associated with AIP. AIP manifests with typical radiologic features, such as "sausage-like diffuse pancreatic swelling with peripancreatic capsule-like rim, and irregular narrowing of the pancreatic duct" along with an elevated serum IgG4 level.[107] Ghazale and colleagues[108] showed that in AIP, an IgG4 greater than 140 mg/dL had a sensitivity and specificity of 76% and 93%, respectively, and when the cutoff was raised to 280 mg/dL, the sensitivity and specificity were 53% and 99%, respectively. However, 9% of patients with PSC may also have elevated IgG4 levels. Patients with IgG4-SC may be associated with hypergammaglobulinemia, positive ANA in 40% to 50% of patients, positive rheumatoid factor in approximately 20%, and eosinophilia in 15%.[108]

The cholangiographic features in IgG4-SC is classified into 4 types[109]

Type 1: stenosis occurs in the lower part of the common bile duct; often misdiagnosed as pancreatic cancer

Type 2: diffuse stenosis involving intrahepatic and extrahepatic bile ducts; closely resembles PSC

Type 3: stenosis involving the hilar region and the lower part of the common bile duct; often misdiagnosed as cholangiocarcinoma

Type 4: stenosis only in the hilar hepatic region; often misdiagnosed as cholangiocarcinoma

Table 6
Differences between PSC and IgG4-SC

	PSC	IgG4-SC
Age	25–45 y	65 y
Male	65%	80%
Association with IBD	Present	Absent
Other organ involvement	No	Pancreas frequently involved
p-ANCA	Positive	Less common
Elevated serum IgG4	7%–9%	70%
Histology	Ductopenia Periductal concentric fibrosis	Abundant IgG4 + plasma cells Periportal fibroinflammatory nodules
Cholangiogram	Multifocal "beaded"; pruned tree appearance of intrahepatic and extrahepatic ducts	Segmental, long strictures with prestenotic dilatation, distal CBD involvement, pancreatic duct involvement
Response to steroid	No	Yes

The gold standard for the diagnosis of IgG4-SC is histology showing the characteristic diffuse lymphoplasmacytic infiltration, infiltration by $IgG4^+$ plasma cells, and obliterative phlebitis, which is distinct from the ductopenia and periductal concentric fibrosis seen in PSC (see **Fig. 2**).[110,111]

Treatment

This disease may be characterized by a spontaneous relapsing and remitting course but is very responsive to corticosteroid therapy, and steroids can induce remission.[111] No consensus exists regarding dose and duration of steroid therapy, but an initial high dose of prednisone, 40 mg/d for 3 to 4 weeks followed by a tapering course guided by biochemical and radiologic response should be considered.[93] Steroid-sparing immunosuppressive therapy with azathioprine, mycophenolate mofetil, and rituximab is sometimes indicated for patients with a relapsing course requiring chronic immunosuppressive therapy.[112]

HEPATIC SARCOIDOSIS

Sarcoidosis is a multisystemic disease of unknown origin characterized by the presence of noncaseating granulomata.[113] Sarcoidosis primarily affects the lungs and lymph nodes but can involve almost every organ, including the liver.[114] Hepatic sarcoid usually affects individuals between 20 and 40 years of age; African Americans have a twofold to threefold increased risk of developing sarcoidosis compared with Caucasians.[115] African Americans also may have a more chronic and severe form of disease.[115]

Clinical Features

Most patients with hepatic sarcoid are asymptomatic, and only 5% to 30% present with symptoms, such as nausea, vomiting, abdominal pain, fever with night sweats, myalgia, and possible weight loss.[116] Approximately 50% to 80% of patients with systemic sarcoidosis have hepatic involvement.[117]

Diagnosis

The most common biochemical abnormality noted in hepatic sarcoid is an elevated AP and GGT, and the extent of elevation may reflect severity of fibrosis.[118] Serum angiotensin-converting enzyme (ACE) level is almost always elevated in hepatic sarcoid and is associated with an active disease process.[118] Other granulomatous conditions have not been associated with significant ACE level elevation.[119] Hepatic nodules are usually diffuse, multiple, and small, usually approximately 1.0 cm in diameter.[120] On CT imaging these nodules generally appear as multiple low-attenuating, non–contrast-enhancing lesions, and on MRI they appear as hypodense lesions on T2-weighed sequence without contrast enhancement.[120,121] The main histologic features in hepatic sarcoid are noncaseating granulomas, which consist of multinucleated giant cells (see **Fig. 2**). Granulomas are typically in the portal and periportal areas.[122] In more advanced cases, chronic cholestasis, ductopenia, and cirrhosis may be evident.[122] Several other conditions may be associated with granulomas, including PBC, lymphoma, and tuberculosis.[123]

Treatment

Corticosteroids is the mainstay of treatment for hepatic sarcoidosis.[124] General consensus exists that treatment is not required in the absence of symptoms or biochemical abnormalities. In patients with symptoms such as fever and abdominal pain, low-dose prednisone, 10–15 mg/d is often associated with clinical response.[125]

Steroid therapy also seems to improve liver tests in patients with mild to moderate enzyme elevation.[124] However, biochemical response does not correlate with histologic response, and progression to cirrhosis may occur.[124] In advanced hepatic sarcoidosis, steroids are unlikely to have any significant benefit.[126] Methotrexate, hydroxychloroquine, azathioprine, and cyclophosphamide have been used as steroid-sparing agents and have shown benefit.[126] UDCA has also proven useful in patients with chronic cholestasis and may improve clinical and biochemical abnormalities.[127]

Portal hypertension (PHT) is a rare complication of hepatic sarcoid and warrants mention. PHT may occur with or without cirrhosis.[128] In the absence of cirrhosis, PHT may be a result of obstruction of portal flow by granulomas; arteriovenous shunts that increase portal blood flow; granulomatous phlebitis causing portal and hepatic vein occlusion, resulting in ischemia; or extrinsic hepatic vein obstruction by granulomas, resulting in Budd-Chiari syndrome.[128,129] Liver transplantation may be the ultimate treatment option in these patients.[130]

PARENTERAL NUTRITION–ASSOCIATED LIVER DISEASE

Parenteral nutrition–induced hepatobiliary disease (PNALD) is more common in children, particularly premature infants, compared with adults.[131] This condition should be suspected in patients on parenteral nutrition who develop hyperbilirubinemia and liver enzyme elevation after ruling out drug-induced liver injury, sepsis, and extrahepatic obstruction. Liver enzyme elevation is usually observed within 1 to 4 weeks after initiation of parenteral nutrition, and in most instances improves despite continued parenteral nutrition.[132] Two patterns of injury may be seen in PNALD: steatosis and steatohepatitis or cholestasis.[133] Steatosis is more common in adults, whereas cholestasis occurs in children.[133] PNALD ranges from mild liver enzyme elevation with resolution after cessation of parenteral nutrition, to steatosis, steatohepatitis, and cholestasis, and, in a few patients, may progress to severe hepatobiliary damage and cirrhosis.[134]

The origin of PNALD is multifactorial. Decreased gallbladder emptying resulting in cholelithiasis; bacterial overgrowth from the unused gut, leading to gut translocation of endotoxins into the portal circulation; or amino acids in PN solution are all thought to contribute to the development of PNALD.[133–135] Immaturity of the biliary secretory system plays a major role in the development of cholestasis in premature infants.[136]

PNALD can be prevented through early resumption of oral or enteral intake, prevention of hypoxia, prompt treatment of sepsis, treatment of hypoproteinemia, and avoidance of hepatotoxic drugs. Using a cyclic parenteral nutrition schedule and decreasing excess amino acids in parenteral nutrition will also likely prevent liver injury.[137]

Treatment

Treatment options for PNALD are limited. UDCA has been shown to be possibly effective in PNALD.[138] Bowel decontamination with antibiotics such as metronidazole may be helpful.[139] Intestinal transplantation, frequently along with liver transplantation, is reserved for patients with short bowel syndrome dependent on parenteral nutrition who develop overt or pending liver failure or other life-threatening complications from parenteral nutrition.[140]

INTRAHEPATIC CHOLESTASIS OF PREGNANCY

Intrahepatic cholestasis of pregnancy (ICP) is defined as pruritus and elevated serum bile acid levels in otherwise healthy pregnant women.[141] ICP usually manifests around

25 to 32 weeks of gestation, resolves after delivery, and tends to recur in 45% to 70% of subsequent pregnancies.[142]

Clinical Features

The main manifestation of ICP is pruritus, which affects all parts of the body and is frequently worse at night. Occasionally patients may present with steatorrhea.[143] Jaundice occurs in fewer than 25% of patients.[144] Hormonal (both estrogen and progesterone), genetic, and environmental factors likely influence the development of ICP.[145] *MDR3* mutations account for approximately 15% of cases of ICP.[146]

Diagnosis

The diagnosis of ICP is one of exclusion, and all other causes of hepatic impairment should be considered first. Prompt resolution of symptoms after delivery favors a diagnosis of ICP. Serum AP will be elevated but is of limited diagnostic value in pregnancy. Aminotransferase enzyme elevation is usually mild to moderate, and patients may infrequently have hyperbilirubinemia, although a serum bilirubin level usually less than 5 mg/dL.[147] Serum bile acid level is a more sensitive and specific biochemical marker of ICP, both for diagnosis and subsequent monitoring.[148] Specifically, serum cholic acid level is increased, resulting in an increased cholic/chenodeoxycholic acid ratio; this is the most sensitive test for diagnosing ICP.[149]

Treatment

UDCA is the preferred treatment for ICP and has been shown to not only control symptoms but also reduce both serum bilirubin and bile acid in maternal and cord blood.[150] More importantly, no maternal or fetal adverse effects have been noted.[150] Dexamethasone is occasionally used but is less effective than UDCA.[151]

CHOLESTASIS RELATED TO SEPSIS

Sepsis is the most common cause of jaundice and cholestasis in the intensive care setting.[152] Cholestatic jaundice may complicate both gram-positive and gram-negative bacteremia, with *E coli* being the commonest organism linked to this condition.[153] This syndrome accounts for a third of neonatal jaundice.[152] Sepsis-induced liver disease may be a primary hepatic dysfunction, which occurs immediately after shock as a consequence of hypotension and/or hypoxia and is manifested by significant elevation in aminotransferase enzymes. Secondary hepatic dysfunction is caused by Kupffer cell activation by bacteria and endotoxins and release of inflammatory mediators.[154]

Intrahepatic cholestasis related to sepsis is characterized by a disproportionate elevation in serum bilirubin compared with serum AP. Serum AP is usually two to three times greater than the upper limit of normal. Serum aminotransferases are usually less than two times the upper limit of normal.[155] Biliary obstruction and hepatobiliary infection should be ruled out before diagnosing sepsis-related cholestasis. Unlike other cholestatic conditions, pruritus is not a major manifestation of cholestasis associated with sepsis. Histologically, bile is seen in bile canaliculi and hepatocytes. Hyperplasia of Kupffer cells and apoptotic bodies may be present on histology.[152]

Aggressive supportive measures and treatment of underlying infection are the mainstay of treatment of sepsis-related cholestasis; currently data are insufficient regarding the use of UDCA.[156]

DRUG-INDUCED LIVER INJURY

Drug-induced liver injury (DILI) is probably the most common cause of cholestatic liver disease and accounts for 40% of adults presenting with hepatitis.[157] Hepatotoxicity can occur after the use of prescription drugs, over-the-counter medications, toxins, and herbal medications, and accounts for approximately 10% of all adverse drug reactions.[158] DILI may manifest as pure cholestasis caused by an abnormality in canalicular bile flow or a mixed hepatocellular cholestatic pattern.[159] The pathogenesis of DILI is poorly understood. In genetically susceptible individuals, a direct injury triggered by a drug or its metabolites may initiate both an innate and adaptive immune response.[160] Certain drugs also directly bind to intracellular proteins or inhibit mitochondrial function, resulting in decreased energy production and, eventually, activation of apoptotic pathways, resulting in programmed cell death.[161] In a subset of patients, inhibition of hepatobiliary transporter systems by a drug may be a major factor in pathogenesis of cholestasis. Studies support the role of mutations in the *ABCB11* and *ABCB4* genes encoding BSEP and MDR3 in DILI.[162] Drugs that affect canalicular membrane transport pumps, such as MDR3, also can interrupt bile flow, causing cholestasis.

Clinical Features

DILI may present with nonspecific symptoms, such as abdominal pain, nausea, and fatigue, or as an acute illness with jaundice.[163] Chronic drug-induced cholestasis may present with pruritus. DILI often resolves after withdrawal of the offending drug but occasionally can cause significant bile duct damage and chronic liver disease.[163] **Table 7** outlines some of the manifestations of DILI. DILI should be suspected in individuals with no known medical illness who present with symptoms and abnormal liver tests shortly after initiation of a medication, with prompt improvement after withdrawal of the drug.

Diagnosis

A temporal relationship between drug exposure and clinical presentation is not always possible to establish. When a single agent is involved, diagnosis may be simple, but most individuals are on multiple medications that have the potential for hepatotoxicity. Furthermore, other liver conditions, such as autoimmune hepatitis or nonalcoholic steatohepatitis, may have a similar clinical presentation. A detailed history should be obtained, including the duration, dose, route of administration, prior exposure to drug, use of over-the-counter medications, and herbal medications. Laboratory studies should be performed to assess degree of liver enzyme elevation and synthetic liver function. A liver biopsy remains an important tool for diagnosis, although it is not always necessary (see **Fig. 2**).[164]

Treatment

Treatment of DILI is early recognition and withdrawal of the offending drug. Specific treatment is limited to acetaminophen and valproic acid overdose, which are treated with the specific antidotes *N*-acetylcysteine and *L*-carnitine, respectively.[165] In individuals with a predominant cholestatic pattern, ursodeoxycholic acid has been used.[166] In this setting, acute liver failure has a mortality rate of more than 80% without liver transplant and should prompt an early transplant referral.

Table 7
Clinical characteristics of drug-induced liver injury

Subclinical ALT <3 × ULN Usually benign Resolves weeks to months after stopping drug eg, sulfonamide, salicylate	Granulomatous hepatitis Noncaseating granulomas Usually asymptomatic Hepatocellular or cholestatic pattern eg, allopurinol, carbamazepine, cephalexin
Acute liver injury Acute hepatitis Resembles viral hepatitis Cytotoxic hepatocellular injury High mortality if acute liver failure develops eg, acetaminophen Cholestatic injury Resembles extrahepatic May take months for jaundice to improve eg, amoxicillin/clavulanate Mixed Increased risk of chronic liver disease eg, phenytoin Acute steatosis Usually microvesicular eg, amiodarone, zidovudine, herbal remedies	Chronic hepatic injury Chronic hepatitis Resembles autoimmune hepatitis Extrahepatic features common (arthralgia, eosinophilia, rash) eg, methyldopa, diclofenac Chronic steatosis Usually macrovesicular eg, valproate, amiodarone Cirrhosis eg, methotrexate, azathioprine, OCP Phospholipidosis High incidence of cirrhosis eg, amiodarone, chloroquine
Chronic cholestasis Chronic intrahepatic Resembles PBC Usually resolves after stopping drug eg, amitriptyline, ampicillin, chlorpromazine Vanishing bile duct syndrome Ductopenia Hepatitis C progress to cirrhosis eg, amoxicillin, clindamycin, carbamazepine Biliary sclerosis Resembles PSC eg, intraarterial infusion 5-flurodexoyuridine	Vascular disease Hepatic vein thrombosis Thrombosis of hepatic vein or inferior vena cava eg, OCP Sinusoidal obstruction syndrome Clinically resemble Budd-Chiari syndrome eg, azathioprine, vitamin A Peliosis hepatis Multiple, small, blood-filled cavities in hepatic parenchyma eg, anabolic steroids, arsenic

Abbreviations: ALT, alanine aminotransferase; OCP, oral contraceptive pill; ULN, upper limit of normal.

EXTRAHEPATIC CHOLESTASIS

Choledocholithiasis and Acute Ascending Cholangitis

Cholelithiasis affects approximately 10% of adults in the United States, and 10% to 20% of patients with symptomatic choleithiasis have concomitant choledocholithiasis.[167] A CBD stone may result in biliary obstruction and bile stasis, resulting in the life-threatening complication of acute ascending cholangitis. Biliary manipulation during ERCP is the second most common cause of acute cholangitis.[168]

Clinical features

Choledocholithaisis may be asymptomatic and one-third of patients may have normal laboratory values.[169] Symptomatic stones can present with right upper quadrant pain, fever, and jaundice. This triad of symptoms is present in 55% to 70% of patients with acute cholangitis.[170] The pentad, which also includes hypotension and altered mental status, is seen in less than 5% to 7%.

Diagnosis

Ninety percent of patients with obstruction from stones will have an elevated AP and GGT.[170] Bile cultures are positive in 80% to 100% of patients who have cholangitis, and blood cultures may be positive in 20% to 70%.[171] TUS remains the initial screening test for CBD stones, with a sensitivity and specificity of 25% to 60% and 95% to 100%, respectively.[172] MRCP has evolved into an accurate noninvasive modality for diagnosing CBD stones, with sensitivity and specificity comparable to ERCP (85% and 93% vs 93%–98% and 97%–100%, respectively).[173] MRCP, however, may be falsely negative in patients with stones smaller than 6 mm. Endoscopic ultrasound is also comparable to ERCP for detecting stones and does not carry the risk of pancreatitis and cholngitis.[173] The main advantage of ERCP over MRCP is that ERCP is both a diagnostic tool but can be used for therapeutic interventions, such as stone retrieval.[169]

Choledochal Cyst

Choledochal cyst is a rare condition characterized by cystic dilatation of intrahepatic ducts, extrahepatic ducts, or both.[174] This condition is more common among Asians than Caucasians, with a female preponderance (4:1)[174] Reflux of pancreatic secretion into CBD results in damage to bile ducts and recurrent cholangitis, pancreatitis, chronic inflammation, and fibrosis.[175]

Clinical features

Most patients are diagnosed in childhood, and the classic triad of abdominal pain, jaundice, and a palpable right upper quadrant abdominal mass is seen in only 10% to 20% of adults.[176]

Diagnosis

No specific laboratory tests help in the diagnosis. TUS is the preferred initial test, although MRI and MRCP are preferred because they delineate the biliary tree, define the extent of involvement of bile ducts, and provide information on surrounding parenchyma.[177] On MRCP, choledochal cysts appear as a markedly dilated CBD with saccular formation. On histology, the cyst wall appears thin and fibrous, and adults may have evidence of biliary cirrhosis.[178] The most dreaded complication of choledochal cyst is cholangiocarcinoma, which occurs in approximately 20% of adults, and therefore surgical resection is recommended, except for type 3 choledochal cyst (choledochocele), which carries a low risk of cholangiocarcinoma.[179,180]

Benign and Malignant Biliary Stricture

Benign biliary stricture may occur in patients with a history of surgery resulting in bile duct injury, history of PSC, recurrent choledocholithiasis, chronic pancreatitis, and history of blunt trauma to the abdomen and following liver transplant. In approximately 30% of patients, the injury to bile ducts during surgery is unrecognized and patients may present many years later with biliary strictures.[181] Anastomotic strictures usually occur 2 to 6 months after liver transplant surgery.[182] Chronic pancreatitis accounts for 9% to 10% of benign strictures that occur in the intrapancreatic section of the CBD.[183]

Pancreatic cancer is the commonest cause of malignant biliary stricture.[184] Other conditions that cause malignant stricture include cholangiocarcinoma, gallbladder tumor, and ampullary tumor. Cholangiocarcinoma or biliary tree cancers can involve the intrahepatic or extrahepatic ducts. Klatskin tumors are cholangiocarcinoma that occurs at the bifurcation of the right and left main bile ducts or proximal hepatic ducts.[185] Malignant strictures can be caused by either a primary bile duct cancer causing narrowing within the bile ducts, or extrinsic compression by a tumor in an adjacent organ, such as the head of the pancreas.

Clinical features

Benign strictures may be asymptomatic, although cholangitis is a common presentation. Patients with pancreatic cancer usually present with painless jaundice. Jaundice is also the commonest symptom in patients with cholangiocarcinoma. Decreased appetite, weight loss, and epigastric pain radiating to the back should raise a suspicion of a malignant process.

Diagnosis

Extrahepatic cholestasis presents with elevated AP and GGT, with normal or near normal aminotransferase enzymes. Hyperbilirubinemia may be significant in patients with pancreatic cancer with serum bilirubin often higher than 20 mg/dL.[186] A serum CA19-9 greater than 100 U/mL has a sensitivity and specificity of 75% and 80%, respectively, for cholangiocarcinoma in patients with PSC.[186] Workup for extrahepatic obstruction includes imaging such as TUS or CT, followed by MRCP or ERCP depending on the clinical situation and need for possibly therapeutic interventions. When malignancy is suspected, brushings of biliary tree for cytology should be obtained during ERCP. Advanced techniques, such as digital image analysis and fluorescence in situ hybridization, have greatly increased sensitivity and specificity for detecting cholangiocarcinoma.[187]

MANAGEMENT OF CHOLESTASIS

Pruritus

Pruritus is a challenging clinical problem that often complicates chronic cholestatic liver disease. Cholestyramine is the first-line agent in patients with moderate pruritus, and the recommended dose is 4 to 16 g/d in divided doses.[188] Cholestyramine is a resin that binds to bile salts in the small intestine, thereby interrupting enterohepatic circulation and decreasing its reabsorption by approximately 90%.[188] Cholestyramine, however, is unpalatable and interferes with absorption of other drugs, such as digoxin, warfarin, and thiazides.[189] Rifampin has also been shown to be useful in the treatment of pruritus. Rifampin decreases hepatic uptake and facilitates renal elimination of bile acids.[190] The recommended dose is 300 to 600 mg/d. Liver tests should be monitored closely while on rifampin, because severe hepatitis may sometimes occur.[191] A few small studies have reported benefit with phenobarbital; however, it is less effective than rifampin and cholestyramine and is therefore not recommended for treatment of pruritus.[192] The antidepressants sertraline and paroxetine have been shown to be useful in a few trials.[193,194] Increased opioidergic neurotransmission in the brain may have a role in the pathogenesis of pruritus. The opioid receptor antagonists naloxone, nalmefene, and naltrexone have been shown to cause substantial relief of symptoms.[191] The main drawback for their use, however, is the potential for opioid withdrawal.[195] The role of UDCA was discussed earlier under specific cholestatic diseases. Plasmapheresis should be reserved for patients with refractory disabling pruritus when all other treatment options are ineffective.[196] Finally, liver transplantation is an indication for severe pruritus secondary to cholestatic liver disease.[197]

Fatigue

No therapy has been found to be effective in the treatment of fatigue. UDCA has not been shown to be useful, and fatigue may persist even after liver transplant, although its intensity may be reduced.[198,199] Central nervous system stimulants such as modafinil and low-dose amitriptyline may be beneficial in some patients.[200]

Osteoporosis

Calcium and vitamin D should be recommended to all patients with chronic cholestatic liver disease to prevent metabolic bone disease. Once osteoporosis is established, bisphosphonates are recommended. In a study comparing etidronate and alendronate, the latter was found to be more effective in increasing bone mass.[201]

Fat-Soluble Vitamin Deficiencies

All patients with chronic cholestatic liver disease should have vitamin A, D, E, and K levels monitored annually and appropriate treatment should be initiated if found to be deficient.

Hyperlipidemia

The efficacy of cholestyramine for the treatment of hyperlipidemia in this group of patients has not been established. UDCA has been shown to significantly reduce total, very-low-density lipoprotein, and low-density lipoprotein cholesterol but has no effect on triglyceride or high-density lipoprotein cholesterol, and the maximum benefit was seen in patients with higher baseline cholesterol and higher serum bilirubin values.[202] Clofibrate, due to an unknown mechanism, results in paradoxic increase in cholesterol in patients with PBC and therefore should not be used for the treatment of hyperlipidemia in these patients.[203] Statins have been shown to be effective in reducing cholesterol with frequent monitoring of liver enzymes and should possibly be avoided in patients with severe cholestatic disease.[204] Plasmapheresis is reserved for patients with extremely high serum cholesterol levels. Approximately 6 g of cholesterol can be removed by a single plasma exchange, resulting in decrease in serum cholesterol levels, resorption of xanthomata, decrease in pain caused by xanthomatous neuropathy, and improvement in pruritus associated with cholestasis.[205]

OUTCOME IN THE REPRESENTATIVE CASE

The patient was started on prednisone, 40 mg once a day, which was slowly tapered based on his clinical response. He experienced complete biochemical response within 3 to 4 months of therapy. The patient is currently on a maintenance dose of 10 mg/d and his AP is 90 IU/ml, alanine aminotransferase is 31 mg/dL, and aspartate aminotransferase is 35 mg/dL.

SUMMARY

Although the causes of cholestasis are numerous, a systematic step-by-step workup starting with a comprehensive history and physical and complemented by laboratory testing and appropriate imaging results in an accurate diagnosis in almost all patients.

ACKNOWLEDGMENTS

The authors would like to acknowledge the help of Dr. Anjali D'Souza in the preparation of this manuscript.

REFERENCES

1. Scharschmidt BF, Goldberg HI, Schmid R. Current concepts in diagnosis. Approach to the patient with cholestatic jaundice. N Engl J Med 1983; 308(25):1515–9.
2. Trauner M, Boyer JL. Bile salt transporters: molecular characterization, function, and regulation. Physiol Rev 2003;83(2):633–71.
3. Hagenbuch B, Dawson P. The sodium bile salt cotransport family SLC10. Pflugers Arch 2004;447(5):566–70.
4. Niemi M, Pasanen MK, Neuvonen PJ. Organic anion transporting polypeptide 1B1: a genetically polymorphic transporter of major importance for hepatic drug uptake. Pharmacol Rev 2011;63(1):157–81.
5. Arrese M, Trauner M. Molecular aspects of bile formation and cholestasis. Trends Mol Med 2003;9(12):558–64.
6. Kipp H, Arias IM. Intracellular trafficking and regulation of canalicular ATP-binding cassette transporters. Semin Liver Dis 2000;20(3):339–51.
7. Gerk PM, Vore M. Regulation of expression of the multidrug resistance-associated protein 2 (MRP2) and its role in drug disposition. J Pharmacol Exp Ther 2002;302(2):407–15.
8. Kullak-Ublick GA, Beuers U, Paumgartner G. Hepatobiliary transport. J Hepatol 2000;32(Suppl 1):3–18.
9. Lazaridis KN, Pham L, Tietz P, et al. Rat cholangiocytes absorb bile acids at their apical domain via the ileal sodium-dependent bile acid transporter. J Clin Invest 1997;100(11):2714–21.
10. Xu G, Shneider BL, Shefer S, et al. Ileal bile acid transport regulates bile acid pool, synthesis, and plasma cholesterol levels differently in cholesterol-fed rats and rabbits. J Lipid Res 2000;41(2):298–304.
11. Rost D, Mahner S, Sugiyama Y, et al. Expression and localization of the multidrug resistance-associated protein 3 in rat small and large intestine. Am J Physiol Gastrointest Liver Physiol 2002;282(4):G720–6.
12. Wang H, Chen J, Hollister K, et al. Endogenous bile acids are ligands for the nuclear receptor FXR/BAR. Mol Cell 1999;3(5):543–53.
13. Ananthanarayanan M, Balasubramanian N, Makishima M, et al. Human bile salt export pump promoter is transactivated by the farnesoid X receptor/bile acid receptor. J Biol Chem 2001;276(31):28857–65.
14. Cheng X, Maher J, Dieter MZ, et al. Regulation of mouse organic anion-transporting polypeptides (Oatps) in liver by prototypical microsomal enzyme inducers that activate distinct transcription factor pathways. Drug Metab Dispos 2005;33(9):1276–82.
15. Gordon T. Factors associated with serum alkaline phosphatase level. Arch Pathol Lab Med 1993;117(2):187–90.
16. Schiele F, Henny J, Hitz J, et al. Total bone and liver alkaline phosphatases in plasma: biological variations and reference limits. Clin Chem 1983;29(4): 634–41.
17. Connell MD, Dinwoodie AJ. Diagnostic use of serum alkaline phosphatase isoenzymes and 5-nucleotidase. Clin Chim Acta 1970;30(2):235–41.

18. McIntyre N. Cholestasis. In: Bircher J, Benhamou J-P, McIntyre N, et al, editors. Oxford textbook of clinical hepatology. 2th edition. Oxford (United Kingdom): Oxford Medical Publications; 1999. p. 1574–9.
19. Maggs JR, Chapman RW. An update on primary sclerosing cholangitis. Curr Opin Gastroenterol 2008;24(3):377–83.
20. Robinson JR, Moyer CA. Methods for differential diagnosis of painless jaundice. Surg Gynecol Obstet 1947;85(4):535–40.
21. Center SA. Diseases of the gallbladder and biliary tree. Vet Clin North Am Small Anim Pract 2009;39(3):543–98.
22. Lillemoe KD. Surgical treatment of biliary tract infections. Am Surg 2000;66(2): 138–44.
23. Bansal V, Schuchert VD. Jaundice in the intensive care unit. Surg Clin North Am 2006;86:1495–502.
24. Cavestro GM, Frulloni L, Cerati E, et al. Progressive familial intrahepatic cholestasis. Acta Biomed 2002;73(3–4):53–6.
25. Fisher DA, Wright TL. Pruritus as a symptom of hepatitis C. J Am Acad Dermatol 1994;30(4):629–32.
26. Jones EA, Bergasa NV. The pathogenesis and treatment of pruritus and fatigue in patients with PBC. Eur J Gastroenterol Hepatol 1999;11(6):623–31.
27. Bergasa NV. Pruritus in chronic liver disease: mechanisms and treatment. Curr Gastroenterol Rep 2004;6(1):10–6.
28. Jones EA, Bergasa NV. The pruritus of cholestasis: from bile acids to opiate agonists. Hepatology 1990;11(5):884–7.
29. Milkiewicz P, Heathcote EJ. Fatigue in chronic cholestasis. Gut 2004;53(4): 475–7.
30. Talwalkar JA, Lindor KD. Primary biliary cirrhosis. Lancet 2003;362(9377):53–61.
31. Walli AK, Seidel D. Role of lipoprotein-X in the pathogenesis of cholestatic hypercholesterolemia. Uptake of lipoprotein-X and its effect on 3-hydroxy-3-methylglutaryl coenzyme A reductase and chylomicron remnant removal in human fibroblasts, lymphocytes, and in the rat. J Clin Invest 1984;74(3):867–79.
32. Crippin JS, Lindor KD, Jorgensen R, et al. Hypercholesterolemia and atherosclerosis in primary biliary cirrhosis: what is the risk? Hepatology 1992;15(5):858–62.
33. Phillips JR, Angulo P, Petterson T, et al. Fat-soluble vitamin levels in patients with primary biliary cirrhosis. Am J Gastroenterol 2001;96(9):2745–50.
34. Isaia G, Di Stefano M, Roggia C, et al. Bone disorders in cholestatic liver diseases. Forum (Genova) 1998;8(1):28–38.
35. Lui P, Ng HS, Teh LB, et al. Ultrasonography in the diagnosis of cholestatic jaundice. Ann Acad Med Singapore 1986;15(2):182–5.
36. Shea JA, Berlin JA, Escarce JJ, et al. Revised estimates of diagnostic test sensitivity and specificity in suspected biliary tract disease. Arch Intern Med 1994; 154(22):2573–81.
37. Balci NC, Befeler AS, Leiva P, et al. Imaging of liver disease: comparison between quadruple-phase multidetector computed tomography and magnetic resonance imaging. J Gastroenterol Hepatol 2008;23(10):1520–7.
38. Varghese JC, Liddell RP, Farrell MA, et al. Diagnostic accuracy of magnetic resonance cholangiopancreatography and ultrasound compared with direct cholangiography in the detection of choledocholithiasis. Clin Radiol 2000; 55(1):25–35.
39. NIH state-of-the-science statement on endoscopic retrograde cholangiopancreatography (ERCP) for diagnosis and therapy. NIH Consens State Sci Statements 2002;19:1–26.

40. Berg PA, Klein R. Antimitochondrial antibodies in primary biliary cirrhosis and other disorders: definition and clinical relevance. Dig Dis 1992;10:85–101.
41. Poupon R, Chazouillères O, Poupon RE. Chronic cholestatic diseases. J Hepatol 2000;32(Suppl 1):129–40.
42. Heathcote J. Autoimmune cholangitis. Gut 1997;40(4):440–2.
43. Strassburg CP, Manns MP. Antinuclear antibody (ANA) patterns in hepatic and extrahepatic autoimmune disease. J Hepatol 1999;31(4):751.
44. Charatcharoenwitthaya P, Lindor KD. Primary sclerosing cholangitis: diagnosis and management. Curr Gastroenterol Rep 2006;8(1):75–82.
45. Kariv R, Konikoff FM. Sclerosing cholangitis–primary, secondary and more. Isr Med Assoc J 2002;4(12):1141–2.
46. Bull LN, Carlton VE, Stricker NL, et al. Genetic and morphological findings in progressive familial intrahepatic cholestasis (Byler disease [PFIC-1] and Byler syndrome): evidence for heterogeneity. Hepatology 1997;26(1):155–64.
47. Strautnieks SS, Kagalwalla AF, Tanner MS, et al. Identification of a locus for progressive familial intrahepatic cholestasis PFIC2 on chromosome 2q24. Am J Hum Genet 1997;61(3):630–3.
48. Jansen PL, Müller MM. Progressive familial intrahepatic cholestasis types 1, 2, and 3. Gut 1998;42(6):766–7.
49. Knisely AS, Strautnieks SS, Meier Y, et al. Hepatocellular carcinoma in ten children under five years of age with bile salt export pump deficiency. Hepatology 2006;44(2):478–86.
50. Jacquemin E, De Vree JM, Cresteil D, et al. The wide spectrum of multidrug resistance 3 deficiency: from neonatal cholestasis to cirrhosis of adulthood. Gastroenterology 2001;120(6):1448–58.
51. Dixon PH, Weerasekera N, Linton KJ, et al. Heterozygous MDR3 missense mutation associated with intrahepatic cholestasis of pregnancy: evidence for a defect in protein trafficking. Hum Mol Genet 2000;9(8):1209–17.
52. Bull LN, Juijn JA, Liao M, et al. Fine-resolution mapping by haplotype evaluation: the examples of PFIC1 and BRIC. Hum Genet 1999;104(3):241–8.
53. van Mil SW, van der Woerd WL, van der Brugge G, et al. Benign recurrent intrahepatic cholestasis type 2 is caused by mutations in ABCB11. Gastroenterology 2004;127(2):379–84.
54. Keitel V, Nies AT, Brom M, et al. A common Dubin-Johnson syndrome mutation impairs protein maturation and transport activity of MRP2 (ABCC2). Am J Physiol Gastrointest Liver Physiol 2003;284(1):G165–74.
55. Colombo C. Liver disease in cystic fibrosis. Curr Opin Pulm Med 2007;13(6): 529–36.
56. Colliton RP, Bason L, Lu FM, et al. Mutation analysis of Jagged1 (JAG1) in Alagille syndrome patients. Hum Mutat 2001;17(2):151–2.
57. Jones DE. Pathogenesis of primary biliary cirrhosis. Gut 2007;56(11):1615–24.
58. Jones DE, Watt FE, Metcalf JV, et al. Familial primary biliary cirrhosis reassessed: a geographically-based population study. J Hepatol 1999;30(3): 402–7.
59. Bloom S, Fleming K, Chapman R. Adhesion molecule expression in primary sclerosing cholangitis and primary biliary cirrhosis. Gut 1995;36(4):604–9.
60. Griem P, Wulferink M, Sachs B, et al. Allergic and autoimmune reactions to xenobiotics: how do they arise? Immunol Today 1998;19(3):133–41.
61. Varyani FK, West J, Card TR. An increased risk of urinary tract infection precedes development of primary biliary cirrhosis. BMC Gastroenterol 2011; 11:95.

62. Gershwin ME, Selmi C, Worman HJ, et al. Risk factors and comorbidities in primary biliary cirrhosis: a controlled interview-based study of 1032 patients. Hepatology 2005;42(5):1194–202.
63. Prince MI, Chetwynd A, Craig WL, et al. Asymptomatic primary biliary cirrhosis: clinical features, prognosis, and symptom progression in a large population based cohort. Gut 2004;53(6):865–70.
64. Newton JL. Fatigue in primary biliary cirrhosis. Clin Liver Dis 2008;12(2):367–83.
65. Levy C, Lindor KD. Management of osteoporosis, fat-soluble vitamin deficiencies, and hyperlipidemia in primary biliary cirrhosis. Clin Liver Dis 2003; 7(4):901–10.
66. Shapiro JM, Smith H, Schaffner F. Serum bilirubin: a prognostic factor in primary biliary cirrhosis. Gut 1979;20(2):137–40.
67. Leung PS, Coppel RL, Ansari A, et al. Antimitochondrial antibodies in primary biliary cirrhosis. Semin Liver Dis 1997;17:61–9.
68. Drebber U, Mueller JJ, Klein E, et al. Liver biopsy in primary biliary cirrhosis: clinicopathological data and stage. Pathol Int 2009;59(8):546–54.
69. Ludwig J, Dickson ER, McDonald GS. Staging of chronic nonsuppurative destructive cholangitis (syndrome of primary biliary cirrhosis). Virchows Arch A Pathol Anat Histol 1978;379(2):103–12.
70. Leuschner U, Fischer H, Kurtz W, et al. Ursodeoxycholic acid in primary biliary cirrhosis: results of a controlled double-blind trial. Gastroenterology 1989;97(5): 1268–74.
71. Poupon RE, Lindor KD, Parés A, et al. Combined analysis of the effect of treatment with ursodeoxycholic acid on histologic progression in primary biliary cirrhosis. J Hepatol 2003;39(1):12–6.
72. MacQuillan GC, Neuberger J. Liver transplantation for primary biliary cirrhosis. Clin Liver Dis 2003;7(4):941–56.
73. Lacerda MA, Ludwig J, Dickson ER, et al. Antimitochondrial antibody-negative primary biliary cirrhosis. Am J Gastroenterol 1995;90(2):247–9.
74. Broome U, Olsson R, Loof L, et al. Natural history and prognostic factors in 305 Swedish patients with primary sclerosing cholangitis. Gut 1996;38(4):610–5.
75. Bargen J. Complications and sequelae of chronic ulcerative colitis. Ann Intern Med 1929;3:335–52.
76. Schrumpf E, Boberg KM. Epidemiology of primary sclerosing cholangitis. Best Pract Res Clin Gastroenterol 2001;15(4):553–62.
77. Mendes FD, Lindor KD. Primary sclerosing cholangitis. Clin Liver Dis 2004;8(1): 195–211.
78. Loftus EV Jr, Sandborn WJ, Tremaine WJ, et al. Primary sclerosing cholangitis is associated with nonsmoking: a case-control study. Gastroenterology 1996; 110(5):1496–502.
79. Bergquist A, Montgomery SM, Bahmanyar S, et al. Increased risk of primary sclerosing cholangitis and ulcerative colitis in first-degree relatives of patients with primary sclerosing cholangitis. Clin Gastroenterol Hepatol 2008;6(8):939–43.
80. Norris S, Kondeatis E, Collins R, et al. Mapping MHC-encoded susceptibility and resistance in primary sclerosing cholangitis: the role of MICA polymorphism. Gastroenterology 2001;120(6):1475–82.
81. van Milligen de Wit AW, van Deventer SJ, Tytgat GN. Immunogenetic aspects of primary sclerosing cholangitis: implications for therapeutic strategies. Am J Gastroenterol 1995;90(6):893–900.
82. Karlsen TH, Franke A, Melum E, et al. Genome-wide association analysis in primary sclerosing cholangitis. Gastroenterology 2010;138(3):1102–11.

83. Krasinskas AM, Yao Y, Randhawa P, et al. Helicobacter pylori may play a contributory role in the pathogenesis of primary sclerosing cholangitis. Dig Dis Sci 2007;52(9):2265–70.
84. Mehal WZ, Hattersley AT, Chapman RW, et al. A survey of cytomegalovirus (CMV) DNA in primary sclerosing cholangitis (PSC) liver tissues using a sensitive polymerase chain reaction (PCR) based assay. J Hepatol 1992;15(3):396–9.
85. Kulaksiz H, Rudolph G, Kloeters-Plachky P, et al. Biliary Candida infections in primary sclerosing cholangitis. J Hepatol 2006;45(5):711–6.
86. Terjung B, Worman HJ. Anti-neutrophil antibodies in primary sclerosing cholangitis. Best Pract Res Clin Gastroenterol 2001;15:629–42.
87. Worthington J, Cullen S, Chapman R. Immunopathogenesis of primary sclerosing cholangitis. Clin Rev Allergy Immunol 2005;28:93–103.
88. Okolicsanyi L, Fabris L, Viaggi S, et al. Primary sclerosing cholangitis: clinical presentation, natural history and prognostic variables: An Italian multicentre study. The Italian PSC Study Group. Eur J Gastroenterol Hepatol 1996;8(7): 685–91.
89. Olsson R, Broome U, Danielsson A, et al. Spontaneous course of symptoms in primary sclerosing cholangitis: relationships with biochemical and histological features. Hepatogastroenterology 1999;46(25):136–41.
90. Ciocirlan M, Ponchon T. Diagnostic endoscopic retrograde cholangiopancreatography. Endoscopy 2004;36(2):137–46.
91. Furmanczyk PS, Grieco VS, Agoff SN. Biliary brush cytology and the detection of cholangiocarcinoma in primary sclerosing cholangitis: evaluation of specific cytomorphologic features and CA19-9 levels. Am J Clin Pathol 2005;124(3): 355–60.
92. Angulo P, Pearce DH, Johnson CD, et al. Magnetic resonance cholangiography in patients with biliary disease: its role in primary sclerosing cholangitis. J Hepatol 2000;33(4):520–7.
93. Burak KW, Angulo P, Lindor KD. Is there a role for liver biopsy in primary sclerosing cholangitis? Am J Gastroenterol 2003;98(5):1155–8.
94. Abdalian R, Heathcote EJ. Sclerosing cholangitis: a focus on secondary causes. Hepatology 2006;44(5):1063–74.
95. Burak K, Angulo P, Pasha TM, et al. Incidence and risk factors for cholangiocarcinoma in primary sclerosing cholangitis. Am J Gastroenterol 2004;99(3):523–6.
96. Charatcharoenwitthaya P, Enders FB, Halling KC, et al. Utility of serum tumor markers, imaging, and biliary cytology for detecting cholangiocarcinoma in primary sclerosing cholangitis. Hepatology 2008;48(4):1106–17.
97. Bergquist A, Ekbom A, Olsson R, et al. Hepatic and extrahepatic malignancies in primary sclerosing cholangitis. J Hepatol 2002;36(3):321–7.
98. Thackeray EW, Charatcharoenwitthaya P, Elfaki D, et al. Colon neoplasms develop early in the course of inflammatory bowel disease and primary sclerosing cholangitis. Clin Gastroenterol Hepatol 2011;9(1):52–6.
99. Mitchell SA, Bansi DS, Hunt N, et al. A preliminary trial of high-dose ursodeoxycholic acid in primary sclerosing cholangitis. Gastroenterology 2001;121(4): 900–7.
100. Imam MH, Sinakos E, Gossard AA, et al. High-dose ursodeoxycholic acid increases risk of adverse outcomes in patients with early stage primary sclerosing cholangitis. Aliment Pharmacol Ther 2011;34(10):1185–92.
101. Lindor KD. Ursodiol for primary sclerosing cholangitis. Mayo Primary Sclerosing Cholangitis- Ursodeoxycholic Acid Study Group. N Engl J Med 1997;336(10): 691–5.

102. Chapman R, Fevery J, Kalloo A, et al. Diagnosis and management of primary sclerosing cholangitis. Hepatology 2010;51(2):660–78.
103. Takuma K, Kamisawa T, Igarashi Y. Autoimmune pancreatitis and IgG4-related sclerosing cholangitis. Curr Opin Rheumatol 2011;23(1):80–7.
104. Sugumar A, Chari ST. Autoimmune pancreatitis. J Gastroenterol Hepatol 2011; 26(9):1368–73.
105. Ghazale A, Chari ST, Zhang L, et al. Immunoglobulin G4-Associated Cholangitis: clinical Profile and Response to Therapy. Gastroenterology 2008;134(3): 706–15.
106. Björnsson E, Chari S, Silveira M, et al. Primary sclerosing cholangitis associated with elevated immunoglobulin G4: clinical characteristics and response to therapy. Am J Ther 2011;18(3):198–205.
107. Sahani DV, Kalva SP, Farrell J, et al. Autoimmune pancreatitis: imaging features. Radiology 2004;233(2):345–52.
108. Ghazale A, Chari ST, Smyrk TC, et al. Value of serum IgG4 in the diagnosis of autoimmune pancreatitis and in distinguishing it from pancreatic cancer. Am J Gastroenterol 2007;102(8):1646–53.
109. Nakazawa T, Ohara H, Sano H, et al. Schematic classification of sclerosing cholangitis with autoimmune pancreatitis by cholangiography. Pancreas 2006;32(2): 229.
110. Zen Y, Fujii T, Sato Y, et al. Pathological classification of hepatic inflammatory pseudotumor with respect to IgG4-related disease. Mod Pathol 2007;20(8): 884–94.
111. Kamisawa T, Shimosegawa T, Okazaki K, et al. Standard steroid treatment for autoimmune pancreatitis. Gut 2009;58(11):1504–7.
112. Hirano K, Tada M, Isayama H, et al. Long-term prognosis of autoimmune pancreatitis with and without corticosteroid treatment. Gut 2007;56(12): 1719–24.
113. Karagiannidis A, Karavalaki M, Koulaouzidis A. Hepatic sarcoidosis. Ann Hepatol 2006;5(4):251–6.
114. Mueller S, Boehme MW, Hofmann WJ, et al. Extrapulmonary sarcoidosis primarily diagnosed in the liver. Scand J Gastroenterol 2000;35(9):1003–8.
115. Rybicki BA, Major M, Popovich J Jr, et al. Racial differences in sarcoidosis incidence: a 5-year study in a health maintenance organization. Am J Epidemiol 1997;45(3):234–41.
116. Baughman RP, Teirstein AS, Judson MA, et al. Clinical characteristics of patients in a case control study of sarcoidosis. Am J Respir Crit Care Med 2001;164:1885–9.
117. Irani SK, Dobbins WO 3rd. Hepatic granulomas: review of 73 patients from one hospital and survey of the literature. J Clin Gastroenterol 1979;1(2):131–43.
118. Cremers J, Drent M, Driessen A, et al. Liver-test abnormalities in sarcoidosis. Eur J Gastroenterol Hepatol 2012;24(1):17–24.
119. Lieberman J. Elevation of serum angiotensin-converting-enzyme (ACE) level in sarcoidosis. Am J Med 1975;59(3):365–72.
120. Farman J, Ramirez G, Brunetti J, et al. Abdominal manifestations of sarcoidosis. CT appearances. Clin Imaging 1995;19(1):30–3.
121. Kessler A, Mitchell DG, Israel HL, et al. Hepatic and splenic sarcoidosis: ultrasound and MR imaging. Abdom Imaging 1993;18(2):159–63.
122. Devaney K, Goodman ZD, Epstein MS, et al. Hepatic sarcoidosis. Clinicopathologic features in 100 patients. Am J Surg Pathol 1993;17(12):1272–80.
123. Geramizadeh B, Jahangiri R, Moradi E. Causes of hepatic granuloma: a 12-year single center experience from southern Iran. Arch Iran Med 2011;14(4):288–9.

124. Kennedy PT, Zakaria N, Modawi SB, et al. Natural history of hepatic sarcoidosis and its response to treatment. Eur J Gastroenterol Hepatol 2006;18(7):721–6.
125. Ayyala US, Padilla ML. Diagnosis and treatment of hepatic sarcoidosis. Curr Treat Options Gastroenterol 2006;9(6):475–83.
126. Baughman RP, Winget DB, Lower EE. Methotrexate is steroid sparing in acute sarcoidosis: results of a double blind, randomized trial. Sarcoidosis Vasc Diffuse Lung Dis 2000;17(1):60–6.
127. Baratta L, Cascino A, Delfino M, et al. Ursodeoxycholic acid treatment in abdominal sarcoidosis. Dig Dis Sci 2000;45(8):1559–62.
128. Ebert EC, Kierson M, Hagspiel KD. Gastrointestinal and hepatic manifestations of sarcoidosis. Am J Gastroenterol 2008;103(12):3184–92.
129. Moreno-Merlo F, Wanless IR, Shimamatsu K, et al. The role of granulomatous phlebitis and thrombosis in the pathogenesis of cirrhosis and portal hypertension in sarcoidosis. Hepatology 1997;26(3):554–60.
130. Casavilla FA, Gordon R, Wright HI, et al. Clinical course after liver transplantation in patients with sarcoidosis. Ann Intern Med 1993;118(11):865–6.
131. Quigley EM, Marsh MN, Shaffer JL. Hepatobiliary complications of total parenteral nutrition. Gastroenterology 1993;104(1):286–301.
132. Grant JP, Cox CE, Kleinman LM, et al. Serum hepatic enzyme and bilirubin elevations during parenteral nutrition. Surg Gynecol Obstet 1977;145(4):573–80.
133. Fisher RL. Hepatobiliary abnormalities associated with total parenteral nutrition. Gastroenterol Clin North Am 1989;18(3):645–66.
134. Chan S, McCowen KC, Bistrian BR, et al. Incidence, prognosis, and etiology of end-stage liver disease in patients receiving home parenteral nutrition. Surgery 1999;126(1):28–34.
135. Touloukian RJ, Seashore JH. Hepatic secretory obstruction with total parenteral nutrition in the infant. J Pediatr Surg 1975;10(3):353–60.
136. Brown MR, Thunberg BJ, Golub L, et al. Decreased cholestasis with enteral instead of intravenous protein in the very low-birth-weight infant. J Pediatr Gastroenterol Nutr 1989;9(1):21–7.
137. Meguid MM, Akahoshi MP, Jeffers S, et al. Amelioration of metabolic complications of conventional total parenteral nutrition. Arch Surg 1984;119(11):1294–8.
138. Beau P, Labat-Labourdette J, Ingrand P, et al. Is ursodeoxycholic acid an effective therapy for total parenteral nutrition-related liver disease? J Hepatol 1994;20(2):240–4.
139. Capron JP, Herve MA, Gineston JL, et al. Metronidazole in prevention of cholestasis associated with total parenteral nutrition. Lancet 1983;1(8322):446–7.
140. Grant D. Current results of intestinal transplantation. The International Intestinal Transplant Registry. Lancet 1996;347(9018):1801–3.
141. Roger D, Vaillant L, Fignon A, et al. Specific pruritic diseases of pregnancy. A prospective study of 3192 pregnant women. Arch Dermatol 1994;130(6):734–9.
142. Geenes V, Williamson C. Intrahepatic cholestasis of pregnancy. World J Gastroenterol 2009;15(17):2049–66.
143. Reyes H, Radrigan ME, Gonzalez MC, et al. Steatorrhea in patients with intrahepatic cholestasis of pregnancy. Gastroenterology 1987;93(3):584–90.
144. Lunzer MR. Jaundice in pregnancy. Baillieres Clin Gastroenterol 1989;3(2):467–83.
145. Leslie KK, Reznikov L, Simon FR, et al. Estrogens in intrahepatic cholestasis of pregnancy. Obstet Gynecol 2000;95(3):372–6.

146. Pauli-Magnus C, Meier PJ, Stieger B. Genetic determinants of drug-induced cholestasis and intrahepatic cholestasis of pregnancy. Semin Liver Dis 2010; 30(2):147–59.
147. Shaw D, Frohlich J, Wittmann BA, et al. A prospective study of 18 patients with cholestasis of pregnancy. Am J Obstet Gynecol 1982;142(6 Pt 1):621–5.
148. Heikkinen J. Serum bile acids in the early diagnosis of intrahepatic cholestasis of pregnancy. Obstet Gynecol 1983;61(5):581–7.
149. Walker IA, Nelson-Piercy C, Williamson C. Role of bile acid measurement in pregnancy. Ann Clin Biochem 2002;39(Pt 2):105–13.
150. Azzaroli F, Mennone A, Feletti V, et al. Clinical trial: modulation of human placental multidrug resistance proteins in cholestasis of pregnancy by ursodeoxycholic acid. Aliment Pharmacol Ther 2007;26(8):1139–46.
151. Hirvioja ML, Tuimala R, Vuori J. The treatment of intrahepatic cholestasis of pregnancy by dexamethasone. Br J Obstet Gynaecol 1992;99(2):109–11.
152. Moseley RH. Sepsis and cholestasis. Clin Liver Dis 1999;3(3):465–75.
153. Tung CB, Tung CF, Yang DY. Extremely high levels of alkaline phosphatase in adult patients as a manifestation of bacteremia. Hepatogastroenterology 2005;52(65):1347–50.
154. Szabo G, Romics L Jr, Frendl G. Liver in sepsis and systemic inflammatory response syndrome. Clin Liver Dis 2002;6(4):1045–66.
155. Brandorg L, Goldman I. Bacterial and miscellaneous infections of the liver. In: Zakim D, Boyer TD, editors. Hepatology, A textbook of the liver. Philadelphia: W.B. Saunders; 1990. p. 1086–98.
156. Lazaridis KN, Gores GJ, Lindor KD. Ursodeoxycholic acid 'mechanisms of action and clinical use in hepatobiliary disorders.'. J Hepatol 2001;35(1): 134–46.
157. Zimmerman HJ. Drug-induced liver disease. Clin Liver Dis 2000;4(1):73–96.
158. Larrey D. Drug-induced liver diseases. J Hepatol 2000;32(Suppl 1):77–88.
159. Geubel AP, Sempoux CL. Drug and toxin-induced bile duct disorders. J Gastroenterol Hepatol 2000;15(11):1232–8.
160. Kaplowitz N. Idiosyncratic drug hepatotoxicity. Nat Rev Drug Discov 2005;4(6): 489–99.
161. Malhi H, Gores GJ. Cellular and molecular mechanisms of liver injury. Gastroenterology 2008;134(6):1641–54.
162. Yoshikado T, Takada T, Yamamoto T, et al. Itraconazole-induced cholestasis: involvement of the inhibition of bile canalicular phospholipid translocator MDR3/ABCB4. Mol Pharmacol 2011;79(2):241–50.
163. Vermillion SE, Gregg JA, Baggenstoss AH, et al. Jaundice associated with bacteremia. Arch Intern Med 1969;124(5):611–8.
164. Ramachandran R, Kakar S. Histological patterns in drug-induced liver disease. J Clin Pathol 2009;62(6):481–92.
165. Papaseit E, Farré M, López MJ, et al. A case of acute valproic acid poisoning treated successfully with L-carnitine. Eur J Emerg Med 2012;19(1):57–8.
166. Wree A, Dechêne A, Herzer K, et al. Steroid and ursodeoxycholic acid combination in severe drug-induced liver injury. Digestion 2011;84(1):54–9.
167. Kratzer W, Mason RA, K'achele V. Prevalence of gallstones in sonographic surveys worldwide. J Clin Ultrasound 1999;27(1):1–7.
168. Lee JG. Diagnosis and management of acute cholangitis. Nat Rev Gastroenterol Hepatol 2009;6(9):533–41.
169. Rosseland AR, Glomsaker TB. Asymptomatic common bile duct stones. Eur J Gastroenterol Hepatol 2000;12(11):1171–3.

170. Wada K, Takada T, Kawarada Y, et al. Diagnostic criteria and severity assessment of acute cholangitis: Tokyo guidelines. J Hepatobiliary Pancreat Surg 2007;14(1):52–8.
171. Sahu MK, Chacko A, Dutta AK, et al. Microbial profile and antibiotic sensitivity pattern in acute bacterial cholangitis. Indian J Gastroenterol 2011;30(5):204–8.
172. Lindsell DR. The diagnostic accuracy of magnetic resonance cholangiopancreatography (MRCP) and ultrasound compared with direct cholangiography in the detection of choledocholithiasis. Clin Radiol 2000;55(7):579.
173. Sugiyama M, Atomi Y. Endoscopic ultrasonography for diagnosing choledocholithiasis: a prospective comparative study with ultrasonography and computed tomography. Gastrointest Endosc 1997;45(3):143–6.
174. Gigot J, Nagorney D, Farnell M, et al. Bile duct cysts: a changing spectrum of disease. J Hepatobiliary Pancreat Surg 1996;3:405–11.
175. Yu ZL, Zhang LJ, Fu JZ, et al. Anomalous pancreaticobiliary junction: image analysis and treatment principles. Hepatobiliary Pancreat Dis Int 2004;3(1):136–9.
176. Shah OJ, Shera AH, Zargar SA, et al. Choledochal cysts in children and adults with contrasting profiles: 11-year experience at a tertiary care center in Kashmir. World J Surg 2009;33(11):2403–11.
177. Huang CT, Lee HC, Chen WT, et al. Usefulness of magnetic resonance cholangiopancreatography in pancreatobiliary abnormalities in pediatric patients. Pediatr Neonatol 2011;52(6):332–6.
178. Dinsmore JE, Murphy JJ, Jamieson D. Pediatric surgical images: MRCP evaluation of choledochal cysts. J Pediatr Surg 2001;36(5):829–30.
179. de Vries JS, de Vries S, Aronson DC, et al. Choledochal cysts: age of presentation, symptoms, and late complications related to Todani's classification. J Pediatr Surg 2002;37:1568–73.
180. Edil BH, Cameron JL, Reddy S, et al. Type III is intraduodenal (choledochocele). Choledochal cyst disease in children and adults: a 30-year single-institution experience. J Am Coll Surg 2008;206(5):1000–5 [discussion: 1005–8].
181. Richardson MC, Bell G, Fullarton GM, et al. Incidence and nature of bile duct injuries following laparoscopic cholecystectomy: an audit of 5913 cases. West of Scotland Laparoscopic Cholecystectomy Audit Group. Br J Surg 1996; 83(10):1356–60.
182. Sharma S, Gurakar A, Jabbour N. Biliary strictures following liver transplantation: past, present and preventive strategies. Liver Transpl 2008;14(6):759–69.
183. Rohrman CA, Baron RL. Biliary complications of pancreatitis. Radiol Clin North Am 1989;27(1):93–104.
184. Deviere J, Cremer M, Baize M, et al. Management of common bile duct stricture caused by chronic pancreatitis with metal mesh self expandable stents. Gut 1994;35(1):122–6.
185. Dixon JM, Armstrong CP, Duffy SW, et al. Factors affecting morbidity and mortality after surgery for obstructive jaundice: a review of 373 patients. Gut 1983;24(9):845–52.
186. Patel AH, Harnois DM, Klee GG, et al. The utility of CA 19-9 in the diagnoses of cholangiocarcinoma in patients without primary sclerosing cholangitis. Am J Gastroenterol 2000;95(1):204–7.
187. Kipp BR, Stadheim LM, Halling SA, et al. A comparison of routine cytology and fluorescence in situ hybridization for the detection of malignant bile duct strictures. Am J Gastroenterol 2004;99(9):1675–81.
188. Datta DV, Sherlock S. Treatment of pruritus of obstructive jaundice with cholestyramine. Br Med J 1963;1(5325):216–9.

189. Carey JB Jr, Williams G. Relief of the pruritus of jaundice with a bile-acid sequestering resin. JAMA 1961;176:432–5.
190. Podesta A, Lopez P, Terg R, et al. Treatment of pruritus of primary biliary cirrhosis with rifampin. Dig Dis Sci 1991;36(2):216–20.
191. Tandon P, Rowe BH, Vandermeer B, et al. The efficacy and safety of bile Acid binding agents, opioid antagonists, or rifampin in the treatment of cholestasis-associated pruritus. Am J Gastroenterol 2007;102(7):1528–36.
192. Bloomer JR, Boyer JL. Phenobarbital effects in cholestatic liver diseases. Ann Intern Med 1975;82(3):310–7.
193. Mayo MJ, Handem I, Saldana S, et al. Sertraline as a first-line treatment for cholestatic pruritus. Hepatology 2007;45(3):666–74.
194. Zylicz Z, Krajnik M, Sorge AA, et al. Paroxetine in the treatment of severe non-dermatological pruritus: a randomized, controlled trial. J Pain Symptom Manage 2003;26(6):1105–12.
195. Bergasa NV, Talbot TL, Alling DW, et al. A controlled trial of naloxone infusions for the pruritus of chronic cholestasis. Gastroenterology 1992;102(2):544–9.
196. Jones EA, Neuberger J, Bergasa NV. Opiate antagonist therapy for the pruritus of cholestasis: the avoidance of opioid withdrawal-like reactions. QJM 2002; 95(8):547–52.
197. Heathcote EJ, Cauch-Dudek K, Walker V, et al. The Canadian multicenter double blind randomized controlled trial of ursodeoxycholic acid in primary biliary cirrhosis. Hepatology 1994;19(5):1149–56.
198. Gross CR, Malinchoc M, Kim WR, et al. Quality of life before and after liver transplantation for cholestatic liver disease. Hepatology 1999;29(2):356–64.
199. Vuoristo M, Farkilla M, Kamonen AL, et al. A placebo controlled trial of primary biliary cirrhosis with colchicines and ursodeoxycholic acid. Gastroenterology 1995;108(5):1470–8.
200. Jones DE, Newton JL. An open study of modafinil for the treatment of daytime somnolence and fatigue in primary biliary cirrhosis. Aliment Pharmacol Ther 2007;25(4):471–6.
201. Guanabens N, Pares A, Ros I, et al. Alendronate is more effective than etidronate for increasing bone mass in osteopenic patients with primary biliary cirrhosis. Am J Gastroenterol 2003;98(10):2268–74.
202. Balan V, Dickson ER, Jorgensen RA, et al. Effect of ursodeoxycholic acid on serum lipids of patients with primary biliary cirrhosis. Mayo Clin Proc 1994; 69(10):923–9.
203. Schaffner F. Paradoxical elevation of serum cholesterol by clofibrate in patients with primary biliary cirrhosis. Gastroenterology 1969;57(3):253–6.
204. Stojakovic T, Putz-Bankuti C, Fauler G, et al. Atorvastatin in patients with primary biliary cirrhosis and incomplete biochemical response to ursodeoxycholic acid. Hepatology 2007;46(3):776–84.
205. Cohen LB, Ambinder EP, Wolke AM, et al. Role of plasmapheresis in primary biliary cirrhosis. Gut 1985;26(3):291–4.

Drug-Induced Liver Disease

Timothy J. Davern, MD

KEYWORDS

• Hepatotoxicity • Liver injury • Hepatotoxins • Hepatitis E virus

Drug-induced liver injury (DILI), also known as hepatotoxicity, refers to liver injury caused by drugs or other chemical agents, and represents a special type of adverse drug reaction. It has been estimated that more than 600 drugs and chemicals have been associated with significant liver injury.[1] To review the entire field of DILI in a detailed and comprehensive fashion is thus beyond the scope of this article. Indeed, twice over the last decade, entire issues of this journal have been devoted to this topic. Many previously published reviews have focused on DILI pathogenesis or have outlined the clinical features of liver injury linked to a litany of different drugs; the current review does neither. Instead, the author briefly touches on several areas that are potentially vexing for both the novice and cognoscenti, with the goal of guiding the consultant through one of the most challenging areas of hepatology. For a comprehensive and up-to-date clinical resource of DILI from hundreds of specific drugs, the consultant is encouraged to access the recently launched LiverTox Web site described in further detail at the end of this article.

CATEGORIES OF DILI

DILI can be categorized in several ways based on its clinical features, the pattern of associated liver biochemistries and/or liver histology, and by the suspected pathogenic mechanisms underlying development of the DILI event. One broad classification of DILI separates drugs into predictable and unpredictable hepatotoxins. Predictable hepatotoxins, such as acetaminophen (Tylenol), cause dose-dependent liver injury. Thus, if any given individual takes enough acetaminophen they will develop severe liver injury and possibly even acute liver failure. Indeed, acetaminophen poisoning is now the single leading cause of life-threatening acute liver failure in the United States and Europe.[2] In contrast to acetaminophen, most of the other drugs that cause DILI do so in an unpredictable or so-called idiosyncratic fashion. The word "idiosyncrasy" comes from Greek (*idios* "one's own" and *sun-krasis* "mixture") and refers to traits peculiar to an individual.[3] A drug that causes idiosyncratic liver injury does so in relatively rare individuals, owing to genetic and environmental characteristics unique to

Department of Transplantation, California Pacific Medical Center, 2340 Clay Street, Room 306, San Francisco, CA 94115, USA
E-mail address: davernt@sutterhealth.org

Clin Liver Dis 16 (2012) 231–245
doi:10.1016/j.cld.2012.03.002
liver.theclinics.com

those individuals. In contrast to liver injury from predictable, dose-dependent hepatotoxins, idiosyncratic reactions tend to be difficult if not impossible to predict, and are usually not dose-dependent, although a certain threshold dose may be required.[4]

DILI may also be classified by the pattern of liver injury observed. There are 2 main patterns. Acute hepatocellular injury is caused by injury primarily to hepatocytes and is characterized by elevated levels of serum alanine aminotransferase (ALT), with minimal elevations of the serum alkaline phosphate. Severe hepatocellular injury may evolve into acute liver failure with hepatic synthetic dysfunction and hepatic encephalopathy, which carries a very poor prognosis and often requires liver transplant for survival.[2] The second pattern, cholestatic injury, is caused by liver injury affecting either the cells lining the bile ducts or the molecular mechanisms involved in the flow of the pigment bilirubin from the blood into the bile. It is characterized by a disproportionately elevated level of alkaline phosphatase, which is synthesized and released by injured bile ducts. Severe cholestatic liver injury, though characterized by troublesome and often lingering, severe pruritus and jaundice, usually does not result in life-threatening liver failure. Occasionally, however, it can evolve into permanent bile duct injury with so-called vanishing bile duct syndrome. Liver injury that has both hepatocellular and cholestatic features is called mixed liver injury. Of note, serum bilirubin may be elevated in all 3 forms of liver injury—hepatocellular, cholestatic, and mixed—and, if so, signifies more severe liver injury.

In the context of clinical trials, detection of milder liver injury that may herald a problem for the drug is conventionally defined as an ALT level of more than 3 times the upper limit of the normal range, a serum alkaline phosphatase level of more than twice the upper limit of normal, or a total bilirubin level of more than twice the upper limit of normal if associated with any elevation of either the ALT or alkaline phosphatase.[1]

MAGNITUDE OF THE DILI PROBLEM

Severe DILI is a life-threatening illness, but many patients who experience mild DILI are completely asymptomatic, and these individuals usually suffer no significant or long-standing liver problems. Once diagnosed, the standard treatment involves quickly stopping and avoiding the implicated drug. For mild to moderate DILI, this is usually sufficient to resolve all signs and symptoms of a liver injury. The problem is that to date there is a growing list of prescription and over-the-counter drugs suspected of causing liver injury, which can be severe and even life-threatening. Herbal and other complementary and alternative medications (CAMs), as well as illicit drugs such as anabolic steroids and amphetamines, have also been implicated with increasing frequency.[5,6]

The problem of DILI is clearly important to patients, physicians, and the pharmaceutical industry, and its importance will likely increase as more drugs are used to prevent and treat disease in the future.

- DILI is obviously important to the individuals affected and their families because severe DILI is a catastrophic, life-threatening illness. Another often unappreciated consequence of DILI for patients is that it may also prevent otherwise promising and important drugs from entering the marketplace, or result in their withdrawal from the market, thus affecting the population as a whole.
- DILI is important to physicians and other health care providers because it represents an unintended, but often severe side effect of therapy that flies in the face of our creed: *Primum non nocere* ("first do no harm"). On a more mundane level, DILI also is important for physicians because affected patients, their families, and

their lawyers may consider DILI an egregious error on the part of the health care system, and DILI may thus have serious legal consequences.

- DILI is very important to the pharmaceutical industry because it is a leading cause of drug withdrawal from the marketplace. Of the 548 drugs approved by the Food and Drug Administration (FDA) between 1975 and 1999, 10 received black-box warnings because of the potential to cause liver injury. Four additional drugs were withdrawn from the market.[7] As discussed below, DILI is often not fully recognized until a drug enters the market and many thousands of people are exposed to the drug, meaning that the substantial costs of drug development, preclinical and clinical testing, and subsequent marketing can be severely jeopardized when a drug is associated with DILI.[8] These substantial financial losses combined with the associated liability risk can be financially devastating for the pharmaceutical companies involved.

Given these issues, a logical question is why are potentially toxic drugs released into the marketplace? The finding of unanticipated liver injury during experiments in preclinical models probably results in the effective termination of many drugs at an early stage in development; drugs that possess intrinsic, dose-dependent liver toxicity are the ones most likely to be identified in this fashion.[7] Unfortunately, preclinical testing does not detect all potentially injurious agents, particularly those that cause liver injury in an idiosyncratic fashion. These agents may enter and successfully complete clinical trials where they again may go unrecognized as possibly toxic.[8] There are several reasons for this. First, severe idiosyncratic DILI is uncommon; for most drugs the reported incidence is between 1 in 10,000 and 1 in 100,000 patients exposed, although this number is difficult to determine accurately because of underreporting. Most clinical trials, which are routinely limited to a few thousand volunteers, are simply not large enough to detect these very rare events.[8] Unfortunately, larger trials that might capture these rare cases are more expensive and take longer to complete, both strong financial disincentives for the pharmaceutical industry. As a result, it is often only when the drug is marketed and many thousands of patients are exposed that the cases of severe DILI tend to appear.[8] Such was the case with troglitazone (Rezulin), the first in a class of novel diabetic drugs called peroxisome proliferator-activated receptor-γ agonists. In clinical trials of troglitazone, the incidence of ALT greater than 3 times the upper limit of normal in patients treated with the drug was 1.8% versus 0.6% in placebo treated controls.[9] Overt jaundice occurred in 2 troglitazone subjects, but there were no episodes of acute liver failure observed during clinical trials of the drug. However, after approval and 2 million patients were treated with troglitazone, nearly 100 cases (1 in 20,000 patients) of acute liver failure were reported to the FDA, which withdrew the drug from the United States market in March of 2000.[9]

Not all potentially hepatotoxic drugs escape clinical trials unrecognized. For example, the FDA recently failed to approve ximelagatran (Exanta), which was poised to replace coumadin as a convenient, effective, and presumably safe oral anticoagulant for deep blood clots, atrial fibrillation, and other conditions. The drug was associated with a serum ALT of greater than 3 times the upper limit of normal in almost 8% of treated patients in clinical trials. More importantly, there were several cases of acute liver failure observed in the clinical trial population of approximately 7000 patients.[7] As a result, the drug was never marketed, undoubtedly much to the chagrin of the pharmaceutical company that invested considerable time and resources into the development of this potential block-buster drug.

On the other hand, some drugs that are well-characterized idiosyncratic liver toxins remain on the market because of practical considerations. For example, isoniazid

(INH) is one of the mainstays for treatment of tuberculosis (TB) but is associated with significant hepatocellular injury in 0.3% to 4.6% of treated adult patients, an increasing risk associated with advancing age. Despite this risk, INH presumably remains on the market because there are no other effective and safe drugs to fill its niche for the treatment of TB, a major public health threat.

BRIEF OVERVIEW OF PATHOGENESIS

In general, the pathogenesis of DILI is poorly understood. However, given the way it functions in the body, it is not surprising that the liver is subject to injury by drugs. Virtually all of the major intra-abdominal organs drain into the liver, so it is exposed to an unusually high concentration of drugs absorbed from the intestine. The liver also extensively metabolizes most of these drugs and indeed, in most cases, liver injury seems to be initiated by reactive metabolites that are generated by metabolism of the drugs in the liver rather than by the drugs themselves.[10] These metabolites can potentially bind to and injure various critical components within liver cells, and begin a series of events culminating in liver injury. In short, the liver may in many if not most cases of DILI produce the very compounds that damage it. Liver injury from the common analgesic acetaminophen is a classic example that is discussed further below.

Given these facts, the real question probably should not be why drugs injure the liver, but rather why such injury is not observed more frequently. The answer probably reflects the impressive array of mechanisms the liver uses for protection, repair, and regeneration. These protective mechanisms probably evolved long ago and enabled our ancestors to survive the numerous threats of prehistoric life, including food-borne botanic toxins.

Deciphering the mechanisms underlying idiosyncratic DILI is challenging, in part because most idiosyncratic reactions as a rule cannot be reproduced in animal models. By contrast, acetaminophen poisoning seems to be broadly similar in humans and mice, and experiments in mice have provided important mechanistic insights into liver injury from acetaminophen in man.[11] When acetaminophen is ingested, a small fraction is metabolized in the liver to a reactive metabolite, *N*-acetyl-*p*-benzoquinoneimine (NAPQI), which is normally rapidly bound to and detoxified by an abundant intercellular compound called glutathione. However, with excessive ingestion of acetaminophen (typically >10–12 g at a single point in time), the production of the reactive metabolite overwhelms and rapidly depletes the available glutathione. With glutathione depleted in liver cells, NAPQI is left free to bind to critical intercellular proteins, possibly leading to liver cell injury and death.[11] Although it was once thought that this was the whole story, it is now very clear from a series of elegant experiments in various animal models that the innate immune system and several cellular signaling pathways also play important roles in modulating acetaminophen toxicity.[11] For example, experimental depletion of natural killer cells, critical to innate immunity, results in significant lessening of acetaminophen toxicity in mice.[11] Likewise, interruption of signaling by interferon-γ and the transcription factor, jun N-terminal kinase (JNK), also markedly attenuate acetaminophen toxicity in mice.[12] These experiments clearly demonstrate that even liver injury from acetaminophen toxicity is far more complicated than was previously appreciated.

Compared with liver injury from acetaminophen poisoning, much less is known about the development of idiosyncratic DILI, in large part because the reactions generally cannot be reproduced in animal models.[10] Like acetaminophen, many drugs that cause idiosyncratic DILI are metabolized in the liver into reactive compounds.

These compounds may bind to cellular components, disrupting their function and initiating a cascade of further liver injury by acting as immune targets and triggering pathways to cell death. Indeed, programmed cell death (apoptosis) appears to be a major mechanism of liver injury from at least some drugs.[10] Some idiosyncratic drug reactions appear to be primarily immune mediated, based on commonly associated clinical features such as rash, the presence of antidrug antibodies, and the rapid onset of liver injury with rechallenge of the drug. In addition, some of these reactions have been associated with specific human leukocyte antigens (HLA types) that have also been associated with autoimmunity. For example, recent studies suggested specific HLA haplotypes are linked to hepatotoxicity from flucloxacillin and amoxicillin-clavulanate.[13,14] Mutations in keratin cytoskeletal proteins have also recently been identified as potentially important in predisposing to acute liver injury from a variety of causes, including hepatotoxicity.[15] These associations aside, however, many of the underlying genetic and environmental factors that account for idiosyncratic DILI have remained elusive.[16] The difficulty in defining the key genetic elements responsible for DILI likely reflects that multiple interacting genetic and environmental factors are required for the DILI phenotype.

DILI PREVENTION

Several strategies potentially can be used to prevent severe liver injury from drugs.

- Patient education Patients taking drugs associated with liver injury should be warned about the symptoms commonly associated with severe liver injury, and should be instructed to stop the medications immediately on developing these symptoms and to contact the prescribing physician. This action is crucial for drugs such as INH that are associated with a relatively high incidence of severe liver injury. Patients should also be educated regarding the possible interaction of other drugs and alcohol with potentially toxic drugs. Finally, patients who suffer significant DILI should be warned to avoid reexposure to the implicated drug and, if appropriate, the reaction should be noted in the medical record as an allergy.
- Liver test screening Periodic screening of liver biochemistries, particularly serum ALT, is recommended for many drugs that have been associated with liver injury. However, whether serum ALT monitoring during drug treatment effectively prevents severe DILI remains controversial. For example, some patients with acute liver failure from troglitazone (an antidiabetic drug pulled from the US market in 2000, as discussed earlier) developed this life-threatening complication despite undergoing the recommended monthly monitoring.[9] Furthermore, ALT monitoring on a frequent basis is costly and cumbersome for both patients and clinicians; consequently, compliance with such surveillance is poor even with drugs for which formal recommendations for surveillance exist. Adding to this problem, the significance of a mildly elevated serum ALT is not always clear, as some patients appear to adapt and liver injury improves despite ongoing use of the medication.[17] However, the finding of a significantly elevated liver test often causes great angst among both clinicians and patients. Indeed, anxiety caused by the detection of abnormal, but asymptomatic, elevated aminotransferases may ultimately result in inappropriate drug withdrawal in some patients.
- Legislation Another way of decreasing the problem of DILI is through effective legislation aimed at restricting or eliminating potentially toxic drugs from the marketplace. Consider, for example, acetaminophen-opiate drugs. Nearly half of all cases of acute liver failure in the United States are currently due to

acetaminophen toxicity. Many of these cases are from intentional acetaminophen overdose in suicidal patients, but a recent, multicenter United States study suggests that as many as 50% of patients accidentally overdose with acetaminophen in an effort to relieve pain.[18] Many of these patients are prescribed acetaminophen-opiate combinations such Vicodin, a combination of the opiate hydrocodone and acetaminophen that is among the most commonly prescribed drugs in the United States. Over time, many patients treated with acetaminophen-opiate drugs for chronic pain appear to become tolerant to the analgesic effect of the opiate and thus take more than is prescribed to achieve adequate pain relief. Eventually, some inadvertently consume so much acetaminophen that severe liver injury and even life-threatening liver failure can ensue. This problem is further compounded by the presence of acetaminophen in many different cold and flu products. To the author, the concept of combining a highly addictive drug (an opiate) and a dose-dependent liver toxin (acetaminophen) into a single tablet defies logic and is at least broadly analogous to mixing candy and poison.[19,20] There is no reason, other than convenience, that these drugs are combined together in a single pill; they can be taken simultaneously as separate tablets, an opiate (eg, hydrocodone) and acetaminophen, with the same analgesic affect. In the author's opinion, patients should not be prescribed acetaminophen-opiate combinations for chronic pain, and all patients taking these drugs should be warned about the potential for severe liver injury. Although patient and physician education is important, the most effective solution will probably be a legislative action on the part of the FDA to uncouple acetaminophen and other drugs, including opiates as well as cold remedies. Such decisive legislation would help save many of the lives lost each year in the United States from unintentional acetaminophen overdoses.[21] Earlier this year, the FDA announced plans to limit the amount of acetaminophen in prescription medications to 325 mg per tablet over the next few years.[22] Short of uncoupling, this nonetheless represents an important step in the right direction.

RISK FACTORS FOR DILI

For most drugs, adults are usually at higher risk for liver injury than children; a notable exception is the antiseizure medication valproate, which appears to cause liver injury in children more commonly than in adults. Women as a group may also be somewhat more susceptible than men to DILI from many drugs, although this may also reflect more frequent drug exposure in women, or their generally smaller size.[23] For some drugs, including acetaminophen, alcohol abuse and malnutrition appear to predispose to liver injury.[24]

Whether preexisting liver disease predisposes to DILI is unclear with most drugs, although there are notable exceptions. For example, patients infected with both human immunodeficiency virus (HIV) and hepatitis C virus (HCV) appear to be at higher risk for liver injury from antiretroviral drugs than those infected with HIV infection alone.[25] Patients with chronic hepatitis may also be more susceptible to liver injury from the antituberculosis drug, INH.[25] Although underlying liver disease may not predispose to DILI in most situations, common sense dictates that patients with chronic liver disease who suffer significant superimposed DILI will have a worse outcome than patients who are otherwise healthy. In addition, the presence of abnormal baseline liver tests may make screening for DILI in the patient with underlying chronic liver disease more challenging. Thus, drugs associated with a significant risk of liver injury should be used with great care, if at all, in patients with chronic liver disease.[26] That being said, it is now quite clear that statins may be used in patients with chronic liver disease, including from HCV and fatty liver disease.[27]

DIAGNOSIS OF DILI: CAUSALITY ASSESSMENT

Many patients who experience mild DILI are completely asymptomatic and are only diagnosed because they have liver tests performed for other reasons. Indeed, DILI is an important cause of abnormal liver biochemistries observed in clinical practice. When symptoms of DILI are present, usually in cases of more severe hepatocellular DILI, they are often similar to viral hepatitis and include malaise, anorexia, nausea and vomiting, right upper quadrant abdominal pain, jaundice, acholic stools, and dark (tea-colored) urine. Patients with cholestatic DILI may also have intense pruritus. Fever and rash are the hallmarks of hypersensitivity that may be present with DILI from some drugs (eg, anticonvulsants such as phenytoin, sulfa drugs such as sulfamethoxazole-trimethoprim), but are absent in DILI caused by most drugs. If a patient with severe hepatocellular DILI develops hepatic encephalopathy, a hallmark of acute liver failure that is characterized in its severe form by severe memory loss, confusion, and even coma, the prognosis is grim without a liver transplant.[2]

Making a diagnosis of DILI is often very challenging because there are generally no reliable diagnostic tests for this problem, perhaps with the exception of acetaminophen-protein adducts for acetaminophen poisoning (see later discussion). A diagnosis of DILI is thus usually made through a process called causality assessment, which is broadly analogous to a criminal investigation, particularly one in which there are no actual witnesses to the crime. In such cases, the judgment of guilt or innocence hinges on the weight of carefully collected, but ultimately circumstantial evidence. During the process of causality assessment, many features of the drug reaction are considered, including:

- Was the drug in the "right place at the right time?" Obviously if the drug was started after the patient developed signs and symptoms of liver injury, the drug essentially has an alibi and it must be exculpated.
- Does the drug have a "prior record?" That is, has it been previously reported to cause liver injury in similar patients?
- Are the characteristics of the DILI event (the "crime") consistent with the known signature, or modus operandi of the implicated drug? For instance, INH, a drug used to treat tuberculosis, characteristically causes hepatocellular injury with elevated serum aminotransferases and, in severe cases, jaundice as well. The alkaline phosphatase, a marker of cholestasis, is typically only minimally elevated. Anticonvulsants, such as phenytoin (Dilantin), can cause liver injury as part of a hypersensitivity reaction so that rash and fever are often prominent features. A peculiar signature of amoxicillin-clavulanic acid (Augmentin), which can cause liver injury in a cholestatic or mixed pattern with jaundice, is that it typically does so only after the drug has been stopped, usually within 2 to 3 weeks. Another antibiotic, nitrofurantoin (Macrobid), characteristically causes a chronic hepatitis after many weeks, months, or even years of therapy, and is often associated with serum antinuclear antibodies (ANA). Signature features such as these can be helpful in a DILI diagnosis, though for most drugs there are no such features, and the fact that typical features are not seen in a given patient does not exclude a particular drug from causing liver injury.
- Are there other explanations for the liver injury? Critical to the diagnosis of DILI is the exclusion of other possible (so-called competing) causes of severe liver

injury, such as viral hepatitis, bile duct obstruction, hepatic ischemia (eg, secondary to shock), autoimmune hepatitis, and so forth. In essence, DILI is a diagnosis of exclusion.

- Is the clinical course of the reaction consistent with DILI? Most cases of DILI, particularly when not very severe, resolve relatively quickly when the drug is discontinued; the tempo of this improvement in the liver tests is called the dechallenge. If the drug is reintroduced the liver injury often returns, sometimes more rapidly and vigorously than with the initial exposure; however, rechallenge of the patient with the suspect drug is not generally advised as a diagnostic test because the liver injury that follows rechallenge can sometimes be quite severe, even life-threatening. Indeed, rechallenging the patient with suspect drug is roughly analogous to letting the suspect criminal out of custody to see if he commits the crime again: risky, to say the least!

The clinician is typically faced with the sometimes daunting task of carefully weighing these various bits of circumstantial evidence in making the DILI diagnosis. Moreover, that diagnosis can almost never be truly definitive because, with very few exceptions, specific diagnostic testing is lacking, and it is almost impossible to exclude every possible competing cause of liver injury. Serologic testing is done to exclude viral hepatitis A, B, C, and sometimes even E (albeit very rare in the United States) in most patients, as are serologic markers of autoimmunity (eg, an ANA, smooth muscle antibody, and γ-globulins). Other tests exclude metabolic and genetic problems, including iron and copper overload (hemochromatosis and Wilson disease, respectively), as well as other disorders (eg, α1-antitrypsin deficiency, celiac disease). In some cases, a careful history is needed to exclude severe hypotension preceding the onset of liver injury, which would suggest "shock liver" as a possible diagnosis if the liver tests suggest this possibility. Alcohol abuse must also be excluded by careful interrogation of the patient. Fatty liver (particularly nonalcoholic steatohepatitis) is a common cause of low-level abnormal liver tests that can be further evaluated by liver imaging, although liver biopsy is often needed for definitive diagnosis. Finally, most patients will also require some type of liver imaging, by ultrasonography, computed tomography, magnetic resonance imaging or, in cases of suspected biliary obstruction, possibly endoscopic retrograde cholangiopancreatography. Liver biopsy is also sometimes very useful in the diagnosis of drug-induced liver injury, but it is rarely diagnostic, because pathologically DILI can mimic virtually the entire spectrum of other causes of liver injury, including viral and autoimmune hepatitis, biliary tract disease and, in some cases, even alcohol abuse. Liver biopsy also carries a small but significant risk of bleeding and other complications.

Despite extensive evaluation to exclude competing causes of liver injury, causality analysis in many cases of liver injury proves challenging. Cases of possible DILI in patients with underlying liver disease or who are taking multiple drugs are particularly vexing. The diagnosis of DILI in such cases is almost always tentative.

Various causality instruments have been developed with the goal of enhancing the reliability of causality assessment. Perhaps the most popular, the Roussel-Uclaf Causality Assessment Method (RUCAM), also referred to as the CIOMS because the Council for International Organizations of Medical Sciences sponsored development of the instrument, uses numerical weighting of key features in 7 domains: temporal relationship (latency and dechallenge), risk factors, concomitant drug use, exclusion of other etiology, prior information about liver injury and the drug, and the response to rechallenge.[28] Each of these domains is given a numerical weight, all of which are added together to generate an overall numerical score intended to reflect the probability of causality. The total score is divided into ranges that represent highly probably (>8), probable (6–8), possible (3–5), unlikely (1–2), and excluded (≤0). The instrument, which has been incorporated into an online calculator (http://farmacologiaclinica.info/scales/CIOMS-RUCAM/), handles hepatocellular and cholestatic/mixed reactions differently with respect to temporal relationship, recognizing that cholestatic reactions may occur with slower kinetics. Although the RUCAM instrument has some attributes, including a check-list for the consultant faced with assessing causality in cases of possible DILI, it has been recently shown to be less reliable than expert opinion.[29–31]

Hepatitis E Virus Masquerading as DILI: Keeping an Open Mind

As already discussed, accurately diagnosing DILI is challenging because accurate biomarkers are currently lacking, and also because the clinical features of DILI may be identical to those associated with acute viral hepatitis as well as other causes of liver injury. The consultant must always keep an open mind to seemingly unlikely diagnostic possibilities. In essence, the diagnosis of DILI requires exclusion of a wide array of other potential causes of liver injury, including viral and autoimmune hepatitis, biliary obstruction, hepatic ischemia, and metabolic disorders. Whereas viral serologies for hepatitis A, B, and C are part of the standard evaluation of possible DILI, testing for hepatitis E virus (HEV) is rarely performed because HEV is generally considered very rare in developed countries, including the United States. Indeed, until recently almost all reported cases of clinically overt hepatitis E in the United States had been described in travelers returning from endemic areas of infection, such as Asia, Northeast Africa, the Middle East, and Mexico. However, increasingly cases of indigenous (also called autochthonous) HEV infection in developed countries, including the United States, are being recognized.[32,33] Indeed, a recent report suggests that in some areas of the United States, up to 20% of blood donors are immunoglobulin G (IgG)–seropositive for HEV, suggesting prior exposure and immunity to the virus, with the highest prevalence in states that are large producers of swine.[34] The human genotype-3 HEV shares homology with swine HEV, and zoonotic transmission of HEV from both domesticated and wild animals, including acute liver failure from HEV following consumption of raw or undercooked pig and wild boar liver, has been described.[35–37]

Because DILI is a diagnosis of exclusion, and hepatitis E is rarely considered in the evaluation of acute liver injury in the United States, it is possible that some cases of apparent DILI may actually represent occult HEV infection. Supporting this hypothesis, a recent publication from Great Britain described 6 cases of previously unrecognized HEV that had apparently been misdiagnosed as DILI.[38] In the absence of specific testing, it is not surprising that hepatitis E and DILI might be confused clinically. The clinical features of hepatitis E are similar to hepatitis A except that the former is more commonly associated with jaundice and overall more severe disease.[39]

A recently published United States study in fact found that a small but significant number of well-characterized DILI cases appear actually to represent occult HEV infection based on positive anti-HEV immunoglobulin M (IgM) serologies.[40] Specifically, among 318 patients with suspected DILI, 50 (16%) tested positive for HEV IgG, and 9 (3%) for HEV IgM; 4 of the 9 HEV IgM–positive patients also tested positive for HEV RNA. HEV IgM–positive patients were typically older men (mean age, 67 years), and 2 were HIV positive.[40] Of note, HEV infection was not considered, and specific HEV testing was not performed a priori in any of these cases. Furthermore, none of these anti-HEV IgM–positive cases was pregnant and none had recent travel to HEV-endemic areas preceding the onset of symptoms. The results of this study, which was conceived, designed, and executed by Drs Jose Serrano and Jay Hoofnagle of the Liver Branch of the National Institute of Diabetes and Digestive and Kidney Diseases (NIDDK) in collaboration with the Drug-Induced Liver Injury Network (DILIN) and the laboratory of Robert Purcell, also at the National Institutes of Health, represents strong support for testing for HEV in certain situations. For example, specific HEV testing should be considered in cases of apparent DILI with hepatocellular features, especially when a drug without an established track record of liver injury is implicated. This test may be particularly relevant to cases of apparent DILI observed during clinical trials of investigational drugs, as the finding of previously occult acute HEV infection in this setting may exculpate the drug, which in turn may have enormous financial and other practical implications. Unfortunately, because well-validated and approved testing for HEV infection is currently lacking, testing for this burgeoning infection in practice can be challenging.[33] It is hoped that growing interest in HEV infection both in developing and developed countries will spur development of increasingly accurate and reliable diagnostics in this area.

Acetaminophen Adducts: A Reliable Biomarker of DILI?

Acetaminophen is an unusual drug in that it a dose-dependent liver toxin, but remains popular as an effective analgesic for mild to moderate pain that is relatively safe as long as it is used in low doses. Although there are undoubtedly idiosyncratic features of acetaminophen toxicity that reflect poorly defined genetic polymorphisms and environmental exposures, when taken in sufficient quantities acetaminophen causes liver injury in essentially everyone. Indeed, acetaminophen toxicity is the most common cause of acute liver failure (ALF) in the United States, and is typically characterized by the rapid onset of markedly elevated serum aminotransferase levels (values over 10,000 IU/L are not unusual), relatively low serum bilirubin levels (usually <2–3 mg/dL at presentation), and often concomitant renal insufficiency (from acute tubular necrosis).[18] Despite this dramatic and seemingly easily recognized presentation, some cases of acetaminophen-related ALF go unrecognized because of several features. First, the history of excessive acetaminophen ingestion, whether acute (typically as part of a suicide attempt) or more chronically (usually for chronic pain), is often either unreliable or unavailable (eg, due to hepatic encephalopathy). Furthermore, the half-life of acetaminophen in blood is relatively short, and thus acetaminophen blood levels are often in the therapeutic range or even undetectable by the time the patient presents for evaluation; as a result, a low acetaminophen level should never be used as grounds for not administering the antidote, *N*-acetylcysteine (NAC).[18]

For cases in which an accurate history is unavailable and the acetaminophen level is not diagnostic, measuring acetaminophen-protein adducts may be very useful. These adducts, which were initially characterized more than 2 decades ago in rodent models of acetaminophen liver injury, appear to represent specific biomarkers of acetaminophen-related ALF. In a study of 66 patients with ALF collected prospectively as part of a multicenter study, including 20 patients with well-characterized acetaminophen-related ALF, 10 patients with ALF owing to other well-defined causes, and 36 patients with ALF of indeterminate etiology, acetaminophen-protein adducts were detected in serum in 100% of known acetaminophen ALF patients and in none of the ALF patients with other defined causes.[41] In tests of daily serial samples, serum adducts decreased in parallel with aminotransferase levels, with a serum half-life of approximately a week, much longer than that of acetaminophen itself. Most interestingly, 7 of 36 (19%) of the indeterminate cases, who had undergone an extensive but ultimately unrevealing prior investigation to determine the cause of ALF, demonstrated adducts in serum, strongly suggesting that acetaminophen toxicity caused or at least contributed to ALF in these patients.[41] Measurement of serum acetaminophen-protein adducts reliably identified acetaminophen toxicity, and may be a useful diagnostic test for cases lacking historical data or other clinical information. As such, this assay represents one of the only reliable biomarkers for DILI available today. Unfortunately, the assay used to measure acetaminophen-protein adducts in its current form is technically somewhat cumbersome, time consuming, and expensive. Thus the development of rapid, inexpensive, point-of-care assays is eagerly awaited.

PROGNOSIS OF DILI

Although it may understandably cause patients some anxiety, mild, asymptomatic DILI usually causes no significant morbidity and long-term consequences. Indeed, in many cases the liver tests improve over time despite continued use of the drug, owing to a poorly understood process called adaptation, which probably reflects the liver's robust response to injury in most individuals. Indeed, it is thought that the relatively rare cases of more severe idiosyncratic DILI may reflect the inability of the liver in affected patients to undergo this essential process in response to injury.

More than 2 decades ago Hyman Zimmerman, a pioneer of DILI research, observed that an elevated serum ALT (>3 × upper limit of normal) accompanied by jaundice due to drug toxicity carried a significant mortality ranging from 10% to 50%, at least 10-fold higher than icteric viral hepatitis. This important observation has been termed Hy's law in honor of Dr Zimmerman, and is regarded by regulatory agencies such as the FDA as a sign of serious DILI.[42–44]

Thus, an increase in serum bilirubin, which reflects impairment in the liver's ability to excrete bilirubin from blood into bile, is associated with a worse prognosis. Likewise, an increase in the prothrombin time (or the international normalized ratio), and a decrease in serum albumin reflect a severe impairment of the liver's protein synthetic function and are also markers of poor outcome. Finally, DILI severe enough to cause hepatic encephalopathy, thus signifying ALF, has a dire prognosis and is associated with a 70% to 80% chance of death without prompt liver transplantation.[2] Early referral to a liver transplant center is imperative in this setting.

Most episodes of DILI are acute. Rarely, an episode of severe acute DILI can appear to lead to a smoldering chronic liver disease.[45] Likewise, there are rare drugs that have been associated with severe liver scarring; methotrexate, used to treat rheumatoid arthritis and psoriasis, can cause cirrhosis in rare individuals, particularly with long-term use, although the risk appears to be relatively low.[46]

TREATMENT OF DILI

The mainstay of therapy for DILI is quickly stopping and avoiding reexposure to the implicated drug. With mild to moderate DILI this is typically sufficient, and results in relatively rapid and complete resolution of all symptoms and signs of liver injury, although cholestatic liver injury may linger, with complete resolution potentially taking many weeks and even months.

In some DILI cases, specific therapies are available. Prompt institution of NAC (Mucomyst) for acetaminophen poisoning is critically important and may be life-saving. Indeed, one recently published multicenter study suggests that NAC may also improve outcomes of patients with early ALF from a variety of other causes as well.[47] Some data suggest that the use of intravenous L-carnitine may be effective for ameliorating the toxicity associated with the anticonvulsant valproate.[48] The use of the ion-exchange resin, cholestyramine (Questran), is recommended for severe toxicity from leflunomide (Arava), probably because this drug has an extensive enterohepatic circulation, which makes it possible for cholestyramine to bind and eliminate the drug in the feces.[49] For cholestatic DILI, ursodeoxycholic acid (Actigal) is safe and may possibly hasten resolution of jaundice and pruritus, although this has not been well studied. Antipruritic agents (eg, cholestyramine) are also used in this setting to relieve itching.

Some controversy surrounds the role of corticosteroid therapy in the treatment of DILI. For DILI from most drugs corticosteroid therapy is probably ineffective, and does carry some risk.[50] Potential side effects of corticosteroids include mood disturbance, glucose intolerance (diabetes), and infection, and with prolonged use accelerated osteopenia, cataracts, and skin thinning. However, a short course of steroids is sometimes used for treatment of DILI, particularly when there are so-called hypersensitivity features such as rash, fever, and eosinophilia.

When hepatocellular liver injury is more severe, ALF may evolve, and the only effective therapy may be liver transplantation. Because of this, patients with severe DILI liver injury should be referred promptly to a liver transplant specialist for further evaluation and care.

FUTURE PROSPECTS FOR DILI

It is clear that we are a long way from really understanding exactly how idiosyncratic DILI develops. A critical question is: what are the traits of the individual, be they genetic or environmental, that increase the risk for idiosyncratic DILI? If we can identify these traits then perhaps we can one day avoid prescribing certain medications to certain patients identified as being at particularly high risk for developing DILI from these drugs. Such testing, if sufficiently robust and accurate, may also allow use of medications safely that would otherwise be removed from the market because of toxicity in rare individuals, and would represent the Holy Grail of research in this field.

In an effort to make inroads into the difficult but important problem of DILI, the NIDDK established in 2003 the Drug-Induced Liver Injury Network, or DILIN (https://dilin.dcri.duke.edu/).[23,51] The DILIN consists of 8 clinical centers as well as a data collection center at Duke University (**Fig. 1**). The primary objective of the network is to advance our understanding of DILI, its causes, clinical features, pathogenesis, and natural history. Because there are currently few robust and accurate preclinical

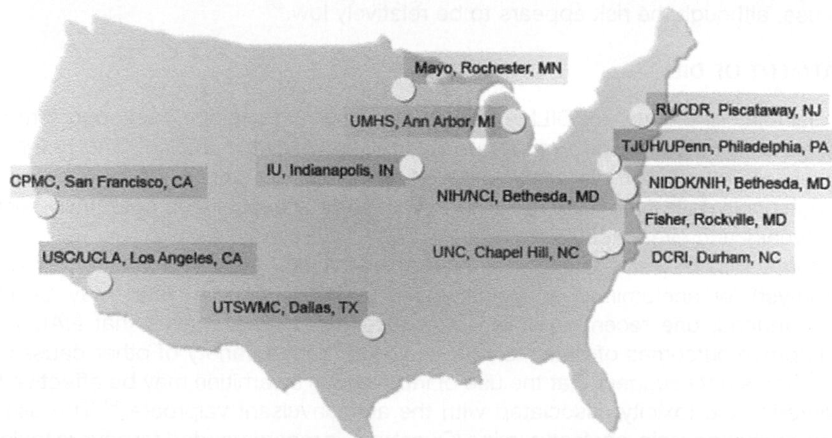

Fig. 1. Centers participating in the Drug-Induced Liver Injury Network (DILIN).

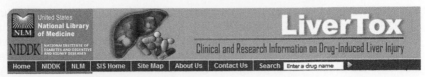

Fig. 2. The LiverTox web site will revolutionize the way information about drug-induced liver injury is accessed and shared in the future.

models of idiosyncratic drug-induced liver injury, the DILIN is developing a comprehensive registry of detailed clinical data, as well as serum, plasma, urine, and DNA from patients who have suffered bona fide idiosyncratic DILI. It is anticipated that investigators around the world who are interested in DILI will exploit this unique resource, which currently includes well over a thousand well-characterized DILI cases, for pharmacogenomic and other studies, to better understand the genetic and environmental factors contributing to the development of DILI and, furthermore, to identify novel biomarkers associated with this important public health problem.

A major development in this field launched by the time this article is in print will be LiverTox (**Fig. 2**), a novel online resource developed as a collaborative effort between the Liver Disease Branch of the NIDDK and the National Library of Medicine, which will include a complete and accurate summary of clinical features, diagnosis, cause, frequency, patterns, and management of DILI associated with an encyclopedic listing of nearly all drugs. LiverTox will represent an easily accessed, up-to-date, accurate, and comprehensive resource for the consultant facing challenging cases of apparent DILI. As such, LiverTox will ultimately render traditional multi-author textbooks on hepatotoxicity, and perhaps even shorter treatments such as this review, essentially obsolete.

REFERENCES

1. Navarro VJ, Senior JR. Drug-related hepatotoxicity. N Engl J Med 2006;354(7): 731–9.
2. Ostapowicz G, Fontana RJ, Schiodt FV, et al. Results of a prospective study of acute liver failure at 17 tertiary care centers in the United States. Ann Intern Med 2002;137(12):947–54.
3. Senior JR. What is idiosyncratic hepatotoxicity? What is it not? Hepatology 2008; 47(6):1813–5.
4. Lammert C, Einarsson S, Saha C, et al. Relationship between daily dose of oral medications and idiosyncratic drug-induced liver injury: search for signals. Hepatology 2008;47(6):2003–9.
5. Watkins PB, Seeff LB. Drug-induced liver injury: summary of a single topic clinical research conference. Hepatology 2006;43(3):618–31.
6. Gordon DW, Rosenthal G, Hart J, et al. Chaparral ingestion. The broadening spectrum of liver injury caused by herbal medications. JAMA 1995;273(6):489–90.
7. Senior JR. Drug hepatotoxicity from a regulatory perspective. Clin Liver Dis 2007; 11(3):507–24.
8. Davern TJ, Chalasani N. Drug-induced liver injury in clinical trials: as rare as hens' teeth. Am J Gastroenterol 2009;104(5):1159–61.
9. Graham DJ, Green L, Senior JR, et al. Troglitazone-induced liver failure: a case study. Am J Med 2003;114(4):299–306.
10. Kaplowitz N. Idiosyncratic drug hepatotoxicity. Nat Rev Drug Discov 2005;4(6): 489–99.

11. James LP, Mayeux PR, Hinson JA. Acetaminophen-induced hepatotoxicity. Drug Metab Dispos 2003;31(12):1499–506.
12. Gunawan BK, Liu ZX, Han D, et al. c-Jun N-terminal kinase plays a major role in murine acetaminophen hepatotoxicity. Gastroenterology 2006;131(1):165–78.
13. Daly AK, Donaldson PT, Bhatnagar P, et al, DILIGEN Study, International SAE Consortium. HLA-B*5701 genotype is a major determinant of drug-induced liver injury due to flucloxacillin. Nat Genet 2009;41(7):816–9.
14. Lucena MI, Molokhia M, Shen Y, et al, Spanish DILI Registry, EUDRAGENE, DILIN, DILIGEN, International SAEC. Susceptibility to amoxicillin-clavulanate-induced liver injury is influenced by multiple HLA class I and II alleles. Gastroenterology 2011;141(1):338–47.
15. Strnad P, Zhou Q, Hanada S, et al, Acute Liver Failure Study Group. Keratin variants predispose to acute liver failure and adverse outcome: race and ethnic associations. Gastroenterology 2010;139(3):828–35.
16. Russmann S, Jetter A, Kullak-Ublick GA. Pharmacogenetics of drug-induced liver injury. Hepatology 2010 Aug;52(2):748–61.
17. Watkins PB, Zimmerman HJ, Knapp MJ, et al. Hepatotoxic effects of tacrine administration in patients with Alzheimer's disease. JAMA 1994;271(13):992–8.
18. Larson AM, Polson J, Fontana RJ, et al, Acute Liver Failure Study Group. Acetaminophen-induced acute liver failure: results of a United States multicenter, prospective study. Hepatology 2005;42(6):1364–72.
19. Davern T. Acetaminophen hepatotoxicity. Hepatology 2004;40(4):1021–2.
20. Available at: http://www.kqed.org/epArchive/R510310737. Accessed March 3, 2012.
21. Available at: http://www.sfgate.com/cgi-bin/article.cgi?f=/c/a/2004/08/15/EDGFT87DK31.DTL. Accessed March 3, 2012.
22. Available at: http://www.fda.gov/NewsEvents/Newsroom/PressAnnouncements/ucm239894.htm. Accessed March 3, 2012.
23. Chalasani N, Fontana RJ, Bonkovsky HL, et al, Drug Induced Liver Injury Network (DILIN). Causes, clinical features, and outcomes from a prospective study of drug-induced liver injury in the United States. Gastroenterology 2008;135(6):1924–34.
24. Thummel KE, Slattery JT, Ro H, et al. Ethanol and production of the hepatotoxic metabolite of acetaminophen in healthy adults. Clin Pharmacol Ther 2000;67(6):591–9.
25. Chalasani N, Björnsson E. Risk factors for idiosyncratic drug-induced liver injury. Gastroenterology 2010;138(7):2246–59.
26. Gupta NK, Lewis JH. The use of potentially hepatotoxic drugs in patients with liver disease. Aliment Pharmacol Ther 2008;28(9):1021–41.
27. Chalasani N, Aljadhey H, Kesterson J. Patients with elevated liver enzymes are not at higher risk for statin hepatotoxicity. Gastroenterology 2004;126(5):1287–92.
28. Bénichou C. Criteria of drug-induced liver disorders. Report of an international consensus meeting. J Hepatol 1990;11(2):272–6.
29. Kaplowitz N. Causality assessment versus guilt-by-association in drug hepatotoxicity. Hepatology 2001;33(1):308–10.
30. Rochon J, Protiva P, Seeff LB, et al, Drug-Induced Liver Injury Network (DILIN). Reliability of the Roussel Uclaf Causality Assessment Method for assessing causality in drug-induced liver injury. Hepatology 2008;48(4):1175–83.
31. Rockey DC, Seeff LB, Rochon J, et al. US Drug-Induced Liver Injury Network. Causality assessment in drug-induced liver injury using a structured expert

opinion process: comparison to the Roussel-Uclaf causality assessment method. Hepatology 2010;51(6):2117–26.
32. Dalton HR, Bendall R, Ijaz S, et al. Hepatitis E: an emerging infection in developed countries. Lancet Infect Dis 2008;8:698–709.
33. Purcell RH, Emerson SU. Hepatitis E: an emerging awareness of an old disease. J Hepatol 2008;48:494–503.
34. Kuniholm MH, Purcell RH, McQuillan GM, et al. Epidemiology of hepatitis E virus in the United States: results from the Third National Health and Nutrition Examination Survey, 1988-1994. J Infect Dis 2009;200:48–56.
35. Yazaki Y, Mizuo H, Takahashi M, et al. Sporadic acute or fulminant hepatitis E in Hokkaido, Japan, may be food-borne, as suggested by the presence of hepatitis E virus in pig liver as food. J Gen Virol 2003;84(Pt 9):2351–7.
36. Matsuda H, Okada K, Takahashi K, et al. Severe hepatitis E virus infection after ingestion of uncooked liver from a wild boar. J Infect Dis 2003;188:944.
37. Wichmann O, Schimanski S, Koch J, et al. Phylogenetic and case-control study on hepatitis E virus infection in Germany. J Infect Dis 2008;198:1732–41.
38. Dalton HR, Fellows HJ, Stableforth W, et al. The role of hepatitis E virus testing in drug-induced liver injury. Aliment Pharmacol Ther 2007;26:1429–35.
39. Chau TN, Lai ST, Tse C, et al. Epidemiology and clinical features of sporadic hepatitis E as compared with hepatitis A. Am J Gastroenterol 2006;101:292–6.
40. Davern TJ, Chalasani N, Fontana RJ, et al, Drug-Induced Liver Injury Network (DILIN). Acute hepatitis E infection accounts for some cases of suspected drug-induced liver injury. Gastroenterology 2011;141(5):1665–72.
41. Davern TJ 2nd, James LP, Hinson JA, et al, Acute Liver Failure Study Group. Measurement of serum acetaminophen-protein adducts in patients with acute liver failure. Gastroenterology 2006;130(3):687–94.
42. Reuben A. Hy's law. Hepatology 2004;39(2):574–8.
43. Björnsson E, Olsson R. Outcome and prognostic markers in severe drug-induced liver disease. Hepatology 2005;42(2):481–9.
44. Senior JR. How can 'Hy's law' help the clinician? Pharmacoepidemiol Drug Saf 2006 Apr;15(4):235–9.
45. Andrade RJ, Lucena MI, Kaplowitz N, et al. Outcome of acute idiosyncratic drug-induced liver injury: long-term follow-up in a hepatotoxicity registry. Hepatology 2006;44(6):1581–8.
46. Kremer JM, Alarcón GS, Lightfoot RW Jr, et al. Methotrexate for rheumatoid arthritis. Suggested guidelines for monitoring liver toxicity. American College of Rheumatology. Arthritis Rheum 1994;37(3):316.
47. Lee WM, Hynan LS, Rossaro L, et al, Acute Liver Failure Study Group. Intravenous N-acetylcysteine improves transplant-free survival in early stage non-acetaminophen acute liver failure. Gastroenterology 2009;137(3):856–64.
48. Lheureux PE, Penaloza A, Zahir S, et al. Science review: carnitine in the treatment of valproic acid-induced toxicity—what is the evidence? Crit Care 2005 Oct 5; 9(5):431–40.
49. Sevilla-Mantilla C, Ortega L, Agúndez JA, et al. Leflunomide-induced acute hepatitis. Dig Liver Dis 2004;36(1):82–4.
50. Marino G, Zimmerman HJ, Lewis JH. Management of drug-induced liver disease. Curr Gastroenterol Rep 2001;3(1):38–48.
51. Fontana RJ, Watkins PB, Bonkovsky HL, et al, DILIN Study Group. Drug-Induced Liver Injury Network (DILIN) prospective study: rationale, design and conduct. Drug Saf 2009;32(1):55–68.

Liver Disease in Pregnancy

Arjmand R. Mufti, MD, MRCP, Nancy Reau, MD*

KEYWORDS

• Liver disease • Pregnancy • Liver biochemical profile

Changes in the liver biochemical profile are normal in pregnancy. However, up to 3% to 5% of all pregnancies are complicated by liver dysfunction.[1] It is important that liver disease during pregnancy is recognized because early diagnosis may improve maternal and fetal outcomes, with resultant decreased morbidity and mortality. Liver diseases that occur in pregnancy can be broadly divided into 3 different groups: liver diseases that are unique to pregnancy, liver diseases that are not unique to pregnancy but can be revealed or exacerbated by pregnancy, and liver diseases that are unrelated to but occur coincidentally during pregnancy (**Box 1**).

LIVER PHYSIOLOGY DURING PREGNANCY

Pregnancy is a time of great metabolic and physiologic changes, and it is essential that any changes in liver function tests are interpreted in this context (**Table 1**). During pregnancy, the body undergoes adaptive changes in physiology, which affect all organ systems including the liver. The plasma volume increases by approximately 50%, there is an increase in venous pressure, and although the absolute hepatic blood flow remains unchanged, the liver receives a lower percentage of the cardiac output.[2] There is also a decrease in the blood pressure and systemic vascular resistance, and these changes mimic the physiologic changes that occur in patients with decompensated chronic liver disease. In addition, serum estrogen and progesterone levels are increased.[3] The resulting hyperestrogenemia is believed to be the cause of spider telengectasias and palmar erythema, signs that are usually seen in chronic liver disease, but are normal during pregnancy and usually resolve after delivery.

The traditional tests of liver function are also affected. Serum alanine aminotransferase (ALT), aspartate aminotransferase (AST) and γ-glutamyl transferase (GGT) levels are within the normal range or marginally reduced secondary to hemodilution.[4–6] In contrast, serum alkaline phosphatase (ALP) increases markedly during the third trimester and levels can be 4 times more than the normal prepregnancy values. This situation is mainly the result of the production of a placental isoenzyme,

Department of Medicine, Section of Gastroenterology, Hepatology and Nutrition, University of Chicago Medical Center, 5841 South Maryland Avenue, MC 4076, Chicago, IL 60637, USA
* Corresponding author.
E-mail address: nreau@medicine.bsd.uchicago.edu

Clin Liver Dis 16 (2012) 247–269
doi:10.1016/j.cld.2012.03.011

Box 1
Classification of liver diseases in pregnancy

Diseases unique to pregnancy
- Hyperemesis gravidarum (HG)
- Intrahepatic cholestasis of pregnancy (ICP)
- Acute fatty liver of pregnancy (AFLP)
- Preeclampsia and eclampsia
- HELLP syndrome

Preexisting underlying liver disease
- Hepatitis B and C
- Autoimmune hepatitis
- Wilson disease
- Primary sclerosing cholangitis (PSC)
- Primary biliary cirrhosis (PBC)
- Cirrhosis

Liver diseases coincident with pregnancy
- Viral hepatitis
- Budd-Chiari syndrome
- Gallstones
- Drug-induced hepatotoxicity
- Liver transplantation
- Sepsis

Table 1
Biochemical changes in liver tests during a normal pregnancy

Test	Alterations Seen
Total bilirubin	No change or slightly decreased
AST	No change or slightly decreased
ALT	No change or slightly decreased
Alkaline phosphatase	Increased 2-fold to 4-fold
Albumin	Decreased
Fibrinogen	Increased by 50%
Factors V, VII, and VIII	Increased
Globulins	Increased α and β globulin; Decrease in γ globulin
Partial thromboplastin and activated partial thromboplastin time	No change
α-Fetoprotein	Increased (especially with twins)
Platelets	No change
Cholesterol and triglycerides	Increased
Ceruloplasmin	Increased
Hemoglobin	Decreased from second trimester
White cell count	Increased

but there is also an increase in production of the bone isoenzyme.[4–6] In pregnant patients, total and unconjugated bilirubin concentrations may be slightly decreased during all 3 trimesters and conjugated bilirubin levels are mildly reduced during the second and third trimesters.[4] There is no difference in the total bile acid concentrations in the pregnant and nonpregnant populations but there is decreased motility of the gallbladder, resulting in increased lithogenicity of the bile.[4] An increase in plasma volume as well as decreased synthesis results in a decrease in serum albumin levels in the first trimester and this becomes more marked as the pregnancy progresses. In contrast, serum triglyceride and cholesterol levels increase by 50% and 200%, respectively, secondary to increased production.[7] There is also an increase in the hepatic synthesis of factors V, VII, VIII, and fibrinogen but there is no change in the range for prothrombin time and activated partial thromboplastin time (APTT). Therefore increased levels of ALT, AST, and serum bilirubin levels should be considered pathologic and further evaluation should be undertaken.

MODALITY OF TESTING IN PREGNANCY

Of course, all modes of evaluation for abnormal liver function should be safe for the fetus and the mother. Ultrasonography remains the safest method to visualize the liver during pregnancy. If further testing is required, according to the American College of Obstetricians and Gynecologists guidelines for diagnostic imaging in pregnancy, exposure to a single diagnostic procedure does not result in harmful fetal effects, and exposure to less than 0.05 Gy is not associated with fetal abnormalities or abortion.[8,9] Nevertheless, the utmost care should be exercised when deciding how to proceed. The embryo and the fetus are particularly sensitive to ionizing radiation, and exposure to increased exposure can be teratogenic, mutagenic, or carcinogenic in nature.[8,9] **Table 2** outlines the different diagnostic techniques that can be used to investigate abnormal liver tests and their related adverse effects.

Table 2
Diagnostic techniques used in pregnancy

Diagnostic Method	Safety Profile
Ultrasonography	Considered safe during pregnancy, with no known adverse effects from in utero exposure
Magnetic resonance imaging	Considered safe during pregnancy, but avoid gadolinium in the first trimester because it crosses the placenta and fetal effects are unknown
Radiograph exposure	Up to 2 weeks' gestation: exposure to high-dose ionizing radiation (>0.10 Gy) may be lethal 2–16 weeks: threshold for radiation is 0.10 Gy 8–15 weeks: highest risk for mental retardation and microcephaly related to abnormalities in neuronal development >16 weeks: threshold for radiation is 0.50–0.70 Gy Low risk of teratogenicity after 25 weeks
Contrast agents	Should be avoided unless risk to the fetus is justified
Liver biopsy	Rarely required but both the ultrasound-guided percutaneous route and transjugular approaches are safe

LIVER DISEASES UNIQUE TO PREGNANCY

Several liver diseases occur only during pregnancy and usually resolve only after delivery. Most liver dysfunction that is seen in pregnancy is caused by diseases that fall into this category.

HG

Nausea and vomiting are common in pregnancy and affects up to 80% of women in the first trimester.[10] HG occurs in 0.3% to 2.0% of pregnant women[11] and is defined as persistent vomiting early in pregnancy that is associated with weight loss of 5% or more of prepregnancy body weight, dehydration, and ketosis.[12] It is a diagnosis of exclusion, and other causes of nausea and vomiting must be ruled out.[13] Hospitalization is usually required for intravenous fluid therapy and symptoms start early in the first trimester of pregnancy, typically between 4 and 10 weeks' gestation and most cases resolve by 20 weeks.[14] However, in approximately 10% of patients, symptoms persist throughout pregnancy and resolve only after delivery.[15,16] The underlying causes of HG are poorly understood, but genetic predisposition, abnormal gastric motility, hormonal factors, immunologic factors, and changes in the autonomic nervous system are postulated to be involved.[17–20] Risk factors include obesity, pre-existing diabetes, molar pregnancy, multiple pregnancies, and psychiatric illness. It is also associated with a biochemical thyrotoxicosis in 60% of cases (increased free tri-iodothyronine [T3] and thyroxine [T4] and suppressed thyroid-stimulating hormone in the absence of clinical hyperthyroidism) and this is believed to be caused by increased human chorionic gonadotrophin levels, which increase thyroid-stimulating activity during pregnancy.[21,22]

Liver involvement is seen in 50% to 60% of cases[23] and a mild increase in aminotransferase levels is the most common biochemical abnormalities seen with ALT levels usually exceeding AST levels.[24] However, more striking derangements are also seen; AST and ALT levels more than 20-times the upper limit of normal have also been reported.[24,25] Jaundice is uncommon and if abnormal chemistries persist, other causes of liver disease such as viral hepatitis or drug-related liver injury should be excluded. A liver biopsy should be performed only if the diagnosis of HG is in doubt and histology is usually normal or shows bland cholestasis and steatosis.[26,27] Treatment is usually supportive and includes intravenous rehydration and nutritional support. Patients should avoid triggers that aggravate nausea, and eat small, frequent, high-carbohydrate, low-fat meals. No medications are currently approved by the US Food and Drug Administration (FDA) for HG, but antiemetics that are safe in pregnancy, such as promethazine, metoclopramide, and ondansetron, may be used.[28,29] Thiamine supplementation is also recommended to prevent Wernike encephalopathy, and parenteral nutrition is occasionally needed in patients who have persistent nausea and are unable to maintain their body weight. Steroid therapy for HG is controversial, because several randomized controlled trials have shown conflicting results, and should be considered only in patients with severe symptoms who are unresponsive to other antiemetic therapy.[14]

ICP

ICP is defined as pruritus and increased bile acid levels that appear in the second and third trimester of pregnancy. ICP typically resolves after delivery, but tends to recur in subsequent pregnancies. It is the second most common cause of jaundice in pregnancy after viral hepatitis. There are clear ethnic differences in the incidence of the disease. The highest incidence has been reported in Bolivia and Chile, with rates ranging from 4% to 28%.[30–32] There seems to have been a decline in the prevalence recently, although the reasons for this are unclear.[31,32] In the United States, the prevalence varies widely according to the ethnic population from 0.3% to 5.6%,[33,34] and in Europe, the incidence ranges from 0.1% to 1.5%.[35] Risk factors include advanced maternal age, women with personal history of cholestasis secondary to the oral contraceptive pill, and a family history of the condition.[36] Maternal outcomes in women with ICP are generally believed to be good. However, a 2006 retrospective, matched cohort study from Finland assessed the risk of liver and biliary diseases in more than 10,000 women with ICP. Several liver and biliary diseases, including hepatitis C, gallstones and cholecystitis, nonalcoholic liver cirrhosis, and nonalcoholic pancreatitis, were found to have a significantly higher incidence in patients with ICP than in controls.[37] The investigators therefore postulated that closer follow-up may need to be considered in patients who are diagnosed with ICP during their pregnancy. However, there is no doubt that ICP can result in significant deleterious effects on the fetus, including chronic placental insufficiency with consequent fetal complications such as fetal distress (20%–40%),[38] preterm labor (60%),[39] prematurity, and intrauterine death (1%).[40,41]

The cause of ICP is multifactorial, with genetic, hormonal, and exogenous factors all believed to play a role in the development of the disease.[42] The cause of ICP remains unclear but is related to deranged biliary transport across the canalicular membrane. Genomic variants in genes coding for several hepatobiliary transporters have been reported in patients with ICP.[43–47] The ABCB4 gene (ATP-binding cassette, subfamily B member 4) encodes the multidrug resistance 3 P-glycoprotein (MDR3), which is the main transporter of phospholipids across the canalicular membrane into bile. In the absence of phospholipids in bile, bile acids can injure the canalicular membrane, leading to cholestasis.[44,45,47] At least 10 different mutations in the ABCB4 gene located on chromosome 7q21.1 have been identified and are implicated in up to 15% of cases of ICP in a White population.[47] Other defects that have been reported include mutations of the ABCB11 gene (ATP-binding cassette, subfamily B member 11) encoding the bile salt export pump (BSEP)[43] and in the ATP8B1 (ATPase, aminophospholipid transporter, class I, type 8B, member 1) gene, which is associated with familial cholestasis.[46] In addition, cyclosporine inhibits BSEP, and its use has also been associated in renal transplant patients with ICP.[48]

The female sex hormones estrogen and progesterone also play a role in the development of ICP. Estrogen is known to be cholestatic because it inhibits the BSEP. In addition, abnormal progesterone metabolism with resultant increased sulfated metabolite levels may saturate the hepatic transport system and precipitate the development of ICP.[49] Exogenous factors also play a role because ICP recurs in only 60% to 70% of patients, with varying intensity. In addition, there is seasonal variability and dietary factors such as selenium deficiency have been postulated to play a role in the high incidence of the disease in Chile.[50]

Pruritus is the main presenting symptom and may initially be more marked in the palms and soles before spreading to the rest of the body. It usually starts at week 25 of gestation, but has been reported in the first trimester as well. Patients can also present with anorexia, fatigue, diarrhea, and steatorrhea caused by fat malabsorption and have a prolonged prothrombin time because of vitamin K deficiency. Supplementation of fat-soluble vitamins may be required.[40,51] Jaundice occurs in less than 10% to 25% of cases, but when present it arises 2 to 4 weeks after the onset of pruritus. If the jaundice precedes the pruritus, other causes of liver disease should also be ruled out.[40,51] The most sensitive and specific marker of the disease is a fasting serum bile acid concentration of greater than 10 μmol/L, and this may be the only biochemical abnormality seen. In particular, cholic acid is increased and chenodeoxycholic acid is decreased.[52] There is a direct correlation between fetal distress and serum bile acid levels; Glantz and colleagues[40] showed that no fetal complications are usually seen until serum bile acid levels reach 40 μmol/L. Aminotransferase levels are usually mildly increased but can be 20 times the upper limit of normal; when this is the case, viral hepatitis should be ruled out. ALP levels are unhelpful because they are normally increased throughout pregnancy and GGT levels are usually normal.[52] Liver biopsy is not usually needed to make a diagnosis of ICP, but histologic findings include mild centrilobular cholestasis with preserved portal tracts, minimal or no inflammation, and bile plugs in hepatocytes.[53]

The treatment of choice for ICP is ursodeoxycholic acid (UDCA) at 10 to 15 mg/kg bodyweight.[54] It has been shown to improve symptoms and biochemical markers of liver function, it does not have any side effects in the mother or fetus, and it reduces the risk of prematurity (**Table 3**).[54] The mechanism of action of UDCA is still being elucidated but it has been shown to increase expression of BSEPs such as ABCB11 as well as increasing placental bile transporters, thereby facilitating improved bile transfer. It also decreases plasma bile acid and sulfated progesterone metabolite levels, which have been implicated in ICP.[55] UDCA is safer and more effective than cholestyramine and *S*-adenosyl-L-methionine, a glutathione precursor, in the treatment of ICP[56,57] and has also been shown to be superior to dexamethasone in

Table 3
Common side effects of some drugs used in pregnancy

Drug	FDA Category	Side Effects
Cyclosporine	C	Generally safe; premature labor, low birth weight
Azathioprine	D	Generally safe; lymphopenia, thymic hypoplasia, and hypogammaglobulinemia
Prednisone	C	Generally safe; cleft palate, intrauterine growth retardation, adrenal insufficiency
Tacrolimus	C	Generally safe; premature labor, low birth weight
Mycophenol ate mofetil	D	Contraindicated; first trimester loss, teratogenecity
Penicillamine	D	Use for Wilson disease because of benefits; birth defects including congenital cutix laxa
Trientine	C	Limited data but likely safe
Zinc acetate	A	No adverse effects reported
UDCA	B	Safe to use
Octreotide	B	Probably safe to use
Lamivudine	C	Crosses placenta; low risk
Entecavir	C	Limited data; not recommended
Tenofovir	B	Bone effects including demineralization
Adefovir	C	Limited data; likely safe to use
Interferon/ ribavirin	C/X in combination with ribavirin	Not recommended; severe fatal toxicity with combination therapy
Nadolol	C: first trimester D: second/third trimesters	Prolonged half-life, risk of intrauterine growth retardation in second/third trimesters

improving pruritus and reducing bile acid levels in patients with concentrations greater than 40 μmol/L.[51] Dexamethasone may be used because it promotes fetal lung maturity in preterm infants with ICP. ICP normally resolves after delivery, but rarely the condition can persist after delivery, leading to fibrosis and even cirrhosis; these cases may represent chronic cholestatic liver diseases with a first presentation during pregnancy.[37]

Preeclampsia and Eclampsia

Preeclampsia is a multisystem disorder characterized by hypertension (systolic blood pressure ≥140 mmHg or diastolic blood pressure ≥90 mmHg) and proteinuria (≥300 mg/24 h) occurring after 20 weeks' gestation in a previously normotensive patient.[58,59] It affects 5% to 10% of all pregnant women and is mild in 75% of cases and severe in 25% of patients.[60] Eclampsia is the term used when seizures or altered consciousness are seen in the setting of preeclampsia or gestational hypertension. Tight control of blood pressure is essential. Risk factors for preeclampsia and eclampsia include previous history of preeclampsia, presence of antiphospholipid antibodies, nulliparity, extremes of maternal age (<18 years and >40 years), gestational and pregestational diabetes, obesity, and family history.[60] Both maternal and fetal/placental factors are believed to contribute to the development of preeclampsia. Abnormalities in the development of placental vasculature secondary to abnormal trophoblast implantation early in pregnancy may result in relative placental ischemia. This situation leads to the release of antiangiogenic factors into the maternal circulation, which causes endothelial dysfunction and the activation of procoagulant factors.[60]

Liver involvement is not common, but when present it signifies severe preeclampsia and should result in immediate delivery. The mechanism of injury involves vasoconstriction of the hepatic vasculature and precipitation of fibrin in the liver. Although biopsy is not necessary for the diagnosis, periportal hemorrhage and fibrin deposition, ischemic lesions, and microvesicular fat deposits are seen histologically.[52] Liver involvement should be suspected clinically with the development of right upper quadrant or epigastric pain. Biochemically, 10-fold to 20-fold increases in aminotransferases as well as increases in ALP levels beyond those normally associated with pregnancy are present. The bilirubin is usually normal, but mild increases to 5 mg/dL may be observed. These biochemical changes usually resolve within 2 weeks of delivery. In the most severe cases, a hematoma may develop beneath the Glisson capsule and result in hepatic rupture, a finding that may indicate the development of HELLP syndrome (hemolysis, elevated liver enzymes, low platelets), which is discussed in more detail in the next section.

HELLP Syndrome

As the name suggests, HELLP syndrome is characterized by hemolytic anemia with a microangiopathic smear, increased liver enzymes, and low platelets. Although the acronym was first coined in 1982, the syndrome was probably first described by Pritchard and colleagues[61,62] in 1954. It complicates 10% to 20% of cases of severe preeclampsia/eclampsia and 0.2% to 0.6% of all pregnancies.[63,64] It was historically believed to be the most extreme clinical manifestation of severe preeclampsia, but up to 20% of patients without hypertension and proteinuria also develop HELLP, resulting in speculation that it may represent a separate disorder that has features in common with preeclampsia.[64,65]

In a prospective cohort study by Sibai and colleagues[65] of 442 pregnancies with HELLP syndrome, the incidence of the syndrome was 20% in patients with preeclampsia. Most patients were diagnosed between 28 and 36 weeks of gestation and 30% presented with the disease in the postpartum period, some as long as 1 week after delivery. Risk factors include advanced maternal age, White ethnicity, and multiparity.[58] There are no pathognomonic clinical features that can distinguish HELLP from preeclampsia. Patients with HELLP syndrome might be asymptomatic or present with right upper quadrant and epigastric pain, nausea, vomiting, malaise, headache, edema, and weight gain. Hypertension and proteinuria are present in up to 80% of cases and jaundice is present in 5% of patients.[66]

As in preeclampsia, hepatic injury is precipitated by hypovolaemia, intravascular fibrin deposition, and increased sinusoidal pressures.[67] Diagnosis is made by the clinical picture and changes in the complete blood count, peripheral smear, and liver function tests. Clinically, because of the hemolysis, patients with HELLP characteristically have increased serum bilirubin and lactate dehydrogenase (LDH) levels but low serum haptoglobin levels.[63,64] Liver aminotransferases are increased and thrombocytopenia is also present. The thrombocytopenia is secondary to consumption of peripheral blood platelets because they aggregate at sites of endothelial damage.[63,64] Various diagnostic criteria for HELLP syndrome have been used, and the 2 most commonly used classifications were developed at the Universities of Mississippi and Tennessee (**Table 4**).[68]

The diagnosis of HELLP must be quickly established because of maternal and fetal risk and the absolute necessity for immediate delivery. Mortality of 3% with the development of HELLP syndrome has been reported.[63,64,69] Patients should be admitted to a high-dependency or intensive care unit, especially if complications such as disseminated intravascular coagulation (DIC), hepatic encephalopathy, and acute renal failure are present. A computed tomography scan of the liver should be performed to evaluate for subcapsular hematomas, intraparenchymal hemorrhage, or hepatic rupture, which is seen in 1% of patients with HELLP.[70] Delivery of the fetus is the definitive treatment of HELLP and should be undertaken at greater than 34 weeks' gestation

Table 4
Mississippi and Tennessee classification systems of HELLP syndromes

HELLP Class	Mississippi Classification	Tennessee Classification
Class 1 (severe)	AST or ALT >70 IU/L LDH >600 IU/L Platelets <50 × 10⁹/L	AST >70 IU/L LDH >600 IU/L or bilirubin ≥1.2 mg/dL Platelets <100 × 10⁹/L Evidence of hemolysis on peripheral blood smear
Class 2 (moderate)	AST or ALT >70 IU/L LDH >600 IU/L Platelets 50–100 × 10⁹/L	
Class 3 (mild)	AST or ALT >40 IU/L LDH >600 IU/L Platelets 100–150 × 10⁹/L	N/A
Partial HELLP	N/A	Severe preeclampsia and one of the following: • ELLP • HEL • EL • LP

Abbreviations: EL, elevated liver enzymes; ELLP, absence of hemolysis; HEL, hemolysis and elevated liver enzymes absent thrombocytopenia; LP, low platelets; N/A, not applicable.

Data from Martin Jr JN, Rose CH, Briery CM. Understanding and managing HELLP syndrome: the integral role of aggressive glucocorticoids for mother and child. Am J Obstet Gynecol 2006;195(4):917.

or if there is evidence of multiorgan failure, including DIC, acute renal failure, abruptio placentae, or if fetal distress is present.[63,64,69] If the fetal gestation age is less than 34 weeks, corticosteroids (such as dexamethasone and betamethasone) that cross the placenta should be administered because they promote fetal lung maturity and result in improved perinatal outcomes.[63,64,71] In the absence of complications, labor can be allowed to proceed naturally but up to 50% require a cesarean section. Hypertension should be treated using vasodilators such as labetalol, hydralazine, and nifedipine, and intravenous magnesium sulfate should be given for seizure prophylaxis.[63,64,69]

Although variable, HELLP syndrome onset and progression is usually rapid (35%–50% decrease in platelets per 24 hours) because LDH and AST and ALT levels increase until 48 hours post partum, when laboratory values begin to normalize.[72] Most patients have rapid, early resolution of HELLP after delivery. However, persistence of thrombocytopenia or hemolysis for more than 72 hours after delivery, worsening hepatic or renal failure, or life-threatening complications should be treated as medically indicated.[63,64,69,72] Indications for liver transplantation include persistent bleeding from a hepatic hematoma, hepatic rupture, or hepatic failure; in 1 case series, the 5-year and 10-year survival rates after liver transplantation were 88% and 65%, respectively.[73] If hepatic rupture occurs, shock usually develops rapidly and rapid surgical intervention allied with supportive measures is advocated. Maternal mortality from hepatic rupture is 50%, and perinatal mortality is 10% to 60%.[74]

If HELLP syndrome develops in the postpartum period, it is managed in the same way as the antepartum phase, with supportive care. As with preeclampsia, the risk of recurrence of HELLP syndrome in subsequent pregnancies is increased, as are the rates of preeclampsia, prematurity, intrauterine growth retardation, and abruptio placentae.[74]

AFLP

AFLP was first described by Stander and Cadden in 1934 in their article entitled "Acute yellow atrophy of the liver in pregnancy". It is histologically characterized by microvesicular fatty infiltration, usually in the third trimester, which results in encephalopathy and hepatic failure. It affects women of all ages and races and there is no distinctive epidemiologic feature that has been related to geographic areas or ethnic groups. Forty percent to 50% of patients are nulliparous and there is a higher incidence in twin pregnancies.[75,76]

It has historically been reported to affect between 1 in 7000 and 1 in 20 000 pregnancies. Traditionally, maternal and fetal mortality had been believed to be between 5% and 25%.[77,78] A large population-based descriptive study using the UK Obstetric Surveillance System, performed in 229 hospitals across the country, identified 57 cases in a total of more than 1.1 million pregnancies with an estimated incidence of 5 per 100 000 pregnancies.[79] Eighteen percent of the women had twin pregnancies and there were a total of 67 deliveries. Seventy-four percent of cases were identified at a median gestation age of 36 weeks and 60% were delivered within 24 hours of diagnosis. The cesarean section rate was 74%. The perinatal mortality was 104 per 1000 births and there was 1 maternal death; 1 woman in the cohort required liver transplantation.[79] This study, the largest of its kind, indicated that the disease incidence may be lower than previously believed and both maternal and fetal outcomes may also be better than the literature states.

AFLP is associated with an inherited defect in mitochondrial fatty acid β-oxidation, which is an important source of energy for skeletal and cardiac tissue.[77,80–82] Beta-oxidation of fatty acids in hepatic mitochondria is a complex process requiring 4 essential enzymes including long-chain 3-hydroxyacyl-CoA dehydrogenase (LCHAD), which catalyzes the formation of 3-ketoacyl-CoA from 3-hydroxyacyl-CoA. This enzyme is part of the mitochondrial trifunctional protein (MTP), which is an important complex associated with the inner mitochondrial membrane. Defects in LCHAD result in the accumulation of 3-hydroxyacyl metabolites produced by the fetus or placenta, which return to the maternal circulation and are then deposited in the liver, resulting in hepatotoxicity.[77,80–82] This association has been borne out in several studies. Treem and colleagues[83] reported on 12 women with a previous episode of AFLP and 8 were heterozygous for LCHAD. These 8 heterozygous patients had 9 pregnancies complicated by fatty liver, and 7 of these pregnancies were also associated with preeclampsia and HELLP. Fetal genotype is also believed to be important in determining fetal and maternal outcomes. In a study looking at 35 families with MTP mutations, Yang and colleagues[84] found that approximately half of women who carried affected fetuses had AFLP and 11% had HELLP syndrome. In addition, 100% of women who developed maternal illness carried fetuses with isolated LCHAD deficiency, and no maternal or fetal complications were associated with heterozygous or wild-type fetal genotypes.

This association between LCHAD deficiency and AFLP has been further defined. The autosomally inherited genetic mutations of LCHAD, especially the G1548C mutation on 1 or both alleles, are most closely associated with AFLP and are associated with a 20-fold increased risk of development of maternal liver disease during pregnancy. This mutation is present on the α subunit of the trifunctional protein, which is associated with the inner mitochondrial membrane and provides the active site for LCHAD enzymatic activity. An LCHAD deficiency in the fetus (either homozygous for the G1528C mutation where glutamic acid is replaced with glutamine [E474Q] or a compound heterozygous mutation when E474Q plus a different mutation on the other allele is present) was associated with a 79% chance of developing maternal AFLP or HELLP. In fetuses with other mutations or with at least 1 wild-type allele, no pregnancy-related liver complications were present.[85] Under stress, infants with LCHAD deficiency are at risk of developing fatal nonketotic hypoglycemia, imitating Reye syndrome, and there is an association with neonatal dilated cardiomyopathy or progressive neuromyopathy.[78,83] These associations with serious outcomes mean it is important to have an accurate and early diagnosis, with a plan for expedited delivery of the fetus. There are no sequelae of chronic liver disease, but mothers who have LCHAD mutations have a chance of recurrence of AFLP in a subsequent pregnancy.[86,87] Testing for the known genetic variants of LCHAD is available and should be performed in affected women and their infants.[88]

The diagnosis of AFLP is usually made clinically based on the presentation, and compatible laboratory and imaging results. AFLP can present in a myriad of ways; patients may have nonspecific symptoms such as nausea, anorexia, headache, and abdominal pain, and this can progress to more localizing signs and symptoms such as hepatic encephalopathy and jaundice. Laboratory findings include increased AST and ALT levels (which can be mildly increased to 20 times the upper limit of normal), increased bilirubin, increased uric acid, and coagulopathy with or without DIC. In addition, patients usually have renal dysfunction, metabolic acidosis, leukocytosis, anemia, and hyperammonemia.[76,89,90] Hypoglycemia is a poor prognostic sign. The differential diagnosis includes HELLP syndrome and acute viral hepatitis such as hepatitis E and herpes simplex infection. Viral serologies should therefore be checked, and although it is rarely required, liver biopsy remains the gold standard for diagnosis. The histologic changes usually seen are microvesicular steatosis, predominantly in zone 3 within hepatocytes with relative sparing of the periportal areas. The fatty deposits around central nuclei give the cytoplasm a foamy appearance.

Prompt delivery is essential in women with AFLP. As in preeclampsia, steroids may be required for lung maturation in preterm fetuses and mothers can develop a long postnatal cholestatic phase, lasting up to 4 weeks. The histologic changes resolve within days to weeks after delivery.[77,78]

PREEXISTING UNDERLYING LIVER DISEASE AND PREGNANCY

Hepatitis B

Approximately 350 million people are chronic carriers of hepatitis B virus (HBV) infection.[88] The prevalence of HBV infection varies greatly and more than 10% of the population is infected in high endemic areas such as China, Africa, and South America.[88] HBV has 2 primary modes of transmission: from an infected mother to newborn during childbirth (vertical transmission) and from an infected sexual or household contact (horizontal transmission).[91] The vertical transmission of HBV from mother to infant occurs in the perinatal period. During childbirth, maternal secretions in the birth canal come into close contact with the baby's mucosal membranes, and in the immediate postpartum period, transmission results from close contact between mother and baby.[91] There is no evidence that cesarean section prevents maternal-infant transmission. Some infants are also infected in utero. In a Chinese study, 3.7% of babies tested hepatitis B surface antigen (HbsAg) positive at birth from in utero infection and this was believed to be related to the ability of the virus to translocate across the placenta from the maternal circulation. Factors that predispose to transplacental infection remain unknown, but high maternal viral load and preterm labor are predisposing factors.[92]

Vertical transmission is associated with chronic infection rates of 85% to 95%, unlike horizontal modes of transmission, which result in chronic infection in only 5% to 10% of cases. There are approximately 43,000 new cases of HBV in the United States every year and only 1000 cases are seen in children.[91,93] Vertical transmission therefore is responsible for only a few cases. However, worldwide the situation is different, because 50% of chronically infected individuals acquired their infection perinatally or in early childhood.[93] Approximately 10% to 20% of neonates born to HBsAg-positive mothers and 90% of those born to both HBsAg-positive and hepatitis B e antigen (HBeAg)-positive mothers become infected with HBV. HbeAg-negative mothers with high viral loads also have high transmission rates of the virus from the mother to the fetus.[94] Hepatitis B viral load is a key factor in transmission, with high viral load being associated with 80% to 90% risk of transmission compared with 10% to 30% transmission rates in patients with undetectable viral load.[94] Universal vaccination of all newborns regardless of maternal HBsAg status is necessary for global eradication of HBV infection and has been adopted by more than 90% of nations worldwide. This strategy has been shown to be a successful way of preventing HBV infection as well as reducing the complications associated with chronic HBV infection.

Screening of all pregnant women for HBsAg is performed routinely in the United States. All neonates born to HBsAg-positive mothers should receive hepatitis B immunoglobulin (HBIG) within 12 hours of birth as well as the first dose of the HBV vaccine at birth. This passive-active immunization is more than 90% effective at preventing transmission in HbeAg-negative mothers.[95] However, this protocol is less effective in cases in which the mother is HBeAg positive or in the setting of high maternal viral loads. The use of lamivudine (pregnancy category C) and telbivudine and tenofovir (pregnancy category B) from 32 weeks of gestation decreases the rate of transmission of HBV in patients with high circulating levels of HBV DNA (10^6–10^8/ml copies).[96,97] There is no consensus on when to stop therapy after delivery but if the only reason for therapy was to reduce vertical transmission, it may be discontinued between 1 and 3 months post partum. Breast-feeding is not contraindicated for HBV-positive mothers and there are no differences in rates of infection between breast-fed and formula-fed babies.[98] The American Academy of Pediatrics guidelines advocate breastfeeding provided the infant has received HBIG and hepatitis B vaccine. Assisted reproduction is also safe in couples in whom only the male partner is affected.[99]

Hepatitis C

The worldwide prevalence of hepatitis C virus (HCV) in pregnant women is between 1% and 8%. In the United States, it ranges from 0.5% to 3% and the prevalence in children is between 0.05% and 0.36%.[100–102] Vertical transmission is believed to be the leading cause of mother-to-baby transmission, with maternal viral load and prolonged time from rupture of membranes to delivery being the major factors determining infectivity. HCV vertical transmission is approximately 5% to 10% in HCV RNA-positive mothers, but can be as high as 22% in human immunodeficiency virus/HCV-coinfected patients. Neonatal transmission is rare.[103,104]

There are conflicting data regarding the effect of HCV infection on the fetus, with some studies showing an association with the development of gestational diabetes mellitus and lower birth weight.[105] There are no studies to determine the safest mode of delivery in HCV-infected mothers but because prolonged time from rupture of membranes is associated with increased infection, the second stage of labor should be kept short.[106] Breast-feeding is safe, although there remains a theoretic risk of HCV transmission because HCV RNA has been detected in breast milk. However, the US Centers for Disease Control and Prevention recommend that HCV-infected women with cracked or bleeding nipples should abstain from breast-feeding.[107] There are no effective interventions to decrease the transmission of HCV from mother to infant. However, children who have been exposed to HCV in utero should undergo testing for HCV RNA because maternal antibodies may result in a false-positive result on serologic testing.[107]

Although the protease inhibitors boceprevir and telaprevir have been designated as category B in pregnant patients, triple therapy with pegylated interferon, ribavirin, and a protease inhibitor has been given a category X designation by the FDA because ribavirin is teratogenic in animal models. Therefore, therapy is not recommended for HCV-infected pregnant women.[107] However, numerous agents are in development for hepatitis C, some of which do not require interferon or ribavirin, and in the next few years, these drugs may be suitable for the pregnant patient.

Cirrhosis in Pregnancy

Pregnancy is rare in cirrhosis because most patients with advanced cirrhosis have amenorrhea and anovulation secondary to derangement of the hypothalamic-pituitary axis. In addition, the prevalence of cirrhosis in women of reproductive age is only 0.0004%, so there is little overlap between the 2 conditions.[108,109] Nevertheless, a successful pregnancy is possible in well-compensated cirrhotic patients with mild portal hypertension, and these patients should be seen by a high-risk obstetrician as well as a hepatologist. Maternal and fetal complications have been reported in 50% of cases, and maternal mortality of up to 10% has been reported.[110,111] Fetal outcomes include prematurity in up to 50% of cases, perinatal death in 18%, and a rate of spontaneous abortion that is double that of the general population (40% vs 20%). The main risk to the mother is from variceal hemorrhage in 15% to 25% of patients with cirrhosis, and in patients with known portal hypertension, the risk is as high as 50%.[26] Amongst patients with preexisting varices, the mortality ranges from

18% to 50%, and up to 80% have variceal bleeding. The risk of bleeding increases with progression of the pregnancy and is highest during labor. All patients with cirrhosis who are planning a pregnancy should have a screening upper endoscopy to look for varices. In pregnant patients who were not screened, upper endoscopy should be performed in the second trimester. A nonselective β-blocker such as nadolol (FDA category C) may be used for primary prophylaxis during the pregnancy, but because nadolol crosses the placenta, newborns should be monitored for hypoglycemia and bradycardia during the first days of life. The use of octreotide for variceal bleeding is controversial despite its classification as a pregnancy category B agent because it causes splanchnic vasoconstriction and may precipitate placental ischemia and abruption.[109,112]

Other maternal complications are hepatic decompensation (24%), especially after variceal bleeding, spontaneous bacterial peritonitis, and hepatic encephalopathy. In addition, splenic artery aneurysm rupture is seen in 2.6% of cases, especially in the third trimester. The cause of the development of these aneurysms is not known but it is believed to be related to the altered hormonal milieu associated with cirrhosis and pregnancy. Vaginal deliveries are preferred except in patients with known large varices. A cesarean section is recommended for these patients to prevent the increases in portal pressure during labor. Postpartum hemorrhage remains a significant source mortality and morbidity in 6% to 10% of cases.[108,110,111]

Autoimmune Hepatitis

Although autoimmune hepatitis predisposes to infertility, adequate control of the disease can result in normal menstruation and successful pregnancies. In patients with autoimmune hepatitis, the major risk is prematurity, and adverse fetal outcomes are directly related to the degree of prematurity. Nevertheless, the outcomes in autoimmune hepatitis are similar to those in the general population with chronic disease.[113,114] If it is clinically appropriate, an attempt should be made to stop immunosuppressive therapy. If this action is not possible, then patients with autoimmune hepatitis need to be on a stable drug regimen throughout their pregnancy. It may be possible to reduce the dose of immunosuppressive therapy because autoimmune hepatitis can improve during the course of the pregnancy. Nevertheless, after delivery, as the blood estrogen levels decrease, flares in the disease have been reported (12%–86%) and patients should resume their normal dose of immunosuppression 2 weeks before their delivery date.[114,115]

Both prednisone and azathioprine, the mainstays of therapy, can be used during pregnancy. Azathioprine has an FDA category D pregnancy rating and is teratogenic in animal models. Birth defects have not been reported in human beings, so the risk is theoretic, but it should nevertheless be used with care in pregnant patients, because other fetal side effects including lymphopenia, hypogammaglobulinaemia, and thymic hypoplasia have been reported. Disease exacerbations during pregnancy are usually treated with oral steroids.[116]

PBC and PSC

PBC and PSC are both chronic cholestatic diseases that lead to the destruction of bile ducts. The course of both these diseases is uncertain during pregnancy because there are limited data available as a result of their negative effects on fertility.[117,118] In PBC, estrogens promote cholestasis and therefore during pregnancy pruritus may become severe even early in the pregnancy and may not resolve in the postpartum stage. If a pregnant patient has PBC, an upper endoscopy should be performed in the second trimester to look for esophageal varices. Otherwise, patients can continue with UDCA at 13 to 15 mg/kg and complications should be managed expectantly.[119]

There are limited data on outcomes in pregnancy in patients with PSC, but fertility does not seem to be reduced compared with normal controls. Pregnancies are often complicated by pruritus and can also be associated with the development of dominant strictures, or choledocholithiasis. UDCA at 10 to 15 mg/kg has been used to improve pruritus in this patient population during pregnancy.[120]

Wilson Disease

Wilson disease is an eponymously named disease that was first described by Samuel Wilson in 1912.[121] It is a multisystem autosomal-recessive disorder of copper metabolism that results from mutations in ATP7B, a gene encoding a P type ATPase involved in copper transport. More than 200 different mutations in this gene located on chromosome 13 have been implicated in the development of Wilson disease and results in defective export of copper.[122,123] It is characterized by the pathologic accumulation of copper in the liver, brain, and other organs, including the kidneys. The worldwide prevalence is between 1 in 30000 and 1 in 50000; patients usually present in young adulthood, but cases have been reported from the age of 3 to 72 years.

Wilson disease can be difficult to diagnose because of the myriad of ways in which it can present, but patients usually have some hepatic, psychiatric, or neurologic manifestations. Wilson disease complicated by liver disease can present as isolated hepatomegaly or splenomegaly with portal hypertension. In addition, patients can present with jaundice, low serum ALP levels, increased aminotransferase levels, compensated or decompensated cirrhosis, and fulminant hepatic failure with or without associated Coombs-negative hemolytic anemia.[122,123] Care should be taken that undiagnosed Wilson disease in the pregnant patient presenting with hemolysis and acute liver failure is not misdiagnosed as HELLP syndrome.

During pregnancy, serum copper levels can increase without treatment and can result in a flare in patients, with fatal outcomes. Wilson disease is treated with chelation with penicillamine. If thee is an adverse reaction to penicillamine, trientine is used in conjunction with zinc acetate and all patients should be on a low-copper diet.[122,124,125] The American Association for the Study of Liver Diseases guidelines recommend continuing with chelation therapy throughout pregnancy, with the caveat that the dose of penicillamine and trientine should be reduced by 25% to 50% in the third trimester to promote better wound healing in the event of a cesarean section.[126]

LIVER DISEASES COINCIDENT WITH PREGNANCY

Viral Hepatitis

In the United States, viral hepatitis accounts for 40% of all cases of jaundice in the pregnant population. The causative agents are hepatitis A, B, C, D, and E virus, herpes simplex virus (HSV), Epstein-Barr virus and cytomegalovirus. The outcome is usually benign, except in acute hepatitis E and HSV hepatitis.[127] Ascites and hypertension can be used to differentiate pregnancy-associated liver diseases such as HELLP from viral hepatitis and should prompt expedited delivery.[128]

Worldwide, acute hepatitis E virus (HEV) is the most common viral hepatitis in pregnancy, unlike hepatitis A, B, and C, which have the same prevalence in pregnant and nonpregnant women. HEV is uncommon in the United States but is endemic to parts of Asia, Africa, the Middle East, and Central America and accounts for up to 50% of all cases of acute hepatitis in these areas.[129,130] In men and nonpregnant women, the disease is usually self-limited and has a case-fatality rate of less than 0.1%. However, hepatitis E has a more severe course in pregnancy, especially in the third trimester, and patients, especially in India, are more likely to develop fulminant liver failure, with mortality of 15% to 25%.[131] The reasons for increased virulence in pregnancy are not fully understood but are believed to be related to the hormonal and immunologic changes seen in pregnancy, including downregulation of nuclear factor (NF-κB) along with host susceptibility factors.[132,133] Management is supportive and delivery of the fetus does not affect outcomes.[134]

Hepatitis A virus (HAV) infection has the same frequency and clinical course in the pregnant and nonpregnant populations.[135] In a retrospective Israeli study of 79,458 pregnant patients, 13 cases of second and third trimester HAV infection were found. Nine of the 13 patients developed gestational complications, including premature contractions, premature rupture of membranes, and vaginal bleeding. Fever and hypoalbuminemia was associated with preterm labor and occurred in 62% of cases.[135] Treatment is supportive, and infection is not associated with adverse long-term maternal outcomes. Vertical transmission of hepatitis A is rare and occurs only with high maternal viral loads. Breast-feeding is not contraindicated in women with HAV infection.

HSV hepatitis is a rare condition, which can be catastrophic when the primary infection occurs in pregnancy, because it is associated with a 40% risk for fulminant liver failure and death.[136] HSV usually presents with a prodrome of fever and upper respiratory tract symptoms and mucocutaneous lesions may be present in 50% of patients.[136,137] Patients are usually anicteric but typically have markedly increased serum aminotransferase levels and prothrombin time as well as thrombocytopenia and leucopenia.[136,137] Early diagnosis should be sought because HSV hepatitis can be treated with intravenous acyclovir.[137] Recurrent HSV infections usually manifest as genital mucocutaneous lesions, and transmission of HSV to the fetus can be as high as 50%. Cesarean section should be considered if lesions are present at delivery.[136]

Gallstones and Biliary Disease

Pregnancy is associated with increased cholesterol secretion in the second and third trimesters, increased lithogenicity of bile caused by decreased hepatic synthesis of chenodeoxycholic acid, and decreased gallbladder contractility.[138] These changes mean that gallstones are more common in pregnancy, and 10% of pregnant patients develop gallstones or biliary sludge compared with 5% at the start of pregnancy.[138] Risk factors include increased prepregnancy body mass index (calculated as weight in kilograms divided by the square of height in meters) and serum leptin levels.[138] Pregnant patients can present with biliary colic, gallstone pancreatitis, acute cholecystitis, and cholangitis and are managed in the same manner as nonpregnant patients.[139] Laparoscopic cholecystectomy for symptomatic cholelithiasis in pregnancy is safe during the second trimester, but is associated with abortion and premature labor in the first and third trimesters, respectively. Endoscopic retrograde cholangiopancreatography can also be performed safely for cholodocholithiasis.[139]

Budd-Chiari Syndrome

Budd-Chiari syndrome is a term denoting outflow obstruction of the hepatic veins, resulting in sinusoidal congestion and necrosis of hepatocytes around the central vein. Clinical manifestations include hepatomegaly, ascites, and abdominal pain. Pregnant patients with Budd-Chiari syndrome often have an underlying predisposing condition, such as factor V Leiden, antithrombin III deficiency, protein C or S deficiency, or the presence of antiphospholipid antibodies.[140] Pregnancy also represents a prothrombotic state because there is relative protein S deficiency. All these factors result in the development of Budd-Chiari syndrome.[140,141] Doppler ultrasonography and magnetic resonance imaging are the diagnostic imaging modalities of choice in pregnancy. Complete anticoagulation throughout pregnancy is required, and liver transplantation may be necessary in the most severe cases.

Pregnancy and Liver Transplantation

Successful organ transplantation often restores fertility,[142] and the first known pregnancy in a liver transplant recipient was reported in 1978.[143] For patients who have undergone a liver transplant, deferral of pregnancy for at least 1 year after transplantation is recommended.[144,145] Approximately 70% of pregnancies in liver transplant patients result in a live birth, and pregnancy before 1 year after transplantation is associated with a higher risk of prematurity, low birth weight, and increased incidence of acute allograft rejection.[144,145] Mycophenolate mofetil should be discontinued in all liver transplant patients planning to get pregnant, but cyclosporine, tacrolimus, and azathioprine may be continued.[146,147]

SUMMARY

Hepatic disorders in the pregnant patient are uncommon, but remain important because of the potential severe ramifications in the mother and fetus. Significant strides have been made in understanding the pathophysiology underlying these disorders as well as in the management of some of the severe sequelae associated with these disorders. These diseases should be managed in specialized centers to ensure the best possible outcome in patients.

REFERENCES

1. Ch'ng CL, Morgan M, Hainsworth I, et al. Prospective study of liver dysfunction in pregnancy in Southwest Wales. Gut 2002;51(6):876–80.
2. Kerr MG, Scott DB, Samuel E. Studies of the inferior vena cava in late pregnancy. Br Med J 1964;1(5382):522.4–33.4.
3. Van Thiel DH, Gavaler JS. Pregnancy-associated sex steroids and their effects on the liver. Semin Liver Dis 1987;7(1):1–7.
4. Bacq Y, Zarka O, Brechot JF, et al. Liver function tests in normal pregnancy: a prospective study of 103 pregnant women and 103 matched controls. Hepatology 1996;23(5):1030–4.
5. Girling JC, Dow E, Smith JH. Liver function tests in pre-eclampsia: importance of comparison with a reference range derived for normal pregnancy. Br J Obstet Gynaecol 1997;104(2):246–50.
6. Valenzuela GJ, Munson LA, Tarbaux NM, et al. Time-dependent changes in bone, placental, intestinal, and hepatic alkaline phosphatase activities in serum during human pregnancy. Clin Chem 1987;33(10):1801–6.
7. Darmady JM, Postle AD. Lipid metabolism in pregnancy. Br J Obstet Gynaecol 1982;89(3):211–5.
8. ACOG Committee on Obstetric Practice. ACOG Committee Opinion. Number 299, September 2004 (replaces No. 158, September 1995). Guidelines for diagnostic imaging during pregnancy. Obstet Gynecol 2004;104(3):647–51.
9. De Santis M, Cesari E, Nobili E, et al. Radiation effects on development. Birth Defects Res C Embryo Today 2007;81(3):177–82.

10. Bashiri A, Neumann L, Maymon E, et al. Hyperemesis gravidarum: epidemiologic features, complications and outcome. Eur J Obstet Gynecol Reprod Biol 1995;63(2):135–8.
11. Goodwin TM. Hyperemesis gravidarum. Obstet Gynecol Clin North Am 2008; 35(3):401–17, viii.
12. Goodwin TM. Hyperemesis gravidarum. Clin Obstet Gynecol 1998;41(3): 597–605.
13. Verberg MF, Gillott DJ, Al-Fardan N, et al. Hyperemesis gravidarum, a literature review. Hum Reprod Update 2005;11(5):527–39.
14. Bottomley C, Bourne T. Management strategies for hyperemesis. Best practice & research. Clin Obstet Gynaecol 2009;23(4):549–64.
15. Gadsby R, Barnie-Adshead AM, Jagger C. A prospective study of nausea and vomiting during pregnancy. Br J Gen Pract 1993;43(371):245–8.
16. Tsang IS, Katz VL, Wells SD. Maternal and fetal outcomes in hyperemesis gravidarum. Int J Gynaecol Obstet 1996;55(3):231–5.
17. Kaplan PB, Gucer F, Sayin NC, et al. Maternal serum cytokine levels in women with hyperemesis gravidarum in the first trimester of pregnancy. Fertil Steril 2003;79(3):498–502.
18. Leylek OA, Toyaksi M, Erselcan T, et al. Immunologic and biochemical factors in hyperemesis gravidarum with or without hyperthyroxinemia. Gynecol Obstet Invest 1999;47(4):229–34.
19. Minagawa M, Narita J, Tada T, et al. Mechanisms underlying immunologic states during pregnancy: possible association of the sympathetic nervous system. Cell Immunol 1999;196(1):1–13.
20. Taskin S, Taskin EA, Seval MM, et al. Serum levels of adenosine deaminase and pregnancy-related hormones in hyperemesis gravidarum. J Perinat Med 2009; 37(1):32–5.
21. Colin JF, Mathurin P, Durand F, et al. Hyperthyroidism: a possible factor of cholestasis associated with hyperemesis gravidarum of prolonged evolution. Gastroenterol Clin Biol 1994;18(4):378–80 [in French].
22. Goodwin TM, Montoro M, Mestman JH. Transient hyperthyroidism and hyperemesis gravidarum: clinical aspects. Am J Obstet Gynecol 1992;167(3):648–52.
23. Hepburn IS, Schade RR. Pregnancy-associated liver disorders. Dig Dis Sci 2008;53(9):2334–58.
24. Conchillo JM, Pijnenborg JM, Peeters P, et al. Liver enzyme elevation induced by hyperemesis gravidarum: aetiology, diagnosis and treatment. Neth J Med 2002;60(9):374–8.
25. Kuscu NK, Koyuncu F. Hyperemesis gravidarum: current concepts and management. Postgrad Med J 2002;78(916):76–9.
26. Hay JE. Liver disease in pregnancy. Hepatology 2008;47(3):1067–76.
27. Su GL. Pregnancy and liver disease. Curr Gastroenterol Rep 2008;10(1):15–21.
28. Nageotte MP, Briggs GG, Towers CV, et al. Droperidol and diphenhydramine in the management of hyperemesis gravidarum. Am J Obstet Gynecol 1996; 174(6):1801–5 [discussion: 1805–6].
29. Seto A, Einarson T, Koren G. Pregnancy outcome following first trimester exposure to antihistamines: meta-analysis. Am J Perinatol 1997;14(3):119–24.
30. Reyes H, Gonzalez MC, Ribalta J, et al. Prevalence of intrahepatic cholestasis of pregnancy in Chile. Ann Intern Med 1978;88(4):487–93.
31. Ribalta J, Reyes H, Gonzalez MC, et al. S-adenosyl-L-methionine in the treatment of patients with intrahepatic cholestasis of pregnancy: a randomized, double-blind, placebo-controlled study with negative results. Hepatology 1991;13(6):1084–9.

32. Rioseco AJ, Ivankovic MB, Manzur A, et al. Intrahepatic cholestasis of pregnancy: a retrospective case-control study of perinatal outcome. Am J Obstet Gynecol 1994;170(3):890–5.
33. Laifer SA, Stiller RJ, Siddiqui DS, et al. Ursodeoxycholic acid for the treatment of intrahepatic cholestasis of pregnancy. J Matern Fetal Med 2001;10(2): 131–5.
34. Lee RH, Goodwin TM, Greenspoon J, et al. The prevalence of intrahepatic cholestasis of pregnancy in a primarily Latina Los Angeles population. J Perinatol 2006;26(9):527–32.
35. Schneider G, Paus TC, Kullak-Ublick GA, et al. Linkage between a new splicing site mutation in the MDR3 alias ABCB4 gene and intrahepatic cholestasis of pregnancy. Hepatology 2007;45(1):150–8.
36. Reyes H. Review: intrahepatic cholestasis. A puzzling disorder of pregnancy. J Gastroenterol Hepatol 1997;12(3):211–6.
37. Ropponen A, Sund R, Riikonen S, et al. Intrahepatic cholestasis of pregnancy as an indicator of liver and biliary diseases: a population-based study. Hepatology 2006;43(4):723–8.
38. Fisk NM, Bye WB, Storey GN. Maternal features of obstetric cholestasis: 20 years experience at King George V Hospital. Aust N Z J Obstet Gynaecol 1988;28(3):172–6.
39. Bacq Y, Sapey T, Brechot MC, et al. Intrahepatic cholestasis of pregnancy: a French prospective study. Hepatology 1997;26(2):358–64.
40. Glantz A, Marschall HU, Mattsson LA. Intrahepatic cholestasis of pregnancy: relationships between bile acid levels and fetal complication rates. Hepatology 2004;40(2):467–74.
41. Turunen K, Sumanen M, Haukilahti RL, et al. Good pregnancy outcome despite intrahepatic cholestasis. Scand J Prim Health Care 2010;28(2):102–7.
42. Arrese M, Macias RI, Briz O, et al. Molecular pathogenesis of intrahepatic cholestasis of pregnancy. Expert Rev Mol Med 2008;10:e9.
43. Dixon PH, van Mil SW, Chambers J, et al. Contribution of variant alleles of ABCB11 to susceptibility to intrahepatic cholestasis of pregnancy. Gut 2009; 58(4):537–44.
44. Eloranta ML, Hakli T, Hiltunen M, et al. Association of single nucleotide polymorphisms of the bile salt export pump gene with intrahepatic cholestasis of pregnancy. Scand J Gastroenterol 2003;38(6):648–52.
45. Floreani A, Carderi I, Paternoster D, et al. Hepatobiliary phospholipid transporter ABCB4, MDR3 gene variants in a large cohort of Italian women with intrahepatic cholestasis of pregnancy. Dig Liver Dis 2008;40(5):366–70.
46. Mullenbach R, Bennett A, Tetlow N, et al. ATP8B1 mutations in British cases with intrahepatic cholestasis of pregnancy. Gut 2005;54(6):829–34.
47. Oude Elferink RP, Paulusma CC. Function and pathophysiological importance of ABCB4 (MDR3 P-glycoprotein). Pflugers Arch 2007;453(5):601–10.
48. Day C, Hewins P, Sheikh L, et al. Cholestasis in pregnancy associated with ciclosporin therapy in renal transplant recipients. Transpl Int 2006;19(12): 1026–9.
49. Dann AT, Kenyon AP, Seed PT, et al. Glutathione S-transferase and liver function in intrahepatic cholestasis of pregnancy and pruritus gravidarum. Hepatology 2004;40(6):1406–14.
50. Reyes H, Baez ME, Gonzalez MC, et al. Selenium, zinc and copper plasma levels in intrahepatic cholestasis of pregnancy, in normal pregnancies and in healthy individuals, in Chile. J Hepatol 2000;32(4):542–9.

51. Glantz A, Marschall HU, Lammert F, et al. Intrahepatic cholestasis of pregnancy: a randomized controlled trial comparing dexamethasone and ursodeoxycholic acid. Hepatology 2005;42(6):1399–405.
52. Knox TA, Olans LB. Liver disease in pregnancy. N Engl J Med 1996;335(8): 569–76.
53. Rolfes DB, Ishak KG. Liver disease in pregnancy. Histopathology 1986;10(6): 555–70.
54. Mazzella G, Rizzo N, Azzaroli F, et al. Ursodeoxycholic acid administration in patients with cholestasis of pregnancy: effects on primary bile acids in babies and mothers. Hepatology 2001;33(3):504–8.
55. Zapata R, Sandoval L, Palma J, et al. Ursodeoxycholic acid in the treatment of intrahepatic cholestasis of pregnancy. A 12-year experience. Liver Int 2005; 25(3):548–54.
56. Kondrackiene J, Beuers U, Kupcinskas L. Efficacy and safety of ursodeoxycholic acid versus cholestyramine in intrahepatic cholestasis of pregnancy. Gastroenterology 2005;129(3):894–901.
57. Roncaglia N, Locatelli A, Arreghini A, et al. A randomised controlled trial of ursodeoxycholic acid and S-adenosyl-l-methionine in the treatment of gestational cholestasis. BJOG 2004;111(1):17–21.
58. Barton JR, Sibai BM. Gastrointestinal complications of pre-eclampsia. Semin Perinatol 2009;33(3):179–88.
59. Sibai B, Dekker G, Kupferminc M. Pre-eclampsia. Lancet 2005;365(9461):785–99.
60. Lindheimer MD, Taler SJ, Cunningham FG. Hypertension in pregnancy. J Am Soc Hypertens 2008;2(6):484–94.
61. Pritchard JA, Weisman R Jr, Ratnoff OD, et al. Intravascular hemolysis, thrombocytopenia and other hematologic abnormalities associated with severe toxemia of pregnancy. N Engl J Med 1954;250(3):89–98.
62. Weinstein L. Syndrome of hemolysis, elevated liver enzymes, and low platelet count: a severe consequence of hypertension in pregnancy. Am J Obstet Gynecol 1982;142(2):159–67.
63. Barton JR, Sibai BM. Diagnosis and management of hemolysis, elevated liver enzymes, and low platelets syndrome. Clin Perinatol 2004;31(4):807–33, vii.
64. Baxter JK, Weinstein L. HELLP syndrome: the state of the art. Obstet Gynecol Surv 2004;59(12):838–45.
65. Sibai BM, Ramadan MK, Usta I, et al. Maternal morbidity and mortality in 442 pregnancies with hemolysis, elevated liver enzymes, and low platelets (HELLP syndrome). Am J Obstet Gynecol 1993;169(4):1000–6.
66. Egerman RS, Sibai BM. HELLP syndrome. Clin Obstet Gynecol 1999;42(2): 381–9.
67. Benjaminov FS, Heathcote J. Liver disease in pregnancy. Am J Gastroenterol 2004;99(12):2479–88.
68. Martin JN Jr, Rose CH, Briery CM. Understanding and managing HELLP syndrome: the integral role of aggressive glucocorticoids for mother and child. Am J Obstet Gynecol 2006;195(4):914–34.
69. Mihu D, Costin N, Mihu CM, et al. HELLP syndrome–a multisystemic disorder. J Gastrointestin Liver Dis 2007;16(4):419–24.
70. Shames BD, Fernandez LA, Sollinger HW, et al. Liver transplantation for HELLP syndrome. Liver Transpl 2005;11(2):224–8.
71. van Runnard Heimel PJ, Franx A, Schobben AF, et al. Corticosteroids, pregnancy, and HELLP syndrome: a review. Obstet Gynecol Surv 2005;60(1): 57–70 [quiz: 73–4].

72. Sibai BM. Diagnosis, controversies, and management of the syndrome of hemolysis, elevated liver enzymes, and low platelet count. Obstet Gynecol 2004; 103(5 Pt 1):981–91.
73. Zarrinpar A, Farmer DG, Ghobrial RM, et al. Liver transplantation for HELLP syndrome. Am Surg 2007;73(10):1013–6.
74. Sibai BM, Ramadan MK, Chari RS, et al. Pregnancies complicated by HELLP syndrome (hemolysis, elevated liver enzymes, and low platelets): subsequent pregnancy outcome and long-term prognosis. Am J Obstet Gynecol 1995; 172(1 Pt 1):125–9.
75. Bacq Y, Riely CA. Acute fatty liver of pregnancy: the hepatologist's view. Gastroenterologist 1993;1(4):257–64.
76. Fesenmeier MF, Coppage KH, Lambers DS, et al. Acute fatty liver of pregnancy in 3 tertiary care centers. Am J Obstet Gynecol 2005;192(5):1416–9.
77. Browning MF, Levy HL, Wilkins-Haug LE, et al. Fetal fatty acid oxidation defects and maternal liver disease in pregnancy. Obstet Gynecol 2006;107(1):115–20.
78. Reyes H, Sandoval L, Wainstein A, et al. Acute fatty liver of pregnancy: a clinical study of 12 episodes in 11 patients. Gut 1994;35(1):101–6.
79. Knight M, Nelson-Piercy C, Kurinczuk JJ, et al. A prospective national study of acute fatty liver of pregnancy in the UK. Gut 2008;57(7):951–6.
80. Schoeman MN, Batey RG, Wilcken B. Recurrent acute fatty liver of pregnancy associated with a fatty-acid oxidation defect in the offspring. Gastroenterology 1991;100(2):544–8.
81. Treem WR, Rinaldo P, Hale DE, et al. Acute fatty liver of pregnancy and long-chain 3-hydroxyacyl-coenzyme A dehydrogenase deficiency. Hepatology 1994;19(2):339–45.
82. Wilcken B, Leung KC, Hammond J, et al. Pregnancy and fetal long-chain 3-hydroxyacyl coenzyme A dehydrogenase deficiency. Lancet 1993;341(8842): 407–8.
83. Treem WR, Shoup ME, Hale DE, et al. Acute fatty liver of pregnancy, hemolysis, elevated liver enzymes, and low platelets syndrome, and long chain 3-hydroxyacyl-coenzyme A dehydrogenase deficiency. Am J Gastroenterol 1996; 91(11):2293–300.
84. Yang Z, Zhao Y, Bennett MJ, et al. Fetal genotypes and pregnancy outcomes in 35 families with mitochondrial trifunctional protein mutations. Am J Obstet Gynecol 2002;187(3):715–20.
85. Ibdah JA, Bennett MJ, Rinaldo P, et al. A fetal fatty-acid oxidation disorder as a cause of liver disease in pregnant women. N Engl J Med 1999;340(22): 1723–31.
86. Visconti M, Manes G, Giannattasio F, et al. Recurrence of acute fatty liver of pregnancy. J Clin Gastroenterol 1995;21(3):243–5.
87. MacLean MA, Cameron AD, Cumming GP, et al. Recurrence of acute fatty liver of pregnancy. Br J Obstet Gynaecol 1994;101(5):453–4.
88. Goldstein ST, Zhou F, Hadler SC, et al. A mathematical model to estimate global hepatitis B disease burden and vaccination impact. Int J Epidemiol 2005;34(6): 1329–39.
89. Castro MA, Fassett MJ, Reynolds TB, et al. Reversible peripartum liver failure: a new perspective on the diagnosis, treatment, and cause of acute fatty liver of pregnancy, based on 28 consecutive cases. Am J Obstet Gynecol 1999; 181(2):389–95.
90. Ibdah JA. Acute fatty liver of pregnancy: an update on pathogenesis and clinical implications. World J Gastroenterol 2006;12(46):7397–404.

91. McMahon BJ, Alward WL, Hall DB, et al. Acute hepatitis B virus infection: relation of age to the clinical expression of disease and subsequent development of the carrier state. J Infect Dis 1985;151(4):599–603.
92. Xu DZ, Yan YP, Choi BC, et al. Risk factors and mechanism of transplacental transmission of hepatitis B virus: a case-control study. J Med Virol 2002;67(1):20–6.
93. Alter MJ. Epidemiology of hepatitis B in Europe and worldwide. J Hepatol 2003;39(Suppl 1):S64–9.
94. Burk RD, Hwang LY, Ho GY, et al. Outcome of perinatal hepatitis B virus exposure is dependent on maternal virus load. J Infect Dis 1994;170(6):1418–23.
95. Noto H, Terao T, Ryou S, et al. Combined passive and active immunoprophylaxis for preventing perinatal transmission of the hepatitis B virus carrier state in Shizuoka, Japan during 1980-1994. J Gastroenterol Hepatol 2003;18(8):943–9.
96. Han GR, Cao MK, Zhao W, et al. A prospective and open-label study for the efficacy and safety of telbivudine in pregnancy for the prevention of perinatal transmission of hepatitis B virus infection. J Hepatol 2011;55(6):1215–21.
97. Shi Z, Yang Y, Ma L, et al. Lamivudine in late pregnancy to interrupt in utero transmission of hepatitis B virus: a systematic review and meta-analysis. Obstet Gynecol 2010;116(1):147–59.
98. Gartner LM, Morton J, Lawrence RA, et al. Breastfeeding and the use of human milk. Pediatrics 2005;115(2):496–506.
99. Englert Y, Lesage B, Van Vooren JP, et al. Medically assisted reproduction in the presence of chronic viral diseases. Hum Reprod Update 2004;10(2):149–62.
100. Alter MJ, Kruszon-Moran D, Nainan OV, et al. The prevalence of hepatitis C virus infection in the United States, 1988 through 1994. N Engl J Med 1999;341(8):556–62.
101. Costa ZB, Machado GC, Avelino MM, et al. Prevalence and risk factors for Hepatitis C and HIV-1 infections among pregnant women in Central Brazil. BMC Infect Dis 2009;9:116.
102. Schwimmer JB, Balistreri WF. Transmission, natural history, and treatment of hepatitis C virus infection in the pediatric population. Semin Liver Dis 2000;20(1):37–46.
103. Conte D, Fraquelli M, Prati D, et al. Prevalence and clinical course of chronic hepatitis C virus (HCV) infection and rate of HCV vertical transmission in a cohort of 15,250 pregnant women. Hepatology 2000;31(3):751–5.
104. Mast EE, Hwang LY, Seto DS, et al. Risk factors for perinatal transmission of hepatitis C virus (HCV) and the natural history of HCV infection acquired in infancy. J Infect Dis 2005;192(11):1880–9.
105. Pergam SA, Wang CC, Gardella CM, et al. Pregnancy complications associated with hepatitis C: data from a 2003-2005 Washington state birth cohort. Am J Obstet Gynecol 2008;199(1):38.e1–9.
106. Ghamar Chehreh ME, Tabatabaei SV, Khazanehdari S, et al. Effect of cesarean section on the risk of perinatal transmission of hepatitis C virus from HCV-RNA+/HIV- mothers: a meta-analysis. Arch Gynecol Obstet 2011;283(2):255–60.
107. Recommendations for prevention and control of hepatitis C virus (HCV) infection and HCV-related chronic disease. Centers for Disease Control and Prevention. MMWR Recomm Rep 1998;47(RR-19):1–39.
108. Aggarwal N, Sawnhey H, Suril V, et al. Pregnancy and cirrhosis of the liver. Aust N Z J Obstet Gynaecol 1999;39(4):503–6.
109. Russell MA, Craigo SD. Cirrhosis and portal hypertension in pregnancy. Semin Perinatol 1998;22(2):156–65.
110. Steven MM. Pregnancy and liver disease. Gut 1981;22(7):592–614.

111. Steven MM, Mackay IR. Prognosis of pregnancy in chronic liver disease. Gastroenterology 1980;78(5 Pt 1):1116–7.
112. Mahadevan U. Fertility and pregnancy in the patient with inflammatory bowel disease. Gut 2006;55(8):1198–206.
113. Candia L, Marquez J, Espinoza LR. Autoimmune hepatitis and pregnancy: a rheumatologist's dilemma. Semin Arthritis Rheum 2005;35(1):49–56.
114. Heneghan MA, Norris SM, O'Grady JG, et al. Management and outcome of pregnancy in autoimmune hepatitis. Gut 2001;48(1):97–102.
115. Schramm C, Herkel J, Beuers U, et al. Pregnancy in autoimmune hepatitis: outcome and risk factors. Am J Gastroenterol 2006;101(3):556–60.
116. Manns MP, Czaja AJ, Gorham JD, et al. Diagnosis and management of autoimmune hepatitis. Hepatology 2010;51(6):2193–213.
117. Gossard AA, Lindor KD. Pregnancy in a patient with primary sclerosing cholangitis. J Clin Gastroenterol 2002;35(4):353–5.
118. Poupon R, Chretien Y, Chazouilleres O, et al. Pregnancy in women with ursodeoxycholic acid-treated primary biliary cirrhosis. J Hepatol 2005;42(3):418–9.
119. Lindor KD, Gershwin ME, Poupon R, et al. Primary biliary cirrhosis. Hepatology 2009;50(1):291–308.
120. Wellge BE, Sterneck M, Teufel A, et al. Pregnancy in primary sclerosing cholangitis. Gut 2011;60(8):1117–21.
121. Compston A. Progressive lenticular degeneration: a familial nervous disease associated with cirrhosis of the liver, by S. A. Kinnier Wilson, (From the National Hospital, and the Laboratory of the National Hospital, Queen Square, London) Brain 1912:34;295–509. Brain 2009;132(Pt 8):1997–2001.
122. Brewer GJ, Yuzbasiyan-Gurkan V. Wilson disease. Medicine 1992;71(3):139–64.
123. Mak CM, Lam CW. Diagnosis of Wilson's disease: a comprehensive review. Crit Rev Clin Lab Sci 2008;45(3):263–90.
124. Brewer GJ, Johnson VD, Dick RD, et al. Treatment of Wilson's disease with zinc. XVII: treatment during pregnancy. Hepatology 2000;31(2):364–70.
125. Walshe JM. The management of pregnancy in Wilson's disease treated with trientine. QJM 1986;58(225):81–7.
126. Roberts EA, Schilsky ML. Diagnosis and treatment of Wilson disease: an update. Hepatology 2008;47(6):2089–111.
127. Fiore S, Savasi V. Treatment of viral hepatitis in pregnancy. Expert Opin Pharmacother 2009;10(17):2801–9.
128. Devarbhavi H, Kremers WK, Dierkhising R, et al. Pregnancy-associated acute liver disease and acute viral hepatitis: differentiation, course and outcome. J Hepatol 2008;49(6):930–5.
129. Clemente-Casares P, Pina S, Buti M, et al. Hepatitis E virus epidemiology in industrialized countries. Emerg Infect Dis 2003;9(4):448–54.
130. Rein DB, Stevens G, Theaker J, et al. The global burden of hepatitis E virus. Hepatology 2011. [Epub ahead of print].
131. Aggarwal R. Clinical presentation of hepatitis E. Virus Res 2011;161(1):15–22.
132. Kumar RM, Uduman S, Rana S, et al. Sero-prevalence and mother-to-infant transmission of hepatitis E virus among pregnant women in the United Arab Emirates. Eur J Obstet Gynecol Reprod Biol 2001;100(1):9–15.
133. Mateos Lindemann ML, Morales JG, Fernandez-Barredo S, et al. Fulminant hepatitis E in a woman taking oral contraceptive medication. Am J Trop Med Hyg 2010;82(1):12–5.
134. Teshale EH, Hu DJ, Holmberg SD. The two faces of hepatitis E virus. Clin Infect Dis 2010;51(3):328–34.

135. Elinav E, Ben-Dov IZ, Shapira Y, et al. Acute hepatitis A infection in pregnancy is associated with high rates of gestational complications and preterm labor. Gastroenterology 2006;130(4):1129–34.
136. Ehsanipoor RM, Major CA. Herpes simplex and HIV infections and preterm PROM. Clin Obstet Gynecol 2011;54(2):330–6.
137. Klein NA, Mabie WC, Shaver DC, et al. Herpes simplex virus hepatitis in pregnancy. Two patients successfully treated with acyclovir. Gastroenterology 1991; 100(1):239–44.
138. Ko CW, Beresford SA, Schulte SJ, et al. Incidence, natural history, and risk factors for biliary sludge and stones during pregnancy. Hepatology 2005; 41(2):359–65.
139. Mendez-Sanchez N, Chavez-Tapia NC, Uribe M. Pregnancy and gallbladder disease. Ann Hepatol 2006;5(3):227–30.
140. Khuroo MS, Datta DV. Budd-Chiari syndrome following pregnancy. Report of 16 cases, with roentgenologic, hemodynamic and histologic studies of the hepatic outflow tract. Am J Med 1980;68(1):113–21.
141. Rautou PE, Plessier A, Bernuau J, et al. Pregnancy: a risk factor for Budd-Chiari syndrome? Gut 2009;58(4):606–8.
142. Douglas NC, Shah M, Sauer MV. Fertility and reproductive disorders in female solid organ transplant recipients. Semin Perinatol 2007;31(6):332–8.
143. Walcott WO, Derick DE, Jolley JJ, et al. Successful pregnancy in a liver transplant patient. Am J Obstet Gynecol 1978;132(3):340–1.
144. Armenti VT. Pregnancy after liver transplantation. Liver Transpl 2006;12(7): 1037–9.
145. Christopher V, Al-Chalabi T, Richardson PD, et al. Pregnancy outcome after liver transplantation: a single-center experience of 71 pregnancies in 45 recipients. Liver Transpl 2006;12(7):1138–43.
146. Jain AB, Reyes J, Marcos A, et al. Pregnancy after liver transplantation with tacrolimus immunosuppression: a single center's experience update at 13 years. Transplantation 2003;76(5):827–32.
147. Kainz A, Harabacz I, Cowlrick IS, et al. Review of the course and outcome of 100 pregnancies in 84 women treated with tacrolimus. Transplantation 2000;70(12): 1718–21.

Evaluation of Liver Lesions

Alan Bonder, MD, Nezam Afdhal, MD*

KEYWORDS

• Liver lesion • Benign lesion • Malignant lesion • Liver imaging

Focal liver lesions are defined as solid- or liquid-containing masses, foreign to the normal anatomy of the liver, that may be differentiated from normal liver by using cross-sectional imaging techniques. The causes of focal liver lesions are diverse, and may range from benign lesions with an indolent clinical course to aggressive malignant tumors. They are common findings as a result of the increasing use of cross-sectional imaging techniques in patients with nonspecific abdominal complaints.

Clinical evaluation and noninvasive radiologic imaging are critical for decision making in the management of most patients with asymptomatic liver lesions. Knowledge of the natural history of the common lesions allows for a conservative approach to lesions that are benign and an aggressive approach to those that are malignant and still localized (**Tables 1** and **2**).

CLINICAL PRESENTATION

Liver lesions are usually clinically silent and detected as unexpected or as incidental findings in patients undergoing evaluation for unrelated symptoms. Large lesions may cause pain in the abdomen or right upper quadrant secondary to stretching of the liver capsule. Compression symptoms from left-lobe lesions, such as early satiety, are extremely rare. Clinical signs may include tender hepatomegaly, fever of unknown origin, abnormal liver function tests, and, very rarely, jaundice.

The clinical circumstances, such as the patient's age, gender, use of oral contraceptives, history of chronic liver disease, and recent travel, in which a liver lesion is identified may provide clues to the cause of the lesion; however, liver masses frequently pose a diagnostic challenge for clinicians.[1]

The presence of underlying chronic liver disease, either suspected or proven by clinical and/or laboratory features, as well as the time of detection of a mass provide a different dimension to the nature and relevance of the lesion. A mass lesion seen

Financial disclosures: Alan Bonder: no financial disclosures. Nezam Afdhal: no financial disclosures.

Department of Medicine, Liver Center, Beth Israel Deaconess Medical Center, Harvard Medical School, 110 Francis street, Suite 8E, Boston, MA 02215, USA
* Corresponding author.
E-mail address: nafdhal@bidmc.harvard.edu

Clin Liver Dis 16 (2012) 271–283
doi:10.1016/j.cld.2012.03.001

Table 1 Classification of hepatic tumors	
Benign	**Malignant**
Hepatic adenoma	Hepatocellular carcinoma
Regenerative nodules	Fibrolamellar carcinoma
Nodular regenerative hyperplasia	Hepatoblastoma
Focal nodular hyperplasia	Cholangiocarcinoma
Bile duct adenoma	Cystadenocarcinoma
Biliary cystadenoma	Angiosarcoma
Hemangioma	Primary lymphoma
Angiolipoma	Metastases

in a patient with hepatitis B or C infection, particularly when associated with features of chronic liver disease, should raise the threshold for suspicion of a malignancy, such as hepatocellular carcinoma (HCC) (**Fig. 1**).

The size of the liver lesion is extremely important in guiding the evaluation. Lesions less than 1.0 cm are commonly benign incidental findings, representing cysts, hemangiomas, or biliary hamartomas.[2]

Radiologic imaging initially characterizes lesions as solid (benign or malignant tumors) or cystic (cysts, abscesses). The vascular re-enhancement of the lesion further defines the potential cause. Characteristically, tumors with arterial hypervascularization may be benign, adenomas or focal nodular hyperplasia (FNH), or malignant, such as HCC, and metastases from neuroendocrine tumors or hypernephroma.[2,3] Abdominal computed tomography (CT) with intravenous (IV) contrast and magnetic resonance imaging (MRI) with vascular (gadolinium) or ferric (ferumoxides) contrast media have replaced radionuclide tests, and often are adequate for diagnosis and decision making without the need for histologic confirmation.

SIMPLE CYSTS

Simple cysts are congenital lesions affecting 2% to 7% of the population. They can be single or multiple and consist of serous contents lined by cuboidal, biliary-type

Table 2
Clinical and radiological characteristics of common benign lesions

Characteristics	Hemangioma	Focal Nodular Hyperplasia	Adenoma
Age (y)	30–50	20–40	All ages
Gender	Female>male	Female ~ male	Female>>male
Ultrasonography	Hyperechoic	Varied	Varied
Computed tomography	Strongly enhances	Central scar	Capsule
Magnetic resonance imaging	Cerebrospinal fluid intensity	Liver intensity	Liver intensity
Angiogram	Hypervascular	Hypervascular	Hypervascular
Calcification	Yes	No	No
Rupture	Rare	No	Yes

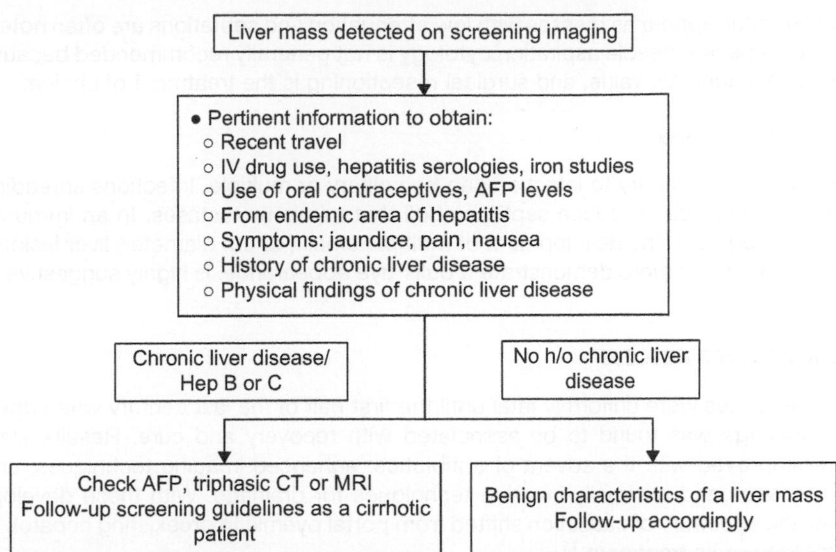

Fig. 1. Diagnostic strategy for a focal liver lesion.

epithelium with no communication with the bile ducts. Usually their size is less than 10 mm.[4,5] Simple cysts tend to occur more frequently in the right hepatic lobe and are more prevalent in women; complex cysts tend to occur more frequently in women as well. Adult-onset cysts are different from autosomal dominant polycystic liver disease, a familial disorder associated with multiple hepatic and renal cysts with or without chronic renal failure. Most simple cysts of the liver tend to be asymptomatic and are diagnosed incidentally on abdominal imaging.

Ultrasonography (US) is the most useful diagnostic test for simple cysts, which appear as anechoic fluid-filled spaces without clear walls and with posterior acoustic enhancement.[4] CT scan reveals well-demarcated water attenuation within cystic lesions that do not enhance after the administration of IV contrast.

Aspiration is not required to diagnose simple cysts, given their typical radiographic appearance. Most simple cysts do not require treatment or follow-up. The presence of symptoms or an increase in the size of the cyst should raise concern for a cystadenoma or cystadenocarcinoma[6]; such patients require surgical intervention.[7] Extremely large cysts (>7 cm) can be symptomatic, and several approaches have been taken including radiological drainage with alcohol obliteration or laparoscopic surgical de-roofing, which is the preferred modality.

CYSTADENOMA AND CYSTADENOCARCINOMA

The most commonly encountered primary cystic neoplasms of the liver are cystadenoma and cystadenocarcinoma, ranging from 2 cm to 28 cm in size and occurring at extremes of age, although they usually present in the fourth decade of life.[8] Most of them are found incidentally on abdominal imaging; however, patients may present with abdominal pain and anorexia.[9]

Cystadenomas can be differentiated from simple cysts based on the appearance on US or recurrence after surgery. Cystadenomas appear as hypoechoic lesions with irregular walls and septations, a feature not present in simple cysts.[4] On CT, cystadenomas appear as masses with low attenuation and septations are often noted. Percutaneous fine-needle aspiration cytology is not generally recommended because it has little diagnostic value, and surgical resectioning is the treatment of choice.

HEPATIC INFECTIONS

Liver masses secondary to infection can be solitary or multiple. Infections spreading hematogenously can produce septic emboli that mimic metastases. In an immunocompromised host, the development of multiple small (<2 cm diameter) liver lesions, especially if one or more demonstrate a bulls-eye appearance, is highly suggestive of candidiasis.[10]

PYOGENIC LIVER ABSCESS

Liver abscesses were uniformly fatal until the first half of the last century when operative drainage was found to be associated with recovery and cure. Results were further improved with the advent of antibiotics, enhanced imaging techniques, and percutaneous and minimally invasive techniques for drainage. With these developments, the spectrum of causation shifted from portal pyemia to preexisting hepatobiliary disease or its treatment.[11]

Pyogenic liver abscess secondary to appendicitis, diverticulitis, or other intra-abdominal infective processes has decreased dramatically because of the improvements in the treatment of the primary condition, which includes source control and early initiation of antibiotics. Nonetheless, these diagnoses may still be relevant in patients with delayed treatment or those residing in the underdeveloped countries of the world. Biliary obstruction (benign or malignant), stenting, or instrumentation is now a more common cause.[12] Hematogenous spread from other sources, such as bacterial endocarditis and IV drug abuse, are also important. Patients who are immunocompromised or diabetic are especially prone, with a 3.6-fold increased risk for developing liver abscess.[13]

Modern treatments for hepatic neoplasms with radiofrequency or microwave ablation and chemoembolization may be complicated by an abscess. Hepatic trauma, especially if associated with necrosis, intrahepatic hematoma, and bile leak, may become secondarily infected and lead to a liver abscess.[14] Vascular thrombosis complicating hepatic transplantation is a serious event, with the parenchyma becoming secondarily predisposed to infection with bacteria and fungi.[15,16]

Plain abdominal and chest radiography are usually nonspecific, unless a coexistent pleural effusion, collapse of lung, or elevation of diaphragm is present. Gas-forming organisms may cause an air/fluid level within the dilated biliary tree. Appearance on US varies according to disease stage. The abscess may be hyperechoic and indistinct; but with maturation and pus formation, it becomes hyperechoic with a distinct margin. Abscess with thick pus or multiple small lesions might be confused with solid lesions. Evaluating an abscess on the dome of the liver may have some limitations. US may highlight the pathologic condition (gallstones, ductal dilation, or solid lesions) of the biliary tract and has a sensitivity of 75% to 95%.[17]

CT is more accurate, especially with contrast enhancement. Peripheral enhancement of the abscess wall is virtually diagnostic in the appropriate clinical setting; moreover, by allowing imaging of the abdomen, the CT may also show the likely cause in approximately 70% of the cases.[18]

MRI does not seem to have any specific advantage over CT[18]; however, it may further delineate previously unsuspected lesions of the liver or intraductal pathologic condition, while investigating the biliary tract noninvasively. Liver abscesses may be single or multiple. Cryptogenic abscesses are more likely to be single (70% on the right side), whereas multiple small abscesses tend to be secondary to an underlying biliary pathologic condition or from metastatic seeding (eg, bacterial endocarditis, IV drug abuse). A lesion less than 2 cm in diameter is described as a microabscess. Multiple microabscesses have been reported as having 2 distinct imaging characteristics: the first, diffuse miliary, is associated with staphylococcal infection, and the second, cluster, which seems to coalesce, is more likely to be secondary to infections from coliform organisms.

Treatment includes empiric parenteral antibiotics and percutaneous drainage. In addition, culture of purulent material for aerobic and anaerobic organisms helps to guide the antibiotic treatment. The results of cultures and determination of antibiotic sensitivities help to further modify antibiotic therapy. Antibiotic therapy may be needed for 4 to 6 weeks. Parenteral antibiotics are recommended initially, and if a patient responds to therapy, treatment can be switched to oral antibiotics to complete the course of treatment. Although antibiotics with percutaneous drainage are the recommended course of therapy, surgical drainage is sometimes necessary and is best done with the input of a hepatobiliary surgeon. Patients with abscesses larger than 5 cm require surgical drainage, but monitoring the response to antibiotics and the patient's clinical course is very important when determining the need for emergency surgical intervention compared with percutaneous drainage.

HYDATID CYST

Hydatid cysts are caused by the zoonotic parasites, *Echinococcus granulosus* or *E multilocularis*. The lifecycle of the echinococcus parasite requires a definitive host, which is often a dog, and an intermediate host, which is commonly a sheep. Humans become accidental intermediate hosts when they get infected from dogs. The disease occurs principally in sheep-grazing areas of the world and is endemic in many Mediterranean countries, the Middle East and Far East, South America, Australia, and East Africa. The incidence in these areas depends on the level of health care and veterinary control. In the Western Hemisphere, immigrants from endemic areas have a greater incidence of hydatid diagnosis.

Small (<5 cm) cysts are usually asymptomatic and are sometimes detected incidentally. The expansion of larger cysts or the inflammatory reaction around the cyst can irritate the surrounding parietal peritoneum and cause moderate pain in the right upper quadrant. Acute pain indicates a purulent cyst or rupture. When the antigenic cyst fluid is released into circulation, it can cause an acute intense allergic manifestation. Extrusion into the biliary tree may cause jaundice, cholangitis, or, rarely, acute pancreatitis. Bronchobiliary fistula resulting from hepatobronchial fistula and ascites, or acute hepatic failure resulting from Budd-Chiari syndrome are other rare but possible complications.

The diagnosis of hydatid cyst is based on the history and likelihood of past exposure but requires imaging and serology. Parasitology of cyst contents confirms the diagnosis. Routine blood tests are usually not helpful, derangement of liver function is unusual, and eosinophilia is only seen in 25% to 40% of patients. Serologic testing for *E granulosus* includes immunoelectrophoresis, enzyme-linked immunosorbent assay, and Western blotting. The sensitivity and specificity of the various tests vary between 60% and 95%.[19] These tests may be used for diagnosis, posttreatment follow-up, and epidemiologic studies.

The World Health Organization developed a classification system based on the appearance to improve uniformity of reporting and judging the effect of different treatment modalities. Although US is the first imaging study that should be performed, CT gives more precise information on the morphology of the cyst. The cyst may have a low signal intensity rim on T2-weighted MRI, which is a characteristic sign of hydatid disease.[20]

AMEBIC LIVER ABSCESS

The protozoan *Entamoeba histolytica* is the causative organism for amebic colitis and hepatic abscess, affecting chiefly individuals living in or visiting tropical and temperate climates. As a causative agent of hepatic abscesses, *E histolytica* burrows through the intestinal mucosal barrier and enters the portal circulation, eventually forming an abscess in the liver. Direct extension or lymphatic spread is not believed to occur. Hepatic involvement is typically silent, and parenchymal necrosis ensues, resulting in the typical anchovy sauce appearance. The lesions are single, large, and loculated.[21]

This disease affects young men, and symptoms last approximately 10 days. Travelers from nonendemic areas may develop the disease between 2 and 5 months after becoming infected.[22] Usually, abrupt abdominal pain and fever occurs. Active colitis and liver abscess occur rarely together. Occasionally, diarrhea may be present. Complications may include secondary bacterial infection, rupture into the peritoneal or thoracic cavity, and pericardial involvement.

Laboratory investigations show leukocytosis without eosinophilia. Liver function tests show moderate increases in alkaline phosphatase, and the prothrombin time is typically elevated. Affected individuals will almost always have positive serum anti-amebic antibodies, which can be confirmed with various serologic tests (eg, indirect hemagglutination). US has a diagnostic accuracy of 90%. CT may not add to the diagnostic accuracy but delineates the morphologic characteristics.[21] The treatment of uncomplicated abscess includes metronidazole, emetine hydrochloride, chloroquine phosphate, or diloxanide furoate. Patients with inconclusive serology, pregnancy, failure of symptom resolution, and imminent rupture should be considered for percutaneous aspiration and drainage if aspiration alone is unsuccessful.

BENIGN SOLID LESIONS

Hemangioma

Most hemangiomas are small and asymptomatic, detected as an incidental mass on abdominal imaging.[23] Hepatic hemangiomas are the most common benign tumors in the liver.[23] Large autopsy series have reported an incidence of 0.35% to 7%. A recent carefully performed autopsy study described an incidence of cavernous hemangiomas in 20% of adult men.[1] Some may present with pain or fullness in the right upper quadrant. Other symptoms include nausea, vomiting, and early satiety, which may result from compression of adjacent organs. Pain may be secondary to infarction, hemorrhage, and torsion or distention of the Glisson capsule.

Large or cavernous hemangiomas represent a separate entity and are usually initially diagnosed by US, in which it appears as a hyperechoic mass that is homogenous with well-defined margins and posterior enhancement.[24] Nelson and Chezmar[25] reviewed the literature and concluded that only a small number of hemangiomas meet all these criteria. For instance, approximately 67% to 70% of hemangiomas are hyperechoic, 58% to 73% are homogenous, 77% to 92% are well defined, and only 37% demonstrate obvious posterior acoustical enhancement whereas 40% demonstrate slight enhancement. Using these data, then 70% of hemangiomas are hyperechoic, 51% are hyperechoic and homogenous, 47% hyperechoic, homogenous, and well defined, and only 36% meet all the classic criteria with any degree of acoustic enhancement.[26] Detection of obvious enhancement limits the number to 17% of hemangiomas. In additon the fact that metastatic lesions are also frequently hyperechoic makes the diagnosis of these atypical hemangioma more complex.[27]

The first choice of imaging for abdominal pain is abdominal US, in which hemangiomas are usually shown as well-defined, homogenous hyperechoic lesions. However, different variations of the usual images are seen in large lesions because of thrombosis, fibrosis, hemorrhage, or calcifications, resulting in a heterogeneous or sometimes hypoechoic appearance. Intralesional features, such as thrombosis, fibrosis, hemorrhage, or calcifications, could be responsible for certain giant hemangiomas lacking centripetal enhancement on CT.

On non–contrast-enhanced CT, liver hemangiomas are well-defined, homogenous hypodense lesions, compared with surrounding liver parenchyma. After injecting IV contrast, a characteristic peripheral nodular enhancement occurs during the arterial phase with subsequent progressive centripetal enhancement on portal venous phase images. The density of enhancement is the same as contrast in blood vessels. On delayed phase images, hemangiomas appear isodense or hyperdense compared with liver parenchyma. The standard approach to hemangiomas that have a nonclassical appearance on US is to move to either CT scan with IV contrast or MRI with gadolinium. The use of tagged red cell scans has fallen out of major clinical practice and is reserved for rare cases in whom MRI or CT fail to make the diagnosis.

Most hepatic hemangiomas remain stable over time and require no treatment. Treatment or follow-up is not indicated for asymptomatic lesions that are less than 5 cm in diameter. Symptomatic and rapidly enlarging hemangiomas, as well as those that are less than15 cm in diameter at initial presentation may need resection.

Focal Fatty Liver and Fatty Sparing

Focal fat in the liver produces an area of low density on CT that can be mistaken for malignant liver lesion. Focal fatty liver has 2 distinctive features. First, focal fatty liver is never spherical in shape. Second, focal fatty liver does not produce a mass effect. Mass effect can be detected on CT either as a bulge in the liver contour if the process is subcapsular, or within the liver parenchyma as a displacement of vessels. However, case reports have demonstrated cases of focal fatty liver with multiple rounded-appearing lesions.[28,29] Therefore, definitive diagnosis of focal fatty liver may require a second imaging test such as MRI with MR spectroscopy, which is diagnostic for both hepatic fat and fatty sparing.

FNH

FNH is the second most common benign solid tumor of the liver, with an estimated prevalence of 2.5% to 8%,[30] which is thought to represent a hyperplastic response of hepatic parenchyma to hyperperfusion by vascular malformations in the liver. In 1985, Wanless and collaborators[31] proposed that FNH is a hyperplastic response of the hepatic parenchyma to a preexisting local arterial spiderlike malformation, likely with a developmental origin. FNH more frequently develops in women (M/F = 1/8) aged between 20 and 50 years. An increased risk linked to oral contraceptive use is still under debate; however, some studies suggest that use of contraceptive pills may increase the size of the nodules.

FNH can be single and multiple and comprises normal hepatocytes arranged in 1- to 2-cell thick plates. Bile ductules are usually found at the interface between hepatocytes and fibrous regions. Increased arterial flow is thought to hyperperfuse the local parenchyma, leading to secondary hepatocellular hyperplasia. FNH is therefore considered the result of a hyperplastic response to increased blood flow, and, accordingly, FNH usually does not bleed or undergo malignant transformation, justifying therapeutic abstention.

Radiological features are characteristic in FNH with the dominant feature being the presence of a central scar. CT scan reveals a hypodense or isodense lesion that homogeneously enhances during the arterial phase of contrast injection. On MRI, the central scar typically presents with high signal intensity on T2-weighted images because of its vascularity.[32–35]

The usual course of FNH is benign and the incidence of complications is low. Lesions generally do not enlarge over time; there is no evidence of malignant transformation. Patients diagnosed with FNH should be managed conservatively; surgery is reserved for the rare, very large (>7 cm), symptomatic FNH lesion and for those in whom the diagnosis is uncertain, despite multiple imaging modalities.

Hepatic Adenoma

In occidental countries, hepatic adenomas (HCAs) are rare tumors that usually develop in women who use oral contraceptives. The relationship between oral contraception and HCA occurrence has been suggested by Baum and collaborators[36] in 1973 and was subsequently confirmed in several case-control studies.[37–39] HCA occurrence may also be related to the use of androgenic-anabolic steroids and glycogen-storage diseases type I and III.[40] HCA is a benign proliferation of hepatocytes in an otherwise normal liver. The HCA nodule, rarely encapsulated, varies from 0.5 to 15 cm in diameter with arterial vascularization. Proliferating hepatocytes usually resemble normal cells that may be steatotic or show glycogen storage. The tumor is also characterized by the lack of frequent mitosis, portal tract, and cholangiolar proliferation. HCA nodules are generally solitary, but 2 or 3 nodules occasionally develop simultaneously. The development of more than 10 HCA nodules is rare and has been specifically defined as adenomatosis by Flejou and collaborators[41] in 1985. HCA development was described to be less significantly related to oral contraception and with women; however, adenomatosis is also described more frequently in women and is also frequently associated with diabetes.

HCA may remain stable, increase in size, or regress. Regression is more frequently described in HCA related to androgenic-anabolic steroids and glycogenosis after hormone withdrawal. HCA occasionally bleeds and this risk increases with the nodule's size more than 7 cm. Malignant transformation in HCC is considered to be extremely rare but has been consistently described. The risk of malignant transformation seems to be more critical in HCA related to androgenic-anabolic steroid exposure or glycogenosis type I.[42,43]

Small lesions (<5 cm) can be managed conservatively by repeated periodic imaging as well as by discontinuing oral contraceptives and steroids. In adenomas that enlarge despite discontinuation of estrogens, as well as those that are symptomatic, therapy should be considered. Surgical options include enucleation, resection, and, rarely, liver transplantation (in the case of glycogen-storage disease or multiple adenomas). Patients are generally advised against pregnancy before resection of adenomas because of the reported increase in size as well as the risk of hemorrhage and rupture. Mortality from elective resection of hepatic adenomas is less than 1%; however, it may increase to 5% to 8% in emergency resection of bleeding or ruptured lesions.[44]

Some typical radiological characteristics have been described: well-demarcated, isointense lesions with peripheral enhancement on CT scan and as hyperintense lesions on T1-weighted MRI because of the presence of glycogen or fat; however, the diagnosis depends on the associated clinical features of female gender, young age, and oral contraceptive use.[3,45]

Differentiation between FNH and adenoma is one of the most difficult diagnostic issues when evaluating liver masses because the demographics and clinical features are very similar. MRI with the newer contrast agents, such as BOPTA, is now the recommended imaging technique replacing technetium sulfur colloid scans.

Nodular Regenerative Hyperplasia

Nodular regenerative hyperplasia (NRH) is a benign proliferative process in which normal hepatic parenchyma is replaced by diffuse regenerative nodules of hepatocytes with minimal associated fibrosis. The prevalence of NRH per autopsy studies is approximately 2%.[46] There is no gender predilection and although NRH mainly affects patients older than 60, cases have been reported in children as well. The nodules vary in size from 1 mm to 1 cm. NRH is associated with lymphoproliferative disorders (through thrombophilia secondary to malignancy, direct invasion of tumor, or chemotherapy), rheumatoid arthritis, primary biliary cirrhosis, bone marrow transplantation, hereditary hemorrhagic telangiectasia, polyarteritis nodosa, Budd-Chiari syndrome, liver transplantation (possibly secondary to postoperative hepatic vascular alterations or the use of azathioprine), amyloidosis, Felty syndrome, and HCC.

Most patients with NRH are asymptomatic; however, patients may present with stigmata of portal hypertension. Most patients with NRH have normal hepatic biochemical tests, although 10% to 25% of patients may have mild elevations, particularly in alkaline phosphatase.[47] Hepatic synthetic function is usually preserved, and fulminant liver failure is rare.

NRH progress slowly and the prognosis reflects the development and progression of portal hypertension. Patients with portal hypertension associated with NRH have a 5-year survival of 90% and 30-year survival of 55%.[48] NRH is not thought to be a premalignant condition, and the association between HCC and NRH is unclear. Treatment of NRH is directed at treating the underlying medical condition and preventing complications of portal hypertension.

HCC

HCC is the fifth most common tumor in the world, and its incidence is expected to increase in the future because of the anticipated increase in cirrhosis secondary to viral hepatitis.[49] The diagnosis of HCC is no longer based on biopsy, especially in patients in whom curative treatment is possible (**Fig. 2**).[50] Approximately 30% of patients are candidates for curative treatments including liver transplantation, liver resection, and percutaneous interventions with a 5-year survival rate between 40% and 75%.[51] Treatment depends on early diagnosis by screening high-risk patients when HCC is small (<5 cm) and remains localized to the liver. The standard screening for HCC includes the monitoring of alpha-fetoprotein level and US.[52] However, the sensitivity of US for HCC detection is low because small nodules can be missed in a cirrhotic liver. CT and MRI have a high sensitivity (55%–91%) and specificity (77%–96%) in diagnosing HCC.[53] Another modality used outside of the United States is contrast-enhanced (bubble) US. According to the European Association for the Study of the Liver (EASL) and the American Association for the Study of Liver Diseases (AASLD), a nodule larger than 2 cm that displays a typical vascular pattern on contrast-enhanced CT or contrast-enhanced MRI can be considered HCC without biopsy. For nodules measuring between 1 and 2 cm, the diagnosis of HCC without biopsy requires a confirmation of the typical vascular pattern on both the imaging modalities. In comparison with EASL and AASLD criteria, the consensus statement from the Asian Oncology Summit from 2009 recommends that for any nodule, regardless of size,

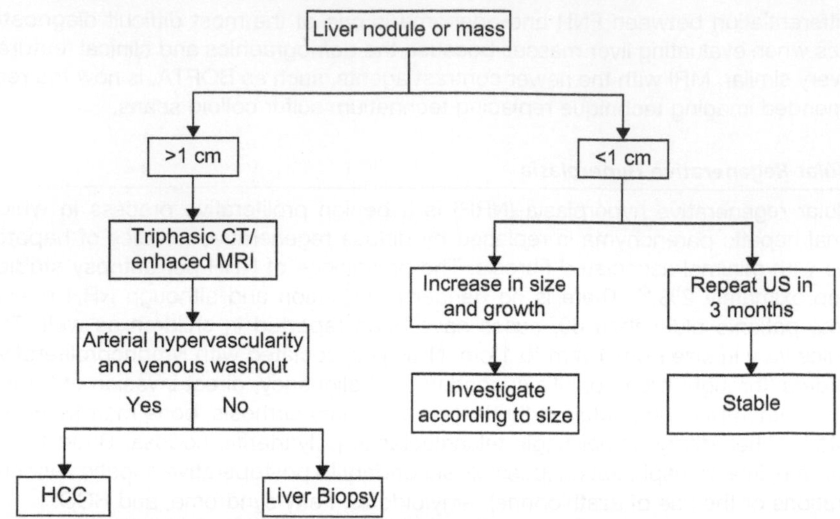

Fig. 2. Diagnostic algorithm for a suspected HCC.

the characteristic features on contrast-enhanced CT or contrast-enhanced MRI is sufficient for diagnosis of HCC, and obviates the need for biopsy.

The imaging criteria used in these recommendations are based exclusively on the vascular findings of HCC after the administration of extracellular contrast agents. A typical enhancement is defined as an early arterial uptake followed by washout in the portovenous or late equilibrium phase. Moreover, the evaluation of the morphologic appearance on unenhanced images together with the evaluation of the vascular features on dynamic contrast-enhanced images enables the radiologist to provide additional information regarding the biomolecular angiogenic activities in HCCs.

SUMMARY

The differential diagnosis of a liver mass is large and requires understanding of the clinical and imaging features of liver lesions. A detailed history, physical examination, hepatic biochemical tests, and imaging studies are all essential in making the diagnosis. Decisions regarding specific imaging modalities for diagnoses, the use of liver biopsy, therapeutic options, and appropriate follow-up are all determined by the presentation of the lesion and associated patient characteristics.

REFERENCES

1. Reddy KR, Kligerman S, Levi J, et al. Benign and solid tumors of the liver: relationship to sex, age, size of tumors, and outcome. Am Surg 2001;67:173–8.
2. Coenegrachts K. Magnetic resonance imaging of the liver: new imaging strategies for evaluating focal liver lesions. World J Radiol 2009;1(1):72–85.
3. Paulson EK, McClellan JS, Washington K, et al. Hepatic adenoma: MR characteristics and correlation with pathologic findings. AJR Am J Roentgenol 1994; 163:113.
4. Spiegel RM, King DL, Green WM. Ultrasonography of primary cysts of the liver. AJR Am J Roentgenol 1978;131:235.

5. Benhamou JP, Menu Y. Non-parasitic cystic diseases of the liver and intrahepatic biliary tree. In: Blumgart LH, editor. Surgery of the liver and biliary tract. 2nd edition. New York: Churchill Livingstone Inc; 1994. p. 1197.
6. Burch JC, Jones HE. Large nonparasitic cyst of the liver simulating an ovarian cyst. Am J Obstet Gynecol 1952;63:441.
7. Taylor BR, Langer B. Current surgical management of hepatic cyst disease. Adv Surg 1997;31:127.
8. Ishak KG, Willis GW, Cummins SD, et al. Biliary cystadenoma and cystadenocarcinoma: report of 14 cases and review of the literature. Cancer 1977;39:322.
9. Gadzijev E, Dragan S, Verica FM, et al. Hepatobiliary cystadenoma protruding into the common bile duct, mimicking complicated hydatid cyst of the liver. Report of a case. Hepatogastroenterology 1995;42:1008.
10. Doyle DJ, Hanbidge AE, O'Malley ME. Imaging of hepatic infections. Clin Radiol 2006;61(9):737–48.
11. Johannsen EC, Sifri CD, Madoff LC. Pyogenic liver abscesses. Infect Dis Clin North Am 2000;14:547–63.
12. Wong WM, Wong BC, Hui CK, et al. Pyogenic liver abscess: retrospective analysis of 80 cases over a 10-year period. J Gastroenterol Hepatol 2002;17:1001–7.
13. Lee KT, Wong SR, Sheen PC. Pyogenic liver abscess: an audit of 10 years' experience and analysis of risk factors. Dig Surg 2001;18:459–65.
14. Pang TC, Fung T, Samra J, et al. Pyogenic liver abscess: an audit of 10 years' experience. World J Gastroenterol 2011;17(12):1622–30.
15. Steinbrück K, Enne M, Fernandes R, et al. Vascular complications after living donor liver transplantation: a Brazilian, single-center experience. Transplant Proc 2011; 43(1):196–8.
16. Nikeghbalian S, Salahi R, Salahi H, et al. Hepatic abscesses after liver transplant: 1997-2008. Exp Clin Transplant 2009;7(4):256–60.
17. K C S, Sharma D. Long-term follow-up of pyogenic liver abscess by ultrasound. Eur J Radiol 2010;74(1):195–8.
18. Alsaif HS, Venkatesh SK, Chan DS, et al. CT appearance of pyogenic liver abscesses caused by *Klebsiella pneumoniae*. Radiology 2011;260(1):129–38.
19. Schweiger A, Grimm F, Tanner I, et al. Serological diagnosis of echinococcosis: the diagnostic potential of native antigens. Infection 2011. [Epub ahead of print].
20. Richter J, Hatz C, Häussinger D. Ultrasound in tropical and parasitic diseases. Lancet 2003;362(9387):900–2.
21. Huch Böni RA, Peter J, Marincek B. Amebic abscess of the liver manifested by "hemoptysis": US, CT, and MRI findings. Abdom Imaging 1995;20(3):214–6.
22. Congly SE, Shaheen AA, Meddings L, et al. Amoebic liver abscess in USA: a population-based study of incidence, temporal trends and mortality. Liver Int 2011; 31(8):1191–8.
23. Karhunen PJ. Benign hepatic tumours and tumour like conditions in men. J Clin Pathol 1986;39:183.
24. Gandolfi L, Leo P, Solmi L, et al. Natural history of hepatic haemangiomas: clinical and ultrasound study. Gut 1991;32:677.
25. Nelson RC, Chezmar JL. Diagnostic approach to hepatic hemangiomas. Radiology 1990;176:11–3.
26. Caseiro-Alves F, Brito J, Araujo AE, et al. Liver haemangioma: common and uncommon findings and how to improve the differential diagnosis. Eur Radiol 2007;17(6):1544–54.
27. Alturkistany S, Jang HJ, Yu H, et al. Fading hepatic hemangiomas on multiphasic CT. Abdom Imaging 2011. [Epub ahead of print].

28. Gariballa SE, Woods DJ, Davidson AR. Case report: focal fatty liver infiltration causing mass effect. Clin Radiol 1997;52(8):630–2.
29. Verhille R, Marchal G, Baert AL, et al. Focal fatty infiltration of the liver associated with important mass effect. J Belge Radiol 1994;77(1):10–2.
30. Craig J, Peters R, Edmundson H. Tumors of the liver and intrahepatic bile ducts, Fasc 26. 2nd edition. Washington DC: Washington, DC Armed Forces Institute of Pathology; 1989. p. 6.
31. Wanless IR, Mawdsley C, Adams R. On the pathogenesis of focal nodular hyperplasia of the liver. Hepatology 1985;5:1194.
32. Cherqui D, Rahmouni A, Charlotte F, et al. Management of focal nodular hyperplasia and hepatocellular adenoma in young women: a series of 41 patients with clinical, radiological, and pathological correlations. Hepatology 1995;22:1674.
33. Carlson SK, Johnson CD, Bender CE, et al. CT of focal nodular hyperplasia of the liver. AJR Am J Roentgenol 2000;174:705.
34. Mattison GR, Glazer GM, Quint LE, et al. MR imaging of hepatic focal nodular hyperplasia: characterization and distinction from primary malignant hepatic tumors. AJR Am J Roentgenol 1987;148:711.
35. Grazioli L, Morana G, Kirchin MA, et al. Accurate differentiation of focal nodular hyperplasia from hepatic adenoma at gadobenate dimeglumine enhanced MR imaging: prospective study. Radiology 2005;236:166–77.
36. Baum JK, Bookstein JJ, Holtz F, et al. Possible association between benign hepatomas and oral contraceptives. Lancet 1973;2(7835):926–9.
37. Sherlock S. Hepatic adenomas and oral contraceptives. Gut 1975;16:753.
38. Klatskin G. Hepatic tumors: possible relationship to use of oral contraceptives. Gastroenterology 1977;73:386.
39. Rooks JB, Ory HW, Ishak KG, et al. Epidemiology of hepatocellular adenoma. The role of oral contraceptive use. JAMA 1979;242:644.
40. Labrune P, Trioche P, Duvaltier I, et al. Hepatocellular adenomas in glycogen storage disease type I and III: a series of 43 patients and review of the literature. J Pediatr Gastroenterol Nutr 1997;24:276.
41. Flejou JF, Barge J, Menu Y, et al. Liver adenomatosis. An entity distinct from liver adenoma? Gastroenterology 1985;89(5):1132–8.
42. Foster JH, Berman MM. The malignant transformation of liver cell adenomas. Arch Surg 1994;129:712.
43. Zucman-Rossi J, Jeannot E, Nhieu JT, et al. Genotype-phenotype correlation in hepatocellular adenoma: new classification and relationship with HCC. Hepatology 2006;43:515–24.
44. Krasinskas AM, Eghtesad B, Kamath PS, et al. Liver transplantation for severe intrahepatic noncirrhotic portal hypertension. Liver Transpl 2005;11:627.
45. Grazioli L, Federle MP, Brancatelli G, et al. Hepatic adenomas: imaging and pathologic findings. Radiographics 2001;21:877.
46. Reshamwala PA, Kleiner DE, Heller T. Nodular regenerative hyperplasia: not all nodules are created equal. Hepatology 2006;44:7.
47. Al-Mukhaizeem KA, Rosenberg A, Sherker AH. Nodular regenerative hyperplasia of the liver: an under-recognized cause of portal hypertension in hematological disorders. Am J Hematol 2004;75:225–30.
48. Faust D, Fellbaum C, Zeuzem S, et al. Nodular regenerative hyperplasia of the liver: a rare differential diagnosis of cholestasis with response to ursodeoxycholic acid. Z Gastroenterol 2003;41:255.
49. El-Serag HB, Mason AC. Rising incidence of hepatocellular carcinoma in the United States. N Engl J Med 1999;340:745–50.

50. Zhang BH, Yang BH, Tang ZY. Randomized controlled trial of screening for hepatocellular carcinoma. J Cancer Res Clin Oncol 2004;130:417–22.
51. Llovet JM, Bruix J, Gores GJ. Surgical resection versus transplantation for early hepatocellular carcinoma: clues for the best strategy. Hepatology 2000;31: 1019–21.
52. Wong LL, Limm WM, Severino R, et al. Improved survival with screening for hepatocellular carcinoma. Liver Transpl 2000;6:320–5.
53. Serste T, Barrau V, Ozenne V, et al. Accuracy and disagreement of CT and MRI for the diagnosis of small hepatocellular carcinoma and dysplastic nodules: role of biopsy. Hepatology 2011. DOI: 10.1002/hep.24746.

Ascites

Fredric D. Gordon, MD[a,b,*]

KEYWORDS

- Ascites • Cirrhosis • Spontaneous bacterial peritonitis
- Hepatorenal syndrome

Ascites is the pathologic accumulation of fluid in the peritoneum. It is the most common complication of cirrhosis, with a prevalence of approximately 10%. Over a 10-year period, 50% of patients with previously compensated cirrhosis are expected to develop ascites.[1] As a marker of hepatic decompensation, ascites is associated with a poor prognosis with only a 56% survival 3 years after onset.[2] In addition, morbidity is increased because of the risk of additional complications, such as spontaneous bacterial peritonitis (SBP) and hepatorenal syndrome. Understanding the pathophysiology of ascites is essential for the proper management of this highly symptomatic and potentially lethal complication of cirrhosis.

PATHOPHYSIOLOGY

Ascites develops in cirrhosis from the complex interaction among the endogenous vasoactive systems, portal hypertension, and renal function. The specific timeline of events and interplay among these abnormally functioning systems is not clearly understood. Nonetheless, three theories have been advanced to explain the development of ascites.

Backward Theory of Ascites Formation

The first theory to explain the development of ascites was the backward theory of ascites formation. This theory states that portal hypertension and ascites formation occur first with subsequent circulatory dysfunction and renal impairment.[3,4] Portal hypertension and hypoalbuminemia lead to increased splanchnic lymph formation. Excessive lymph production overwhelms the ability of the thoracic duct to return lymph to the heart, resulting in extravasation of fluid into the abdominal cavity. These changes impact circulatory and renal function and result in diminished plasma volume and cardiac output and increased peripheral vascular resistance.

The author has nothing to disclose.

[a] Tufts Medical School, Boston, MA, USA; [b] Lahey Clinic Medical Center, 41 Mall Road, 4 West, Burlington, MA 01805, USA
* Lahey Clinic Medical Center, 41 Mall Road, 4 West, Burlington, MA 01805.
E-mail address: Fredric_D_Gordon@lahey.org

Clin Liver Dis 16 (2012) 285–299
doi:10.1016/j.cld.2012.03.004 liver.theclinics.com

Overflow Theory of Ascites Formation

When it became clear that the plasma volume and cardiac output were, in fact, increased and vascular resistance decreased in patients with cirrhosis, the backward theory of ascites formation had to be dismissed. According to the newer overflow theory of ascites formation, the primary event was sodium retention before impairment in the circulatory function.[5] For this hypothesis to be explanatory, sodium retention had to be caused by portal hypertension.[6] These effects would result in increased plasma volume and cardiac output and decreased systemic peripheral vascular resistance, as expected. The arterial hypovolemia and further increase in portal hypertension would induce overflow ascites.[7] Later, this theory was undermined by the fact that arterial vasodilation is not systemic but rather restricted to the splanchnic circulation. Also, according to this theory, one would expect that administration of angiotensin II antagonists would improve arterial pressure and peripheral vascular resistance; however, this does not occur, suggesting that primary sodium retention is not the inciting event.[8,9]

Peripheral Arterial Vasodilation Theory

This hypothesis is the current understanding of the cause of ascites in cirrhosis. The primary abnormality is the impairment in circulatory function characterized by a reduction in systemic vascular resistance (SVR) from arterial vasodilation of the splanchnic circulation caused by portal hypertension.[10] This abnormality has been further evaluated and is attributed to the increased production and activity of vasodilator factors, including nitric oxide, carbon monoxide, and endogenous cannabinoids.[10–17]

In early advanced fibrosis, activation of vasodilatory substances is minimal and the SVR decreases only slightly as the splanchnic arterial vasodilation is compensated by an increase in cardiac output. As the degree of hepatic fibrosis progresses, portal pressure increases. In decompensated cirrhosis, the SVR drops dramatically and overcomes the heart's ability to increase the cardiac output, and underfilling of the arterial circulation develops. Stimulation of baroreceptors causes activation of the renin-angiotensin system and the sympathetic nervous system, and secretion of arginine vasopressin. Portal hypertension causes the spontaneous opening of preexisting portosystemic shunts, diverting both blood and vasodilators from the splanchnic to the systemic circulation.[18] When both portal hypertension and splanchnic arterial vasodilation coexist, capillary permeability and lymph formation in the splanchnic organs markedly increase,[19] constituting the forward theory of ascites formation. Ascites accumulates in the intraabdominal cavity when the rate of production exceeds the rate of absorption, estimated to be 1.4 L/d, ranging from 0.5 L/d to greater than 5 L/d.[20]

An additional subtheory suggests that bacterial translocation may also play a role in the circulatory dysfunction of advanced cirrhosis. Bacteria from the intestinal lumen translocate into the mesenteric lymph nodes, causing an inflammatory response leading to the production of proinflammatory cytokines, which can dilate splanchnic arterial vessels. Evidence supporting this theory includes the finding of increased levels of lipopolysaccharide binding protein or circulating levels of bacterial DNA in patients with cirrhosis.[21,22] Additionally, selective intestinal decontamination with antibiotics has been shown to improve circulatory function.[23]

HEPATORENAL SYNDROME

While attempting to preserve the effect of arterial blood volume and pressure, the body's compensatory mechanisms result in negative effects on renal function, including sodium and free water retention and a reduced glomerular filtration rate (GFR). In severe cases, this combination of findings results in hepatorenal syndrome.[10] The diagnostic criteria for hepatorenal syndrome are shown in **Box 1**. The evolution of hepatorenal syndrome has been divided into five phases.[24]

Phase 1

The first renal abnormality in cirrhosis is impairment in sodium metabolism, which occurs before decompensation and the development of ascites. Typically renal perfusion, GFR, and free water clearance are normal. Nonetheless, stressors such as rapid infusion of intravenous saline result in excessive sodium retention, and possibly the development of ascites or peripheral edema.

Phase 2

As the liver disease progresses, patients become unable to equalize their intake and excretion of sodium. Urinary sodium excretion is reduced but still viable. Renal perfusion, GFR, and free water excretion are preserved. The renin-angiotensin-aldosterone and sympathetic nervous systems are not activated. In this phase, ascites develops when oral sodium intake exceeds the kidney's ability to excrete sodium.

Phase 3

Ultimately urinary sodium excretion decreases to less than 10 mEq/d and endogenous vasoconstrictor systems are activated. Plasma renin activity and plasma concentrations of aldosterone and norepinephrine increase.[25,26] This results in increased sodium resorption throughout the nephron. These homeostatic changes preserve plasma volume, cardiac output, and peripheral vascular resistance; however, precipitous arterial hypotension can easily occur. Renal perfusion remains normal or slightly reduced from the antagonistic effects of angiotensin II, norepinephrine, and antidiuretic hormone (ADH) against intrarenal vasodilators, particularly prostaglandins.[27]

Box 1
Diagnostic criteria for hepatorenal syndrome

The diagnosis of hepatorenal syndrome requires all of the following:

I. Cirrhosis with ascites
II. Serum creatinine >1.5 mg/dL
III. No improvement of serum creatinine (to $\leq$1.5 mg/dL) after at least 2 days with diuretic withdrawal and volume expansion with albumin (1 g/kg body weight up to maximum 100 g/d)
IV. Absence of shock
V. No current or recent treatment with nephrotoxic drugs
VI. Absence of parenchymal kidney disease as indicated by proteinuria >500 mg/d, microhematuria (>50 red blood cells per high-powered field), and/or abnormal renal ultrasonography.

Adapted from Salerno F, Gerbes A, Gines P, et al. Diagnosis, prevention and treatment of the hepatorenal syndrome in cirrhosis: a consensus workshop of the international ascites club. Gut 2007;56:1310–8.

Phase 4

Phase 4 is the development of type 2 hepatorenal syndrome characterized by a steady decrease in renal function over weeks to months. Patients with type 2 hepatorenal syndrome have advanced cirrhosis and circulatory dysfunction attributed to high levels of plasma renin, aldosterone, norepinephrine, and ADH, which results in arterial hypotension and tachycardia.[28] A generalized systemic increase occurs in arterial vasoconstriction with an unsuccessful attempt at intrarenal vasodilation. Sodium resorption in the proximal tubular is excessive, and therefore the sodium content in the distal nephron is minimal, likely accounting for the ineffectiveness of diuretics, which primarily act in the distal tubule. Free water clearance is diminished and hyponatremia and refractory ascites are common.

Phase 5

The final phase is the development of type 1 hepatorenal syndrome characterized by rapid renal failure arbitrarily defined as doubling of the serum creatinine to greater than 2.5 mg/dL in less than 2 weeks. The transition from type 2 to type 1 HRS is usually associated with a triggering event, such as sepsis, SBP, acute hepatitis, gastrointestinal bleeding, or other physiologic stress. Renal function deteriorates precipitously in the kidney already precariously balancing perfusion via vasoconstrictors and vasodilators. The inciting event likely produces further systemic hypotension, leading to renal ischemia. The kidneys then increase production of vasoconstrictors and possibly decrease synthesis of renal vasodilators, causing a further net reduction in renal perfusion. The prognosis of patients with type 1 hepatorenal syndrome is poor, with death expected within 2 weeks after onset.[29]

TREATMENT OF HEPATORENAL SYNDROME

Because patients with hepatorenal syndrome, particularly type 1 hepatorenal syndrome, have a poor prognosis, early recognition is important. Although several measures are available to delay the progression of hepatorenal syndrome, complete reversal with a high chance of patient survival is unusual. Expedited referral to a liver center with expertise in the management of hepatorenal syndrome and the availability of liver transplantation is critical. Patients with suspected type 1 hepatorenal syndrome should be monitored closely in a hospital setting. Because SBP or other systemic infection frequently occurs concomitantly with hepatorenal syndrome, all patients should be screened for sepsis. Adequate rehydration is necessary, but excessive administration of fluids can result in dilutional hyponatremia and pulmonary edema. Diuretics are usually ineffective in removing adequate volume and should be withdrawn during initial evaluation. Early nephrology consultation is also important, because hemodialysis may be required.

Drug Therapies

The most effective pharmaceutical therapy for hepatorenal syndrome involves the administration of vasoconstrictors. In hepatorenal syndrome phase 5, one of the primary inciting events is systemic hypotension, which leads to a compensatory intrarenal vasoconstriction. The vasopressin analogue terlipressin causes vasoconstriction of the splanchnic bed, which ideally would terminate intrarenal vasoconstriction. In a U.S. multicenter, randomized, controlled trial of terlipressin versus placebo in 112 patients with type 1 hepatorenal syndrome, the actively treated group had improved renal function (serum creatinine <1.5 mg/dl on two occasions) compared with placebo, but no survival advantage was seen.[30] A meta-analysis of studies of terlipressin showed a 52% efficacy in reversing hepatorenal syndrome.[31] Terlipressin is currently not available in the United States but is undergoing further study in a randomized controlled trial.

The combination of octreotide, midodrine, and intravenous albumin has been popularized as a treatment option for patients with type 1 hepatorenal syndrome. In the initial study, five patients received 10 to 20 g of intravenous albumin daily for 20 days; octreotide at 200 mcg subcutaneously three times daily; and midodrine titrated to a maximum of 12.5 mg orally three times daily. Eight other patients were treated with intravenous dopamine and albumin. In the albumin/octreotide/midodrine-treated group, three patients were discharged from the hospital, and one subsequently underwent successful transplantation, one recovered renal function, and one died. Overall survival was 67% and transplant-free survival was 33%. Among the dopamine/albumin-treated patients, seven died within the first 12 days (survival, 12.5%) and one recovered renal function and subsequently underwent liver transplantation.[32]

Renal Replacement Therapy

The use of hemodialysis or continuous venous hemofiltration has not been adequately studied in patients with type 1 hepatorenal syndrome. The indications for renal replacement therapy (RRT) are the same as those for patients with chronic kidney disease: life-threatening electrolyte imbalance, metabolic acidosis, and volume overload. RRT can be considered in liver transplant candidates as a bridge to transplantation but cannot be considered appropriate long-term therapy, because other complications of liver failure often result in patient mortality.

Liver Transplantation

Liver transplantation is the preferred treatment for hepatorenal syndrome. Isolated liver transplantation results in return of function in the native kidneys in most patients who do not have underlying kidney disease. Combined liver and kidney transplantation is therefore indicated for patients with underlying kidney disease and those who have been on RRT twice a week for more than 6 weeks.[33]

NONHEPATIC ASCITES

Although cirrhosis and portal hypertension are the primary causes of ascites, other conditions can result in peritoneal fluid accumulation. Congestive heart failure and nephrotic syndrome result in diminished arterial blood volume. Similarly, severe hypothyroidism causes subtle congestive heart failure. Budd-Chiari syndrome can also cause portal hypertension in the absence of cirrhosis. In these cases, the peripheral arterial vasodilation theory applies and ascites may develop.

Chylous ascites can be categorized as traumatic or atraumatic. It is often iatrogenic and caused by surgical transection of the abdominal lymphatics or retroperitoneal lymph node dissection.[34,35] In the pediatric population, a traumatic chylous ascites is most often caused by lymphatic anomalies, such as lymphangiectasia. Malignant lymphoma can also obstruct or rupture lymphatics and is seen almost exclusively in adults.[36] Chylous ascites is, however, commonly caused by cirrhosis as a result of high flow and pressure in the abdominal lymphatics.[37]

Several other conditions cause exudation of protein-rich fluid from the peritoneal lining. Peritoneal carcinomatosis accounts for most cases of nonhepatic ascites. Infections such as tuberculosis, coccidiomycosis, and chlamydia also fall into this category. Peritoneal inflammatory serositis caused by connective tissue disorders such as systemic lupus erythematosus may also result in the development of ascites.

Biliary or pancreatic ascites occurs as a result of inflammation and/or disruption of the pancreatic biliary tree.

Patients undergoing hemodialysis, particularly those with underlying liver disease, are at increased risk of developing nephrogenic ascites. The pathogenesis and cause of nephrogenic ascites are poorly understood, but it is likely caused by an imbalance between fluid exudation and impaired resorption. Cachexia and hypotension during dialysis are also contributing factors.[38]

DIAGNOSIS OF ASCITES

Initial evaluation of patients with ascites includes a detailed history, physical examination, and review of all available laboratory and radiologic data. The history should focus on the risk factors for liver disease and cirrhosis and nonhepatic causes of ascites. Identification of the specific liver disease is necessary, because treatment and control of many diseases can result in improvement in hepatic function and reduction in ascites development. For example, treatment of chronic hepatitis B and hemochromatosis typically result in improved hepatic function and hemodynamics. Although radiologic evaluation is more sensitive and specific for the diagnosis of ascites, a physical examination may be helpful in determining the cause. In addition to the history, a confirmatory physical examination showing spider angiomata, splenomegaly, and prominent superficial abdominal vasculature suggests chronic liver disease. Alternatively, jugular venous distention and anasarca raise the possibility of cardiac or renal disease, and lymphadenopathy suggests malignant disease.

Paracentesis

All patients with new-onset or clinically detectable ascites are recommended to undergo initial diagnostic paracentesis. Additionally, paracentesis should be performed on all patients with ascites on admission to the hospital, because peritonitis is detected in 10% to 27% of hospitalized patients.[39] The classical signs of SBP (diffuse abdominal pain, fever, leukocytosis) are often absent. Paracentesis has virtually no contraindications. In fact, most patients who undergo paracentesis have a prolonged prothrombin time[40] and/or thrombocytopenia. No data support coagulation values to withhold paracentesis nor indications for transfusion of platelets or fresh frozen plasma.[41] In a study of 1100 large-volume paracenteses in patients with platelet counts as low as 19,000 cells/mm (54% had platelets <50,000) and international normalized ratios as high as 8.7 (75% were >1.5 and 26.5% were >2.0) who received no prophylactic transfusions, no hemorrhagic complications were seen.[42]

Fluid Analysis

Initial routine screening tests on ascitic fluid should include a cell count, albumin, total protein level, and culture. Culture should be obtained through bedside inoculation of blood culture bottles. Additional testing such as amylase, bilirubin, triglyceride, glucose, hematocrit, and cytology can be ordered if indicated or the cause of ascites is unknown. On the same day as the paracentesis, a serum albumin level should be obtained so that a serum ascites-albumin gradient (SAAG) can be calculated. Testing on subsequent ascites fluid can be dictated by the clinical situation but should always include a cell count.

The SAAG is an extremely helpful calculation to categorize ascites. Because portal hypertension results in excessively high hydrostatic pressure gradients between the hepatic sinusoids and the peritoneal fluid, one can use the SAAG to differentiate the cause of ascites. Studies have shown that a SAAG of 1.1 g/dL or greater correlates with portal hypertension with 97% accuracy, whereas patients with a SAAG less than 1.1 g/dL likely have ascites from an alternative cause.[43] When the SAAG is 1.1 g/dL or greater, the differential diagnosis includes cirrhosis, alcoholic hepatitis, hepatocellular carcinoma, massive liver metastases, fulminant hepatic failure, cardiac ascites, myxedema, Budd-Chiari syndrome, venoocclusive disease, portal vein thrombosis, and acute fatty liver of pregnancy. When the SAAG is less than 1.1 g/dL, consideration should be given to peritoneal carcinomatosis, tuberculous peritonitis, chlamydia peritonitis, pancreatic ascites, biliary ascites, peritonitis from connective tissue diseases, bowel perforation or infarction, and iatrogenic lymphatic leakage after surgery. A falsely elevated SAAG can be seen in patients with chylous ascites, and a falsely low SAAG in those with peripheral hypotension or elevated serum globulin levels greater than 5 g/dL.[44]

TREATMENT OF ASCITES

Treatment of low SAAG ascites is directed toward management of the underlying disorder. For example, tuberculous and chlamydial ascites respond to antimicrobials, and pancreatic/biliary ascites may respond to endoscopic or surgical treatment. For patients with nephrogenic ascites, aggressive dialysis, ambulatory peritoneal dialysis, peritoneovenous shunt, or kidney transplantation are indicated. Regardless of the cause of low SAAG ascites, therapeutic paracentesis remains the primary treatment. Because portal hypertension is not present, lowering the portal pressure with transjugular intrahepatic portosystemic shunting (TIPS) is ineffective and often contraindicated.

Control of the underlying liver disease in patients with cirrhosis can result in improved hepatic function and diminished portal hypertension, occasionally resulting in control of ascites. Liver diseases that can be treated include alcoholic liver disease, chronic hepatitis B, chronic hepatitis C, autoimmune hepatitis, and hemochromatosis. Spontaneous autolysis of portal vein thrombosis or the development of adequate collateral flow can also resolve ascites.

Dietary Sodium Restriction

Because the development of ascites in cirrhosis is a result of renal sodium retention, dietary sodium restriction is a mainstay of treatment. When dietary sodium intake exceeds urinary and bowel excretion, ascites and peripheral edema may develop. A typical unrestricted American diet contains 4 to 6 g of sodium per day. In patients with ascites, urinary and bowel excretion of sodium is approximately 1.2 and 0.25 g/d, respectively.[45] In patients with ascites and peripheral edema, a negative sodium balance is necessary to achieve control. Limiting sodium intake to 1.5 g/d may be desirable, but the diet is often unpalatable. Therefore, it is important to educate patients to adhere to a more tolerable diet with an intake of 2 g/d of sodium.[43] Reinforcement of this concept is often necessary at each patient contact. Patients should be encouraged to keep a food diary, noting both portion size and sodium content, which can be reviewed by the physician or nutritionist. Twenty-four-hour urine collections to determine sodium excretion can be used in patients with refractory ascites who claim compliance. With strict adherence, approximately 10% of patients will gain control of ascites with only dietary manipulation.[45] Fluid restriction is only indicated in patients with severe hyponatremia, although excessive fluid intake should be avoided.

Nephrotoxic Agents

Patients with ascites should be advised to avoid nephrotoxicity agents, excluding carefully prescribed and controlled diuretics. Muscle cramping and diffuse abdominal pain is common in patients with liver disease, and nonsteroidal anti-inflammatory drugs (NSAIDs) are easily obtained and often prescribed to treat the symptoms. NSAIDs inhibit the production of renal prostaglandins, which lead to further renal vasoconstriction and ultimately to diminished GFR and acute renal failure. Patients with cirrhosis should therefore not receive NSAIDs. Angiotensin-converting enzyme inhibitors and α_1-adrenergic blockers should also be used with caution because of the potential for hypotension and sodium retention. In patients with infection, aminoglycosides can be avoided easily given the plethora of available antibiotics. Finally, the use of intravenous radiocontrast should be given thoughtful consideration before administration; the risk of inducing acute renal failure must be balanced against the benefit of a diagnostic radiologic test.

Diuretics

For most patients with symptomatic ascites, diuretics are needed to control progressive accumulation of abdominal and peripheral fluid. Adequate control of ascites can positively impact the patient's quality of life, mobility, comfort, and nutritional status. Because sodium resorption is a critical component in the development of ascites and occurs throughout the nephron, several diuretics can be used. Most commonly a combination of spironolactone (an aldosterone antagonist) and furosemide (a loop diuretic) are initiated at doses of 100 and 40 mg/d, respectively. This combination avoids excessive use of either diuretic and the inherent potassium-altering side effects. The diuretics can be titrated upward in a stepwise fashion with the goal of maintaining a 100:40 ratio. Initially, success can be defined as loss of 2 to 3 pounds of fluid weight per week, and then later as stabilization of abdominal girth without the need for paracentesis. Diuretics should not be adjusted more frequently than once per week, because the onset of action of spironolactone is approximately 48 hours after ingestion and its peak effect is not seen for 2 weeks. The maximum recommended daily dose of spironolactone is 400 mg/d and furosemide 160 mg/d. Both drugs can be given as single daily doses to avoid inadequate compliance. For patients who develop tender gynecomastia attributed to spironolactone, amiloride starting at 5 mg/d can be substituted, although this regimen is less effective.[46] Other diuretics, such as hydrochlorothiazide and metolazone, are not recommended because of the risk of hyponatremia and profound dehydration. Another potassium-sparing diuretic, eplerenone, has not been adequately studied in this population.

Monitoring Patients on Diuretics

Because of the risk of electrolyte imbalance in patients on diuretics, periodic laboratory assessment of the metabolic profile is necessary, especially after changes in diuretics. These patients are also at risk of overdiuresis and subsequent renal failure. Because the maximum absorptive capacity of the peritoneal cavity is approximately 0.5 L/d,[47] weight loss exceeding 0.5 kg/d in the absence of peripheral edema indicates intravascular volume depletion. Patients with peripheral edema may safely lose up to 1 kg per day. Response to diuretics can be evaluated with a 24-hour urine collection for sodium; daily sodium output should exceed 2 g. Alternatively, a spot urine sodium-to-potassium ratio greater than one predicts a sodium excretion of greater than 1.8 g/d in more than 90% of patients.[48] Diuretics can be increased for patients below this threshold. Patients who are noncompliant with a low-sodium diet will have an adequate 24-hour urinary sodium excretion but will continue to gain fluid weight.

Albumin

The use of intravenous albumin has been shown to improve diuretic response, decrease the need for paracentesis, and reduce the length of hospital stay and need for readmission when used in patients with ascites. These results are not surprising when considering the pathogenesis of ascites. Albumin is a plasma volume expander that improves arterial hypotension. Through this mechanism, albumin has the potential to reverse underfilling of the arterial vasculature, which can then down-regulate the vasoactive systems mentioned earlier. In a study of 100 consecutive patients with cirrhosis and ascites who were given weekly infusions of 25 g of albumin for 1 year then every other week for the second year, in addition to standard diuretics, the median survival was 108 months compared with 36 months in those who did not receive albumin.[49] Despite these promising results, weekly albumin infusions are not practical or cost-effective and therefore have not been accepted as a standard of care.

REFRACTORY ASCITES

Refractory ascites can be defined as peritoneal fluid that is unresponsive to dietary sodium restriction and maximally tolerated diuretics, and requires frequent large-volume paracentesis (LVP).[50] Before categorizing the patient as "refractory," renal failure, NSAID use, and noncompliance must be ruled out. The frequency and volume of the paracentesis requirement can provide insight into the patient's compliance. Ascitic fluid has an approximate sodium concentration of 3 g/L. Hypothetically, patients losing 0.25 g of sodium per day through nonurinary losses but with no urinary sodium excretion and who consume 2 g/d of sodium have a net gain of 1.75 g of sodium daily. A 5-L paracentesis (containing 15 g of sodium) removes approximately 8 days of retained sodium. Therefore, patients who require a 5-L paracentesis more frequently than once per week cannot be compliant with their dietary restrictions.[43]

Ongoing controversy exists regarding the use of plasma expansion with albumin after LVP. Although administration of albumin after LVP has been repeatedly shown to improve electrolytes, plasma renin, and serum creatinine, all patients remain asymptomatic and no study has shown improvement in survival. The exception to this is the use of albumin in the setting of SBP.[51] Despite these findings, both the American Association for the Study of Liver Diseases[43] and European Association for the Study of the Liver guidelines[52] find it "reasonable" or "advisable" to administer albumin for paracentesis larger than 5 L. Both societies acknowledge that further studies are needed.

TIPS

TIPS is a side-to-side portacaval shunt that effectively reduces portal pressure. Several large, multicenter, randomized, controlled trials compared TIPS with serial LVP.[53–56] All reported improved control of ascites in the TIPS groups compared with the paracentesis groups, but also either more frequent or more severe rates of hepatic encephalopathy. Two studies[53,56] showed a statistically significant survival advantage for the TIPS group. Currently, a reasonable approach seems to be to place a TIPS in patients with refractory ascites requiring LVP more often than once per month. Additional criteria to consider include compliance, reversibility of the underlying liver disease, cardiac function, renal function, and transplant candidacy.

SPONTANEOUS BACTERIAL PERITONITIS

SBP occurs in 30% of patients with ascites[57] and has a 20% mortality rate,[58] possibly because of the severity of the underlying cirrhosis. SBP is diagnosed when the ascitic fluid absolute polymorphonuclear cell count is 250 cells/mL or more in the absence of recent surgery.

Empiric Therapy

Empiric therapy should be administered to patients who meet the criteria for SBP. Cell count results from ascitic fluid are rapidly available, whereas culture results may take several days. The administration of broad-spectrum antibiotics is appropriate before a positive fluid culture. Cefotaxime or another third-generation cephalosporin is an appropriate initial choice. Ceftriaxone has the theoretical disadvantage of being highly protein–bound, which may limit its ability to penetrate into ascitic fluid. Oral ofloxacin is as effective as parenteral cefotaxime in patients with SBP who do not exhibit signs of sepsis or hepatic encephalopathy.[59]

An important randomized controlled trial in patients with SBP evaluated the efficacy of intravenous albumin in addition to standard antibiotics. The patients receiving cefotaxime with 1.5 g of albumin per kg body weight within 6 hours of diagnosis on day 1 and 1.0 g per kg on day 3 had decreased in-hospital and 3-month mortality rates (29% vs 10% [*P* = .01] and 41% vs 22% [*P* = .03], respectively) compared with the non–albumin-treated patients. Additionally, renal impairment was seen less frequently in the albumin-treated group (10% vs 33% [*P* = .002]).[60] A more recent study has shown that albumin should be administered only to patients with SBP who have a serum creatinine greater than 1 mg/dL, blood urea nitrogen greater than 30 mg/dL, or total bilirubin greater than 4 mg/dL.[61]

Secondary Prophylaxis of SBP

After an initial episode of SBP, the recurrence rate is approximately 70%, with a 1-year survival of 30% to 50% in patients who do not receive secondary prophylaxis.[62] Hence, prevention of subsequent episodes of SBP is critically important. In a randomized, controlled trial comparing patients who receive norfloxacin at 400 mg daily as secondary prophylaxis for SBP versus placebo, the recurrence rate dropped from 68% to 20%.[63] Subsequent studies have shown efficacy with ciprofloxacin and trimethoprim/sulfamethoxazole.[64,65] It is now standard to provide secondary prophylaxis to all patients after their first episode of SBP. Treatment should continue until ascites is completely resolved or liver transplantation occurs.

Primary Prophylaxis of SBP

Primary prophylaxis of SBP remains controversial. Several studies have addressed this issue with inconclusive results. In the largest study, 109 hospitalized patients without a history of SBP but with a total bilirubin greater than 2.5 mg/dL or ascitic fluid total protein level of 15 g/L or less were randomized to receive norfloxacin at 400 mg daily indefinitely or only during their hospitalization. The incidence of SBP was reduced in the long-term antibiotic group (1.8% vs 16.9%; *P*<.01). Resistance to norfloxacin, however, was significantly higher in the long-term treated group (90% vs 36.3%; *P*<.05).[66] Another study of 68 patients with an ascitic fluid protein level of 15 g/L or less with advanced cirrhosis or renal impairment showed reduced incidence of SBP and improved survival at 3 months in norfloxacin-treated patients. After 1 year, survival no longer differed.[67] Other studies have raised similar concerns about selection of resistant organisms and lack of improvement in survival.[68,69] Currently no recommendation exists to initiate primary prophylaxis for SBP.

Prophylaxis of SBP in Gastrointestinal Bleeding

Patients who have advanced cirrhosis who develop acute gastrointestinal hemorrhage are at increased risk of bacterial infection, which can have a lethal effect in this population. A 2006 study randomized to receive oral norfloxacin at 400 mg twice daily or intravenous ceftriaxone at 1 g daily for 7 days 111 patients with gastrointestinal hemorrhage and at least two of the following conditions: ascites, severe malnutrition, encephalopathy, or bilirubin greater than 3 mg/dL. The risk of developing infection was statistically better in the ceftriaxone-treated group. No difference was seen in hospital mortality.[70] Based on the results of this study, patients with advanced cirrhosis and acute gastrointestinal bleeding are recommended to receive intravenous ceftriaxone prophylaxis. Patients with less-severe liver disease may be treated with norfloxacin twice daily.[43]

SUMMARY

Ascites is often the most limiting chronic complication of cirrhosis in terms of quality of life. It can impact the patient's appearance, risk of infection, mobility, and nutritional status. Progress in understanding the pathophysiology of ascites, specifically the peripheral arterial vasodilation theory, has led to more directed therapy. Differentiating nonhepatic from hepatic causes of ascites is important, and further differentiation using the SAAG is critical. Patients with high SAAG (portal hypertensive) ascites benefit most from sodium restriction and diuretics. Serial paracentesis or TIPS may be needed. The development of ascites is an indicator of poor prognosis, and referral for liver transplantation should be considered. Hepatorenal syndrome is a feared sequela of refractory ascites with limited treatment options. Future treatments will be directed toward maintaining adequate arterial volume, limiting the kidney's exposure to injury, and better infection prophylaxis.

REFERENCES

1. Gines P, Quintero E, Arroyo V, et al. Compensated cirrhosis: the natural history and prognostic factors. Hepatology 1987;7:122–8.
2. Planas R, Montoliu S, Balleste B, et al. Natural history of patients hospitalized for management of cirrhotic ascites. Clin Gastroenterol Hepatol 2006;4:1380–94.
3. Atkinson M, Losowsky MS. The mechanism of ascites formation in chronic liver disease. Q J Med 1961;30:153–66.
4. Sherlock A, Shaldon S. The aetiology and management of ascites in patients with hepatic cirrhosis: a review. Gut 1963;4:95–105.
5. Lieberman FL, Ito S, Reynolds TB. Effective plasma volume in cirrhosis with ascites. Evidence that decreased volume does not account for renal sodium retention, a spontaneous reduction in glomerular filtration rate (GFR), and a fall in GFR during drug-induced diuresis. J Clin Invest 1969;48:975–81.
6. Kostreva DR, Castaner A, Kampine JP. Reflex effects of hepatic baroreceptors on renal and cardiac sympathetic nerve activity. Am J Physiol 1980;238: R390–4.
7. Liebermann FL. Overflow theory of ascites formation. Gastroenterology 1989;96:274.
8. Schroeder ET, Anderson GH, Goldman SH, et al. Effect of blockade of angiotensin II on blood pressure, renin and aldosterone in cirrhosis. Kidney Int 1976; 9:511–9.
9. Arroyo V, Bosch J, Mauri M, et al. Effect of angiotensin-II blockade on systemic and hepatic haemodynamics and on the rennin-angiotensin-aldosterone system in cirrhosis with ascites. Eur J Clin Invest 1981;11:221–9.
10. Schrier RW, Arroyo V, Bernardi M, et al. Peripheral arterial vasodilation hypothesis: a proposal for the initiation of renal sodium and water retention in cirrhosis. Hepatology 1988;8:1151–7.

11. Arroyo V, Gines P, Gerbes AL, et al. Definition and diagnostic criteria of refractory ascites and hepatorenal syndrome in cirrhosis. Hepatology 1996;23:164–76.
12. Martin PY, Gines P, Schrier RW. Nitric oxide as a mediator of hemodynamic abnormalities in sodium and water retention in cirrhosis. N Engl J Med 1998;339: 533–41.
13. Wattanasirichaigoon S, Gordon FD, Resnick RH. Hyperdynamic circulation in portal hypertension: a comparative model of arteriovenous fistula. Med Hypotheses 2000;55:77–87.
14. Bosch J, Abraldes JG, Berzigotti DA, et al. Portal hypertension and gastrointestinal bleeding. Semin Liver Dis 2008;28:3–25.
15. Iwakiri Y, Groszmann RJ. The hyperdynamic circulation of chronic liver diseases: from the patient to the molecule. Hepatology 2006;43:S121–31.
16. Ros J, Claria J, To-Figueras SJ, et al. Endogenous cannabinoids: a new system involved in the homeostasis of arterial pressure and experimental cirrhosis in the rat. Gastroenterology 2002;122:85–93.
17. MacAllister RJ, Calver AL, Collier J, et al. Vascular and hormonal responses to arginine: provision of substrate for nitric oxide or nonspecific effect? Clin Sci 1995;89:183–90.
18. Cannaziga M, Salerno F, Vistentin S, et al. Increased flow-mediated vasodilation in cirrhotic patients with ascites: relationship with renal resistant index. Liver Int 2008;28:1396–401.
19. Korthuis RJ, Kinden DA, Brimer GE, et al. Intestinal capillary filtration in acute and chronic portal hypertension. Am J Physiol 1988;254:G339–45.
20. Henriksen JH, Lassen NA, Parving HH, et al. Filtration as the main transport mechanism of protein exchange between plasma and the peritoneal cavity and hepatic cirrhosis. Scand J Clin Lab Invest 1980;40:503–13.
21. Albillos A, de la Hera A, Gonzalez M, et al. Increased lipopolysaccharide binding protein in cirrhotic patients with marked immune and hemodynamic derangement. Hepatology 2003;37:208–17.
22. Frances R, Zapater P, Gonzalez Navajas JM, et al. Bacterial DNA in patients with cirrhosis and noninfected ascites mimics the soluble immune response established in patients with spontaneous bacterial peritonitis. Hepatology 2008;47: 978–85.
23. Rasaratnam B, Kaye D, Jennings G, et al. The effect of selective intestinal decontamination on the hyperdynamic circulatory state in cirrhosis: a randomized trial. Ann Intern Med 2003;139:186–93.
24. Arroyo V, Colmenero J. Ascites and have had a renal syndrome in cirrhosis: pathophysiological basis of therapy and current management. J Hepatol 2003;38: S69–89.
25. Bosch J, Arroyo V, Betriu A, et al. Hepatic hemodynamics in the renin-angiotensin-aldosterone system in cirrhotics. Gastroenterology 1980;78:92–9.
26. Bichet DG, Van Putten VJ, Schrier RW. Potential role of increased sympathetic activity in impaired sodium and water excretion in cirrhosis. N Engl J Med 1982;307:1552–7.
27. Laffi G, La Villa G, Pinzani M, et al. Arachidonic acid derivatives and renal function in liver cirrhosis. Semin Nephrol 1997;17:530–48.
28. Bataller R, Gines P, Guevara M, et al. have had a renal syndrome. Semin Liver Dis 1997;17:233–47.
29. Gines A, Escorsell A, Gines P, et al. Incidence, predictive factors, and prognosis of the hepatorenal syndrome in cirrhosis with ascites. Gastroenterology 1993; 105:229–36.

30. Sanyal A, Boyer T, Garcia-Tsao G, et al. A prospective, randomized, double-blind, placebo-controlled trial of terlipressin for type 1 hepatorenal syndrome (HRS). Gastroenterology 2008;134:1360–8.
31. Fabrizi F, Dixit V, Martin P. Meta-analysis: terlipressin therapy for hepatorenal syndrome. Aliment Pharmacol Ther 2006;24:935–44.
32. Angeli P, Volpin R, Gerunda G, et al. Reversal of type 1 hepatorenal syndrome with the administration of midodrine and octreotide. Hepatology 1999;29:1690–7.
33. Charlton MR, Wall WJ, Ojo AO, et al. international liver transplantation expert panel. Report of the first international liver transplantation Society expert panel consensus conference on renal insufficiency in liver transplantation. Liver Transpl 2009;15:S1–34.
34. Brown MW, Berk RF. Development of intractable ascites following upper abdominal surgery in patients with cirrhosis. Am J Gastroenterol 1986;80:879–83.
35. Miedema EB, Bissada NK, Finkbeiner, et al. Chylous ascites complicating retroperitoneal lymphadenectomy for testis tumors: management with peritoneovenous shunting. J Urol 1978;120:377–82.
36. Steinemann DC, Dindo D, Clavien PA, et al. Atraumatic chylous ascites: systematic review on symptoms and causes. J Am Coll Surg 2011;212:899–905.
37. Rector WG. Spontaneous chylous ascites of cirrhosis. J Clin Gastroenterol 1984;6:369–72.
38. Hammond TC, Takiyyuddin MA. Nephrogenic ascites: a poorly understood syndrome. J Am Soc Nephrol 1994;5:1173–7.
39. Guarner C, Runyon BA. Spontaneous bacterial peritonitis: pathogenesis, diagnosis, and management. Gastroenterologist 1995;3:311–28.
40. Runyon BA. Paracentesis of ascitic fluid: a safe procedure. Arch Intern Med 1986;146:2259–61.
41. Runyon BA. Management of adult patients with ascites caused by cirrhosis. Hepatology 1998;27:264–72.
42. Grabau CM, Crago SF, Hoff LK, et al. Performance standards for therapeutic abdominal paracentesis. Hepatology 2004;40:484–8.
43. Runyon BA, AASLD practice guidelines. management of adult patients with ascites due to cirrhosis: an update. Hepatology 2009;49:2087–107.
44. Yu AS, Hu KQ. Management of ascites. In: Gish RG, editor. Clinics in liver disease: current and future treatment therapies for liver disease. Philadelphia: WB Saunders Company; 2001. p. 541–68.
45. Leung W, Wong F. Medical management of ascites. Expert Opin Pharmacother 2011;12:1269–83.
46. Angeli P, Della Pria M, De Bei E, et al. randomized clinical study of the efficacy of amiloride and potassium canrenoate in nonazotemic cirrhotic patients with ascites. Hepatology 1994;19:72–9.
47. Shear L, Ching S, Gabuzda GJ. Compartmentalization of ascites and edema in patients with hepatic cirrhosis. N Engl J Med 1970;282:1391–6.
48. Pinto-Marques P, Vieira A. Urinary sodium/potassium ratio on random sample as a useful tool to assess diuretic induced natriuresis on chronic liver disease-associated ascites. Am J Gastroenterol 2007;102:212–3.
49. Romanelli RG, La Villa G, Barletta G, et al. Long-term albumin infusion improves survival in patients with cirrhosis and ascites: an unblinded randomized trial. World J Gastroenterol 2006;12:1403–7.

50. Crenshaw WB, Gordon FD, McEniff NJ, et al. Severe ascites: efficacy of the transjugular intrahepatic portosystemic shunt in treatment. Radiology 1996;200:185–92.
51. Haynes GR, Navickis RJ, Wilkes MM. Albumin administration – what is the evidence of clinical benefit? a systematic review of randomized controlled trials. Eur J Anaesthesiol 2003;20:771–93.
52. European Association for the Study of the Liver. EASL clinical practice guidelines on the management of ascites, spontaneous bacterial peritonitis, and hepatorenal syndrome in cirrhosis. J Hepatol 2010;53:397–417.
53. Rossle M, Ochs A, Gulberg V, et al. A comparison of paracentesis and transjugular intrahepatic portosystemic shunting in patients with ascites. N Engl J Med 2000;342:1701–7.
54. Gines P, Uriz J, Calahorra B, et al. Transjugular intrahepatic portosystemic shunting versus paracentesis plus albumin for refractory ascites in cirrhosis. Gastroenterology 2002;123:1839–47.
55. Sanyal AJ, Genning C, Reddy RK, et al. The North American study for the treatment of refractory ascites. Gastroenterology 2003;124:634–41.
56. Salerno F, Merli M, Riggio O, et al. Randomized controlled study of TIPS vs. paracentesis plus albumin in cirrhosis with severe ascites. Hepatology 2004;40:629–35.
57. Wong F, Bernardi M, Balk R, et al. Sepsis in cirrhosis: report on the seventh meeting of the International Ascites Club. Gut 2005;54:718–25.
58. Tandon P, Garcai-Tsao G. Bacterial infections, sepsis, and multiorgan failure in cirrhosis. Semin Liver Dis 2008;28:26–42.
59. Navasa M, Follo A, Llovet JM, et al. Randomized, comparative study of oral ofloxacin versus intravenous cefotaxime in spontaneous bacterial peritonitis. Gastroenterology 1996;111:1011–7.
60. Sort P, Navasa M, Arroyo V, et al. Effect of intravenous albumin on renal impairment and mortality in patients with cirrhosis and spontaneous bacterial peritonitis. N Engl J Med 1999;341:403–9.
61. Sigal SH, Stanca CM, Fernandez J, et al. Restricted use of albumin for spontaneous bacterial peritonitis. Gut 2007;56:597–9.
62. Garcia-Tsao G. current management of complications of cirrhosis and portal hypertension: variceal hemorrhage, ascites, and spontaneous bacterial peritonitis. Gastroenterology 2001;120:726–48.
63. Gines P, Rimola A, Planas R, et al. Norfloxacin prevents spontaneous bacterial peritonitis recurrence in cirrhosis: results of a double-blind, placebo-controlled trial. Hepatology 1990;12:716–24.
64. Rolachon A, Cordier L, Bacq Y, et al. ciprofloxacin and long-term prevention of spontaneous bacterial peritonitis: results of a prospective controlled trial. Hepatology 1995;22:1171–4.
65. Singh N, Gayowski T, Yu VL, et al. Trimethoprim-sulfamethoxazole for the prevention of spontaneous bacterial peritonitis in cirrhosis: a randomized trial. Ann Intern Med 1995;122:595–8.
66. Novella M, Sola R, Soriano G, et al. Continuous versus inpatient prophylaxis of the first episode of spontaneous bacterial peritonitis with norfloxacin. Hepatology 1997;25:532–6.
67. Fernandez J, Navasa M, Planas R, et al. Primary prophylaxis of spontaneous bacterial peritonitis delays hepatorenal syndrome and improves survival in cirrhosis. Gastroenterology 2007;133:818–24.
68. Grange JD, Roulot D, Pelletier G, et al. Norfloxacin primary prophylaxis of infections in patients with ascites: a double-blind randomized trial. J Hepatol 1998;29:430–6.

69. Terg R, Fassio E, Guevara M, et al. Ciprofloxacin in primary prophylaxis of spontaneous bacterial peritonitis: a randomized, placebo-controlled study. J Hepatol 2008;48:774–9.
70. Fernandez J, Ruiz del Arbol L, Gomez C, et al. Norfloxacin vs ceftriaxone in the prophylaxis of infections in patients with advanced cirrhosis and hemorrhage. Gastroenterology 2006;131:1049–105.

Hepatic Encephalopathy

Vandana Khungar, MD, MSc[a,b,*], Fred Poordad, MD[a,c]

KEYWORDS

- Hepatic encephalopathy • Minimal hepatic encephalopathy
- Overt hepatic encephalopathy • Treatment

Hepatic encephalopathy (HE) represents a continuum of transient and reversible neurologic and psychiatric dysfunction, varying from subtly altered mental status to deep coma. It is a reversible state of impaired cognitive function or altered consciousness in patients with liver disease or portosystemic shunting.[1] HE is not a single clinical entity and may reflect reversible metabolic encephalopathy, brain atrophy, brain edema, or a combination of these factors. Various hypotheses have been set forth to explain the pathophysiology. HE can be categorized into 3 types: type A, which occurs in acute liver failure (ALF); type B, which occurs in patients with bypass shunts; and type C, which occurs in patients with chronic liver disease.[2,3] Type C HE is of great importance given the increasing burden of cirrhosis in the United States and the world. Approximately 5.5 million people in the United States have hepatic cirrhosis.[4] It is difficult to estimate the true incidence of HE, but most patients with cirrhosis develop a degree of encephalopathy at some point during their disease. Overt HE (OHE) occurs in at least 30% to 45% of patients with cirrhosis and 10% to 50% of patients with transjugular intrahepatic portosystemic shunts.[5,6] Minimal HE (MHE), characterized by deficits in attention, reaction time, working memory, visuoconstructive abilities, and fine motor performance, occurs in 60% of patients with cirrhosis. The subtle cognitive abnormalities of MHE are sometimes detectable only on psychometric or neuropsychologic testing but can nevertheless impair daily functioning and quality of life, including the ability to drive.[7,8]

HE imposes a significant burden on patients, their families, and health care resources.[4,9] A recent 104-patient cross-sectional study in 2 transplant centers revealed that previous HE and cognitive dysfunction are associated with worse employment, financial status, and caregiver burden. Patients with previous HE had 87.5% unemployment versus 19% ($P = .00001$), lower financial status, and posed a higher caregiver

[a] Department of Medicine, Cedars-Sinai Medical Center, 8635 West Third Street, Suite 1060, Los Angeles, CA 90048, USA; [b] Department of Medicine, David Geffen School of Medicine at UCLA, Los Angeles, CA, USA; [c] Department of Surgey, Cedars-Sinai Medical Center, 8635 West Third Street, Suite 1060, Los Angeles, CA 90048, USA

* Corresponding author. Department of Medicine, Cedars-Sinai Medical Center, 8635 West Third Street, Suite 1060, Los Angeles, CA 90048.

E-mail address: vandana.khungar@gmail.com

Clin Liver Dis 16 (2012) 301–320
doi:10.1016/j.cld.2012.03.009

burden. Cognitive performance and the Model for End-Stage Liver Disease (MELD) score were significantly correlated with employment and caregiver burden.[10] Based on the Zarit-short form, the caregivers are at similar stress levels compared with caregivers of patients with Alzheimer disease (score 15 ± 10) and advanced cancer (score 12 ± 8.5) but at a lower level compared with caregivers with acute brain injury (score 21.7 ± 10.1).[11]

OHE is a particularly pressing problem. Episodes can occur without warning and often require inpatient hospitalization. In 2005, more than 50,000 patients required hospitalization for HE.[9] Increases in the frequency and severity of episodes of HE predict an increased risk of death.[12,13] Data presented at the 2011 annual meeting of the European Association for the Study of the Liver (EASL) by Bajaj and colleagues[14] showed that deficits in working memory, psychomotor speed, attention, and response inhibition increase with the number and severity of episodes of OHE. It is possible that the metabolic derangements that produce OHE cause chronic neurologic injury that is not readily reversible.[14,15] For patients with severe HE who are hospitalized, 1- and 3-year survival rates are less than 50% and less than 25% respectively.[16]

PATHOPHYSIOLOGY OF HE

The pathophysiology of HE is incompletely elucidated at present. Historically, there has been a focus on the accumulation of various toxins in the bloodstream and brains of animals and human patients to explain HE.[17] The accumulation of ammonia, mostly derived from the intestine, still plays a central role in current hypotheses, but HE truly is multifactorial in nature. Gut flora, particularly urease-producing species, including Klebsiella, proteus, and clostridium species, are important sources of ammonia in humans. The deamination of glutamine in small intestinal mucosa and renal and muscle synthesis also contribute to ammonia production. Impaired hepatic clearance caused by hepatocellular clearance or portosystemic shunting causes increased accumulation of ammonia. Decreased clearance of gut-derived neurotoxins plays a central role in the development of HE. Finally, the catabolic state of cirrhosis leads to atrophy of skeletal muscles and can reduce the ability to synthesize glutamine and reduce ammonia.[18] Ammonia is truly only one piece of the puzzle in HE.

It has long been thought that ammonia in the body is derived from colonic bacteria with urease enzyme activity. The urease breaks down urea from the bloodstream into ammonia and carbon dioxide. Although the intestinal flora are a significant source of ammonia, evidence from animal models shows that bacteria are not required for the development of hyperammonemia. Enterocytes in the small bowel can generate ammonia via intestinal glutaminase, turning glutamine into glutamate and ammonia. This endogenous production of ammonia may even exceed production by fecal flora.[19] Neomycin is thought to have some activity against the intestinal glutaminase. The gene for glutaminase has been shown to be upregulated in patients with cirrhosis, particularly those with MHE.[20] In rats, an increase in expression of intestinal glutaminase was seen following the insertion of a portacaval shunt, which may explain the increased risk of HE in patients following the procedure. After enterocytes and colonic bacteria generate ammonia, it goes to the liver via the splanchnic circulation for detoxification via the urea cycle in zone 1 and, to a lesser extent, via conversion to glutamine in zone 3 hepatocytes.[21] Hyperammonemia occurs secondary to a reduction in the metabolic capacity of the liver's urea cycle and shunting of blood around the hepatic sinusoids. These shunts can occur in the form of extrahepatic portosystemic collaterals, surgically created shunts, such as transjugular intrahepatic portosystemic shunts (TIPS), or intrahepatic spontaneous shunts.

The kidneys contribute to ammonia flux. This renal contribution includes excretion and production and is affected by the acid-base status. Ammonia can be excreted in the urine in the form of ammonium or in the form of urea. The proximal tubular cells of the kidney generate ammonia by metabolizing glutamine via glutaminase into ammonia, bicarbonate, and glutamate. These processes contribute to acid-base homeostasis because bicarbonate is also produced during the reaction. Ammonia formation in the renal system buffers systemic acidosis by releasing hydrogen ions in the urine in the form of ammonium. With a normal pH, 30% to 50% of renal ammonia is excreted in the urine and the remainder is returned to systemic circulation via the renal vein. With systemic acidosis, the kidneys increase the amount of ammonium released into the urine severalfold to autoregulate pH.[22–24] Alkalosis causes a significant decrease in urinary loss of ammonia and can cause hyperammonemia. Hyperammonemia is also caused by the reduced excretion of ammonia and urea in patients with reduced perfusion and decreased glomerular filtration rates. This state can occur in those who are dehydrated and develop prerenal azotemia secondary to the overzealous administration of diuretics or lactulose, with resultant diarrhea. In patients with gastrointestinal bleeding (GI), ammoniagenesis by the kidneys increases up to 6-fold and accounts for most of the hyperammonemia in this setting.[25] In the setting of hypokalemia, hydrogen ions are moved into the cells, leading to intracellular acidosis, which allows for more ammonia and bicarbonate generation from glutamine to balance the acid-base status.

Skeletal muscle is another organ important for regulating ammonia flux.[2] Myocytes in skeletal muscles incorporate ammonia into glutamine via glutamine synthetase. The glutamine produced is recirculated and only temporarily detoxifies ammonia but does not significantly increase ammonia excretion. Muscle wasting and cachexia may only partially contribute to the body's ability to metabolize ammonia. Rather, catabolism itself and the release of excessive glutamine into the circulation, which leads to ammonia production, causes worsening of HE.

Ammonia toxicity affects astrocytes in the brain with development of Alzheimer type II astrocytosis. Cerebral edema is thought to contribute to neurologic dysfunction. Glutamine, produced by the metabolism of ammonia via glutamine synthetase, attracts water into the astrocytes, leading to swelling and induces oxidative dysfunction of the mitochondria. The low-grade edema seen in type C HE causes neurologic dysfunction directly as opposed to an increase in intracranial pressure seen in ALF or type A HE.[26,27]

Molecules other than ammonia have been implicated in HE. Neurosteroids, including allopregnenalone, are produced in the brain and are elevated in patients with HE. They modulate gamma-aminobutyric (GABA)-A receptors in the brain, leading to a decreased state of alertness.[28,29] Endogenous and exogenous benzodiazepines also modulate GABA receptors and trigger astrocyte swelling. Neuronal acetylcholinesterase (AChE) is increased in the brains of patients with cirrhosis and animals with type C HE. AChE inhibitors are being studied in HE.[30–32]

Hyponatremia is common in patients with cirrhosis and portal hypertension because of the activation of antidiuretic hormone secondary to decreased effective arterial volume. Chronic hyponatremia depletes intracellular organic osmolytes, including myoinositol, which regulates intracellular water content. Osmolytes in astrocytes prevent intracellular swelling. Chronic hyponatremia may allow astrocyte osmolytes to be depleted, allowing for intracellular swelling, low-grade cerebral edema, oxidative and nitrosative stress, and astrocyte dysfunction. Hyponatremia is a predictor of the development of OHE in patients with cirrhosis.[33,34]

Inflammation, in concert with hyperammonemia or other neurotoxic molecules, may precipitate HE. The inflammation may be secondary to infection, GI bleeding, obesity, or changes in fecal flora with translocation and increased bacterial overgrowth. Proinflammatory cytokines act synergistically with ammonia in causing cerebral edema.[35–37] Neutrophils with a large amount of degranulation activity and increased production of inflammatory cytokines may augment this process. The many contributing factors to systemic and brain inflammation are complex, and we are just beginning to understand possible mechanisms for HE related to inflammatory cytokines.

It is known that increased levels of gut-derived endotoxin and sensitivity to endotoxin have been noted in patients with cirrhosis.[38–40] Treatment with synbiotics improved serum bilirubin, albumin, and prothrombin activity. Probiotics also reduced endotoxemia and improved Child-Pugh status to a lesser extent. Treatment with paromomycin and neomycin for 3 to 6 months improved serum albumin levels and the Child-Pugh score, mainly through the decreased incidence of ascites and encephalopathy. Preliminary data from a trial of 8 weeks of rifaximin for intestinal decontamination in patients with cirrhosis showed significantly reduced plasma endotoxin levels, increased serum albumin, and decreased serum total bilirubin levels and international normalized ratio. The effects of rifaximin on endotoxin may be multifactorial in nature and may contribute to decreases in inflammation.

High circulating levels of endotoxin and cytokines, such as interleukin 1 (IL-1), interleukin 6 (IL-6), and tumor necrosis factor-α (TNF-α), are thought to occur in cirrhosis because of bacterial overgrowth and translocation.[39,41,42] A new mechanism has been postulated whereby endotoxemia reduces peripheral blood platelet counts in patients with cirrhosis either directly or through the release of cytokines.[43] Kalambokis and colleagues[44] recently demonstrated that rifaximin improves cirrhosis-related thrombocytopenia, presumably because of the reduction of endotoxemia. The severity of thrombocytopenia was correlated significantly with the level of endotoxin and IL-6. The thrombocytopenia may be mediated by platelet toll-like receptors[24] or increased platelet-associated immunoglobulin G giving rise to idiopathic thrombocytopenic purpura.[45,46] Other postulated mechanisms include endotoxin, IL-1, and TNF-α triggering disseminated intravascular coagulation[47,48] or an altered activity of IL-6 in patients with cirrhosis. Endotoxemia and the same inflammatory cytokines implicated in thrombocytopenia likely play a role in the pathogenesis of HE.

DIAGNOSIS OF HE

OHE is diagnosed clinically based on 2 types of symptoms: impaired mental status, as defined by the West Haven criteria (Conn score), and impaired neuromotor function.[4,18,49] The Working Party on Hepatic Encephalopathy recommends the Conn score for assessment of OHE in clinical trials.[3] More recently, the Hepatic Encephalopathy Scoring Algorithm has been used.[50] Examples of neuromotor impairment include hyperreflexia, rigidity, myoclonus, and asterixis.[49,51,52] OHE can be further subdivided into episodic or persistent and precipitated or spontaneously occurring.

The diagnosis of MHE can be slightly more challenging. The working party commissioned by the World Congress of Gastroenterology (WCOG) suggests the following for diagnostic criteria: The number connection test, the digit symbol test, and the block design test should be included as neuropsychological testing because they have high specificity for diagnosing MHE.[53] Some practitioners are also investigating the use of computerized psychometry and other tests, such as the critical flicker frequency test. Neuropsychological symptoms are associated with subcortical impairment, and it is known that MHE has a negative socioeconomic impact and is associated with poor quality of life.[54] A suggested algorithm from Stewart and colleagues[55] recommends that after ruling out other metabolic encephalopathies and neurologic disorders, a brief formal mental status assessment, such as the Mini-Mental State Examination, should be used. If the score is less than 24, then a diagnosis of MHE is probable. If greater than 24, then a report of behavioral change by patients, families, or friends should lead to neuropsychological testing with a battery similar to what is recommended by the WCOG working group. A decrease of 2 standard deviations in studied domains or tests of visuospatial, attention, and processing speed is suggestive of MHE. Deficits of MHE are mainly in the attention and visuospatial domains, whereas language and verbal skills are largely spared.[56] Memory deficits are thought to be short term and are caused by impairment of attention.[57]

MHE has been shown to lead to OHE.[58] Given the relationship between OHE and decreased survival, it is critical to identify MHE to prevent the development of OHE. Testing all patients with cirrhosis may help to treat MHE at the early stages to prevent decreased quality of life and OHE with its resultant debility. It would also identify patients who are unable to drive or those who work in a profession whereby such impairment could pose a risk to themselves or others. The spectrum of neurocognitive impairment in cirrhosis may help to provide a continuum along which to place patients rather than having to place them in the categories of normal, MHE, and OHE.[59] The awareness of MHE exists among physicians, as evidenced by the fact that most physician respondents to an American Association for the Study of Liver Diseases survey thought that MHE constitutes a significant medical problem in need of treatment. Only half of those physicians routinely treated MHE according to the same survey, underscoring the need for a commitment to standardized treatment recommendations for MHE.[60]

THERAPY FOR HE

Treatment goals and strategies should be tailored to the severity and acuity of HE. The burden of OHE is clearly great and the diagnosis fairly simple. Clinicians must ensure that patients have OHE, treat precipitating factors if necessary, triage patients to an intensive care unit versus floor bed, decide if intubation is necessary to protect the airway, and treat with appropriate pharmacotherapy. Following an episode of OHE, prophylactic therapy with lactulose or rifaximin is recommended for an indefinite period of time or until liver transplantation. The currently available treatment strategies for HE are presented in **Table 1**.

Clinical guidelines for OHE were published 10 years ago, and many physicians have developed great comfort with older therapies.[61] As new therapies are discovered, practice patterns should change. The first step in treatment is identifying and treating precipitating causes, including but not limited to hypovolemia, GI bleeding, infection, dehydration secondary to diuretic use, diarrhea, vomiting, hyponatremia, hypokalemia or hyperkalemia, alkalosis, surgery, renal failure, TIPS, constipation, benzodiazepine use, narcotic use, hypoxemia, hepatoma, and noncompliance with lactulose therapy.[62]

Therapy is generally focused on treating episodes after they occur. Many agents currently available reduce the nitrogenous load in the gut to reduce the accumulation of ammonia.[9,63] The 2 key therapies used to reduce circulating ammonia are nonabsorbable disaccharides and oral antibiotics. Both reduce intestinal production and absorption of NH4.[64] The standard of care has been nonabsorbable disaccharides (lactitol or lactulose), which decrease the absorption of ammonia through cathartic effects and by altering colonic pH.[61] Oral antibiotics have also proven to be useful in reducing ammonia-producing enteric bacteria.[61,65,66] The long-term use of some oral antibiotics is not recommended because of nephrotoxicity, ototoxicity, and

Table 1
Therapeutic approaches for the treatment of HE

General supportive care	Fall precautions in disoriented patients Prevention of infections: changing IV lines, prevent aspiration pneumonia, isolation Monitor fluid status Maintain normoglycemia and electrolytes Correct alkalosis
Nutritional support	Energy intake of 35–40 kcal/kg BW/d and protein intake of 1.2–1.5 g/kg BW/d Consider addition of BCAAs, zinc, consider eliminating wheat and milk proteins
Treating precipitating events	
GI bleeding	Octreotide, IV PPI, endoscopic or angiographic therapy Blood transfusions, correction of coagulopathy NG lavage to remove blood from stomach
Infection	Antibiotic therapy
Sedating medications	Discontinue benzodiazepines, narcotics, consider flumazenil or naloxone
Electrolyte abnormalities	Discontinue diuretics, perform serial paracentesis if needed Correct hypokalemia or hyperkalemia, hyponatremia
Constipation	Provide laxatives and enemas
Renal failure	Discontinue diuretics Albumin administration Discontinue nephrotoxic medications
Ammonia excretion	Lactulose enemas
Ammonia production	Antibiotics: neomycin, paromomycin, metronidazole, vancomycin Minimally absorbed antibiotics: rifaximin Nonabsorbable disaccharides: lactulose, lactitol Probiotics: lactobacillus, bifidobacterium Ammonia scavengers: sodium benzoate, sodium phenylacetate, sodium phenylbutyrate AST-120, L-ornithine-L-aspartate, L-ornithine phenylacetate, or OCR-002 α-glucosidase inhibitors: acarbose Closure of spontaneous portal systemic shunt Liver transplantation Artificial liver support
Gut-derived cytokines	Nonabsorbable disaccharides: lactulose, lactitol Minimally absorbed antibiotics: rifaximin

Abbreviations: BCAAs, branched-chain amino acids; BW, body weight; IV, intravenous; NG, nasogastric; PPI, proton pump inhibitor.

peripheral neuropathy. Rifaximin, a minimally absorbed oral antibiotic, has great promise in the treatment of OHE. A recent review recommended that treatment strategies should focus on the management of precipitating factors, reduction of ammonia and other toxins, modulation of fecal flora, modulation of neurotransmission, correction of nutritional deficiencies, and reduction of inflammation.[2] Serial measurements of ammonia levels do not provide additional information beyond clinical assessment of the mental status and may not correlate well with clinical outcomes.[67,68]

The treatment of MHE is evolving. Treatment is directed almost exclusively at reduction of gut-derived ammonia with nonabsorbable disaccharides (lactulose), probiotics, or rifaximin. Lactulose has been shown to improve cognitive function, and probiotics have improved performance on the number connection test.[69,70] Treatments are based on those used for OHE, but astrocyte swelling may not be the primary mechanism of injury in MHE. MCPhail and colleagues[71] presented data at the 2011 EASL meeting that demonstrated that core metabolic and structural regions of the brain showed altered function on functional magnetic resonance imaging following treatment with L-ornithine-L-aspartate (LOLA). This function was associated with improved psychometric performance, but there was no change in regional brain volume, suggesting a mechanism other than low-grade cerebral edema. The Rifaximin in Minimal Hepatic Encephalopathy (RIME) trial recently demonstrated that rifaximin improves psychometric performance and health-related quality of life in patients with MHE. In this 281-person trial, reversal of MHE was achieved in 75.5% in the rifaximin group versus 20.0% in the placebo group. A significant reduction in the mean number of abnormal neuropsychometric tests was also seen in the rifaximin group. The mean total Sickness Impact Profile score improved significantly in the rifaximin group compared with the placebo group.[72]

Bajaj and colleagues[7] recently published data demonstrating that rifaximin improves driving simulator performance in a randomized controlled trial (RCT) of patients with MHE. In this 42-patient study, driving simulation tests were performed at baseline and at 8 weeks into therapy. Cognitive abilities, quality of life (using the Sickness Impact Profile), serum levels of ammonia, levels of inflammatory cytokines, and MELD scores were also collected. Patients taking rifaximin made significantly greater improvements than those on placebo in avoiding total driving errors (76% vs 31%, $P = .13$), speeding (81% vs 33%, $P = .005$), and illegal turns (62% vs 19%, $P = .01$). Ninety-one percent of patients taking rifaximin improved their cognitive performance compared with 61% of patients given placebo ($P = .01$). Patients in the rifaximin group also had increased levels of the antiinflammatory cytokine IL-10.[7]

Management of Precipitating Factors

Breakthrough episodes of HE can be either precipitated by an identifiable event or occur spontaneously. Infection is the most commonly identified precipitant when there is one.[73,74] GI bleeding, both immediately after and for several days following the bleed, can precipitate HE, occult GI bleeding can also lead to HE.[75] Dehydration resulting from aggressive diuresis with volume contraction alkalosis and electrolyte disturbances commonly causes HE in patients with ascites and edema. Patients who have had a TIPS procedure and whose medications are not appropriately adjusted after the procedure often develop HE. This type of HE responds well to fluid resuscitation and electrolyte repletion.[76] Albumin is particularly helpful in these patients, whereas other colloids are not as useful.[77]

The risk of infection in hospitalized patients with cirrhosis is approximately 5 times higher than hospitalized patients without cirrhosis.[2] An aggressive investigation to find the infectious source must be conducted in patients with HE. Some begin empiric antimicrobial therapy while body fluid analyses and cultures are pending, particularly when there are clinical features, such as fever, or laboratory changes, such as leukocytosis. A diagnostic paracentesis should be performed for any patient with ascites who presents with HE to rule out spontaneous bacterial peritonitis.

A generalized inflammatory state exists in patients with cirrhosis even without infection, with elevated levels of endotoxin, TNF-α, inflammatory cytokines, and toll-like receptors. The increase in inflammation may be due to bowel wall edema from portal hypertension or delayed transit time with subsequent translocation of bacteria or endotoxin into the systemic circulation. Antibiotics given to patients with cirrhosis who have

HE may reduce this proinflammatory state. Other therapies with antiinflammatory activity are pentoxifylline (anti–TNF-α) and the activated charcoal product AST-120. Pentoxifylline has not yet been studied as a therapy for HE. AST-120 may bind very small molecules in the gut, such as TNF-α, lipopolysaccharide, or endotoxin, and block their absorption. It is being evaluated in trials for the treatment of HE.[2]

Overzealous administration of lactulose can lead to hypokalemia from diarrhea, exacerbating HE. Repletion of electrolytes, particularly potassium, is crucial in treating HE. Potassium deficiency exacerbates hyperammonemia by upregulating renal glutaminase and the production of ammonia.[2] Constipation is also thought to be a cause of HE, possibly by increasing the amount of time available for ammonia to be absorbed from the GI tract. Hyponatremia can precipitate HE but can also cause neurologic dysfunction, which may be difficult to differentiate clinically from HE. For patients with hypovolemia, treatment of hyponatremia is with intravenous saline, whereas for those who are euvolemic or hypervolemic, water restriction or vasopressin antagonists are used.

An often-overlooked clinical scenario, particularly in the inpatient setting, is the use of sedating or hypnotic medications. Because patients with cirrhosis have a higher incidence of anxiety, depression, pain disorders, and a disrupted sleep-wake cycle, they are often given benzodiazepines or opiates, which can trigger HE.

Reduction of Ammonia by Nonabsorbable Disaccharides

Because ammonia is thought to be a key player in the development of HE, it is the target of the most widely used HE therapies, and decreased ammonia is used as a significant endpoint in many clinical trials assessing HE treatments. The degree of ammonia elevation has been associated with the stage of HE, although this is not as clear outside of research settings.[78,79] This finding is particularly noted in type A HE whereby cerebral edema and death have been correlated with the degree of hyperammonemia.

Ammonia is derived from both intestinal flora and other sources, such as enterocytes in the small bowel and colon, which produce ammonia when they metabolize glutamine.[80] Ammonia may cause neurologic dysfunction by its effect on cerebral edema. Glutamine is produced within astrocytes in the brain from glutamate and ammonia. Glutamine in turn attracts water and causes the swelling of astrocytes. Ammonia can then directly cause oxidative stress, upregulating cytokine production, inflammatory responses, and impaired intracellular signaling. Ammonia can also be broken down by skeletal muscle, so in patients with cirrhosis with a large degree of muscle wasting, it is more difficult to clear ammonia. For this reason, it is clinically appropriate to increase protein intake in patients with cirrhosis to slow the rate of muscle loss. Testosterone levels can also be repleted when low.

The standard approach for reducing ammonia levels in type C HE has been to administer nonabsorbable disaccharides, such as lactulose (β-galactoside-fructose) in the United States or lactitol (β-galactoside-sorbitol) in Europe. They are thought to reduce ammonia levels by several mechanisms. They acidify and speed passage of the fecal stream through the colon and promote the growth of beneficial acid resistant, non–urease-producing bacteria. On entering the colon, lactulose is cleaved into monosaccharides by the bacterial flora. Some bacteria, including *Lactobacilli* and *Bifidobacteria*, can incorporate the monosaccharides into subsequent generations of bacteria, conferring a growth advantage. The unincorporated monosaccharides are also used as fuel for the bacteria. The fermentation generates lactic acid and hydrogen ions, acidifying the fecal stream and causing protonation of the ammonia molecules (NH_3) into ammonium ions (NH_4^+). The charged ammonium ions are difficult for colonocytes to absorb and remain trapped in the colonic lumen. The protonation also allows for movement of NH_3 from the bloodstream into the colonic lumen. Lactulose is also thought to transform fecal flora, with a reduction in urease-producing bacteria that are not given a growth advantage and an increase in the proteolytic species, *Lactobacilli* and *Bifidobacteria*. The cathartic action of excessive amounts of lactulose can also promote the elimination of ammonia, although excessive diarrhea leads to dehydration, which can worsen HE.[81]

A Cochrane database systematic review of RCTs from 2004 did not show a significant survival benefit with the use of nonabsorbable disaccharides for the treatment of HE and showed that they were less effective than antibiotics for improving HE.[66,82] However, in a 125-patient open-label, single-site study, Sharma and colleagues[83] showed that lactulose was more effective than placebo in the secondary prevention of overt HE in the outpatient setting (19.6% vs 46.8%, $P = .001$).

Compliance with lactulose therapy is a concern because many of the side effects are difficult to tolerate. The most common side effects include an unpleasant sweet taste, bloating, flatulence, nausea, vomiting, and severe diarrhea leading to dehydration, hypokalemia, hypernatremia, and other electrolyte disturbances. Dehydration may worsen HE, lead to acute kidney injury, and precipitate hepatorenal syndrome. The dosages of lactulose in HE are 30 to 45 mL (20–30 g) 3 to 4 times daily. This amount should be titrated to produce 2 to 3 soft stools per day. Hourly doses should not be used to induce diarrhea as was common practice in years past, primarily because of the risk of exacerbating volume contraction and rapid shifts in electrolytes. A study of lactulose dosing at a large tertiary care center specialized in liver disease showed great variability in dosing of lactulose. Inpatient orders for lactulose were retrospectively reviewed for 1 year, with a total of 5107 orders. Inappropriate dosing in the form of standing orders, single-dose orders, and as-needed orders was noted, suggesting that a standardized dosing order set may help to prevent complications from inappropriate dosing.[61,84] Lactulose can be administered via enema when patients are too obtunded for oral intake. Enema administration can be difficult for nursing staff and has variable efficacy because of the variation in dwell times and the level of exposure to medication. It can, however, be a safe and effective method for obtunded patients if oral administration is not possible.

Reduction of ammonia levels by ammonia scavengers and activated charcoal

Intravenous sodium benzoate and sodium phenylacetate or the phenylacetate prodrug oral sodium phenylbutyrate can combine with glycine or glutamine to form water-soluble compounds excreted through the kidneys. The US Food and Drug Administration has not yet approved these agents for this use; they depend on normal renal function for ammonia excretion, and the large therapeutic doses confer a significant sodium load, which can increase fluid retention. Newer ammonia scavengers and orally ingested activated charcoal are being studied currently.[2,85] Glycerol phenylbutyrate (HPN-100) is a new compound that is a prodrug of sodium phenylbutyrate with much lower therapeutic doses needed. It is being evaluated for type C HE and has done well in trials for urea cycle disorders.

Orally ingested, activated charcoal is also being explored for the treatment of HE. AST-120 is a spherical carbon adsorbent being studied in patients with mild HE and patients with cirrhosis who have pruritus. The molecule adsorbs small molecules (ammonia, lipopolysaccharides, and cytokines), all of which may contribute to HE. A pilot study shows equal efficacy to lactulose and fewer adverse events.[77] In animal models, the administration of AST-120 caused a reduction in ammonia and cerebral edema. The AST-120 Used to Treat Hepatic Encephalopathy (ASTUTE) trial, a human study of AST-120 in patients with mild type C HE, has recently been completed and results are pending.

Modulation of fecal flora with oral antibiotics, prebiotics, probiotics, and acarbose
The gut microbiome plays a significant role in the pathogenesis of HE. The gut flora can be modified through antibiotics, probiotics, or prebiotics to alter the disease course. Prebiotics include lactulose and fermentable fibers and enhance the growth of bacterial strains that are potentially beneficial to the host and reduce more harmful flora, such as the urease producing species.[70,86,87] Probiotics are not as useful in OHE but have been used with some success in MHE. The species that are most efficacious are *Lactobacilli* and *Bifidobacteria.* Probiotics may also reduce bacterial translocation and subsequent endotoxemia and ameliorate the hyperdynamic circulation.

Oral antibiotics have proven efficacy in treating OHE by reducing the number of ammonia-producing bacteria present in the gut. Neomycin has been used, but because of concerns over nephrotoxicity and ototoxicity of aminoglycosides, the use of this medication has been limited. This toxicity is considered cumulative such that hearing loss, in particular, can occur slowly over time and is not reversible. The doses of neomycin used in most clinical trials was 3 to 4 g daily, which is much higher than what most clinicians are accustomed to using in practice. Similarly, metronidazole is effective in treating HE but concerns over resistance and peripheral neuropathy have limited its use.[88,89] Paromomycin and vancomycin have also been used but there are concerns with their long-term use and bacterial resistance.

Acarbose, an α-glucosidase inhibitor, may be useful in the treatment of HE. By reducing glucose absorption from the gut, the survival of saccharolytic bacteria is favored over proteolytic bacteria, reducing the generation of ammonia. A randomized double-blind crossover trial of acarbose in patients with diabetes with mild HE showed a decrease in ammonia levels and improvement in HE grade. However, this data are not yet compelling enough to adopt the use of this compound.

Rifaximin

Rifaximin has low systemic bioavailability, is concentrated in the GI tract, and has broad-spectrum in vitro activity against gram-positive and gram-negative aerobic and anaerobic enteric bacteria, with a low risk of bacterial resistance, making it a better choice for long-term treatment.[90–92] Its preferred site of action is the small bowel because it has enhanced solubility in bile. In the small bowel, it lowers the bacterial load 100 to 1000 fold, but it is less effective in the colon. One possible mechanism of action of rifaximin in HE is the correction of small intestinal bacterial overgrowth. The benefit of antibiotics may result from the change in bowel flora, their antiinflammatory effects, or downregulation of intestinal glutaminase activity. Rifaximin has been shown to be more efficacious than nonabsorbable disaccharides and equivalent efficacy to other antibiotics used in the treatment of acute HE. It has also been shown to improve health-related quality of life (HRQOL). In an assessment of 219 patients randomized to rifaximin or placebo, most of whom were on concomitant lactulose, Sanyal and colleagues[93,94] assessed quality of life. The Chronic Liver Disease Questionnaire was administered every 4 weeks and rifaximin significantly improved HRQOL in patients with cirrhosis and recurrent HE. A lower HRQOL may also predict recurrence of HE.[93,94] In the 299-patient randomized, double-blind, placebo-controlled, multinational phase 3 trial of rifaximin for remission from HE, Bass and colleagues[95] showed that rifaximin plus lactulose is superior to lactulose alone in the secondary prophylaxis of HE. The primary endpoint was the time to the first breakthrough episode of HE. The key secondary endpoint was the time to the first hospitalization involving

HE. Rifaximin significantly reduced the risk of an episode of OHE as compared with placebo over a 6-month period. The hazard ratio with rifaximin was 0.42, with a 95% confidence interval (CI) of 0.28 to 0.64, $P<.001$. In 22.1% of the rifaximin group versus 45.9% of the placebo group, a breakthrough episode of HE occurred. Hospitalizations involving HE occurred in 13.6% of the rifaximin group and 22.6% of the placebo group, with a hazard ratio of 0.50 (95% CI, 0.29–0.87). In both groups, more than 90% of patients received concomitant lactulose therapy. The number needed to treat (NNT) to prevent one episode of HE is 4 and the NNT to prevent one hospitalization is 9. Adverse events (AEs) and serious adverse events (SAEs) were similar in the 2 groups.[95] Of note, rifaximin has not been studied in patients with MELD scores greater than 25 and 9% of patients in the trial had MELD scores greater than 19. There is a slightly higher systemic exposure of the drug in patients with Child-Pugh C scores because of the biliary excretion of the drug. It is still a low exposure rate overall, and these patients can likely safely take the drug.

In an abstract presented at the 2011 EASL meeting, Mullen and colleagues[96] demonstrated the long-term efficacy and survival in patients treated with rifaximin for the maintenance of remission from OHE. This study was an open-label maintenance extension of the phase 3 trial by Bass and colleagues. The study included 322 patients: 70 from the RCT who continued rifaximin, 82 from the RCT who crossed over from the placebo arm, and 170 new patients. The average follow-up was 16 months, and some patients had up to 3 years of exposure. Across both the RCT and the current open-label study, the mean duration of drug exposure among rifaximin-treated patients was 476 days, for a total of 510 person-exposure years. HE event rates (number of events per person-exposure years of the study drug) ranged from 0.24 to 0.40 in patients on rifaximin to 1.6 in those on placebo. In a pooled analysis, rifaximin was associated with a significant reduction in rates of hospitalization for any cause (0.45 events per person-exposure years with rifaximin vs 1.31 with placebo; $P<.0001$) and rates of HE-related hospitalizations (0.21 vs 0.72, $P<.0001$). Rifaximin was associated with a lower AE rate compared with placebo (0.71 vs 2.8), lower drug-related AE rate (0.11 vs 0.74), lower SAE rate (0.48 vs 1.4), and lower rate of discontinuations caused by AEs (0.25 vs 0.98). Rifaximin was not associated with increased mortality rates.[96]

The results of a case-control study on the long-term administration of rifaximin for patients with alcohol-related decompensated cirrhosis were presented at the 2011 EASL meeting. Vlachigiannakos and colleagues[97] showed that in a population of patients with alcohol-related cirrhosis who had been abstinent from alcohol for at least 6 months, during a follow-up period of 5 years, HE occurred in 31.5% in the rifaximin group versus 47.0% in the placebo group ($P = .034$). More importantly, there were significantly fewer cases of portal hypertension-related events, such as variceal bleeds, spontaneous bacterial peritonitis, and hepatorenal syndrome. As a result, there was a significantly higher survival in patients treated with rifaximin. The probable mechanism of this change in portal hypertension-related events is caused by a change in gut-derived bacterial cytokines, with resultant changes in hepatic venous gradient pressures. Another study by Leise and colleagues[98] revealed a 2-year survival advantage in more than 300 patients with cirrhosis with moderate to severe HE treated with rifaximin compared with more than 6500 patients on the US transplant wait list. These studies need to be validated but are intriguing and may help further clarify the true mechanism of action of rifaximin.

Modulation of Neurotransmission

HE is associated with upregulation of GABA neuroinhibitory receptors and N-methyl-D-aspartic acid-glutamate excitatory receptors, resulting in confusion between inhibitory and excitatory signals. Trials have been completed with flumazenil, naloxone, bromocriptine, levodopa, and AChE inhibitors, but none have had a large degree of success. In comatose patients with HE and benzodiazepine or opiate ingestion, a trial of flumazenil or naloxone is appropriate, with careful monitoring for seizures.[99,100] A pilot study of the AChE inhibitor, rivastigmine, in patients with moderate HE demonstrated an improvement in psychometric testing.[32]

Protein Restriction

Dietary protein restriction was once thought to reduce the nitrogenous load entering the gut, thereby reducing ammonia production and absorption and subsequent HE. Protein restriction has now fallen out of favor as malnutrition from such restriction in patients with cirrhosis has occurred. An RCT of protein-restricted to normal-protein diets in patients with cirrhosis with HE revealed no difference in the course of HE in the 2 groups. Higher protein breakdown was documented in the protein-restricted group.[101] Because poor nutritional status is a risk factor for mortality in patients with cirrhosis, it is now recommended that patients with cirrhosis with HE be given regular-protein diets and medical therapy for HE.[101,102]

An abstract presented at the 2011 EASL meeting from Balzola and colleagues[103] suggested that a wheat- and milk-protein-free diet may be considered as an adjunctive treatment of HE. Diets free of wheat or milk proteins have been shown to reduce blood concentrations of exogenous opioid peptides, which have a direct central morphinelike action. In this prospective study, patients with untreatable chronic HE awaiting liver transplantation were given a normal-protein diet that was free of wheat and milk proteins. After 4 weeks, 87% of patients had consistent clinical improvement. After 3 months, complete resolution of HE was maintained in these patients. The significant improvements in global cognitive status with the diet were not associated with significant electroencephalographic (EEG) changes, and rechallenge with a wheat and milk diet led to an HE event in 1 patient.

Correction of Nutritional Deficiencies

Poor dietary absorption of fat-soluble vitamins; poor intake secondary to confusion, weakness, or ascites; and a baseline hypercatabolic state contribute to poor nutritional status in patients with cirrhosis. Zinc serves as a cofactor in the urea cycle; zinc deficiency, which is common in patients with cirrhosis, may decrease efficiency of the urea cycle. A randomized, open-label trial showed potential benefit in HE with zinc supplementation.[104]

Outside the United States, LOLA is frequently used for HE. LOLA is thought to act by supplying substrates for the urea cycle and glutamine synthesis that are sometimes depleted in patients with cirrhosis with protein malnutrition and amino acid deficiencies. A meta-analysis of 3 trials demonstrated significant benefit in patients with grades I to II HE.[105] L-ornithine phenylacetate (LOPA), or OCR-002, is similar to LOLA and is being developed and tested in HE. It may increase the amount of ornithine available in the urea cycle, enhancing the incorporation of ammonia into glutamine. Ammonia is scavenged by conjugating phenylacetate with glutamine to form phenylacetylglutamine, which is then excreted in the urine. A phase II trial will begin in 2011.[106]

The Fischer ratio is the balance between branched-chain amino acids (BCAA) and aromatic amino acids (AAA). The ratio is usually 3:1 in the healthy population but is reversed in patients with cirrhosis. BCAA, valine, leucine, and isoleucine are necessary for protein production and for the prevention of catabolism. The AAAs are precursors of false neurotransmitters, octopamine or phenylethylamine, and have been implicated in

HE because they can inhibit neurotransmission via the competitive blockade of receptors. Supplementing diets with BCAA may allow adequate protein intake, reduced catabolism, and muscle breakdown and prevent synthesis of false neurotransmitters. A meta-analysis of BCAA supplementation showed improved rate of recovery from episodic HE but no survival advantage.[107]

One Italian center has reported its experience with L-carnitine or acetyl-L-carnitine. A double-blind placebo-controlled RCT performed by this group demonstrated a significant improvement in EEG, cognitive deficits, and reduction of ammonia in the treated group for severe HE.[108]

Extracorporeal Liver Devices

The use of extracorporeal devices for liver dialysis is now being considered. The one system clinically available in the United States is the molecular adsorbent recirculating system (MARS, Gambro, Sweden), otherwise known as albumin dialysis, and is indicated for acute liver toxicity. An RCT in the United States for patients with severe HE not responding to standard care showed quicker improvements in HE but no benefit in mortality.[109–118] Bioartificial machines with hepatocytes have been studied for HE but are not currently available in the United States.

Shunting

Some patients with persistent HE despite removal of precipitating factors and treatment with currently available medical therapies may have extensive portosystemic shunting. These shunts may be embolized via percutaneous catheterization, but this is not yet commonplace in the United States.

SUMMARY

Given the many targets of treatment and lack of a clear singular cause of HE, there is no consensus on a single best treatment. In the case of MHE, there also lacks a clear set of diagnostic criteria that physicians currently adhere to. A major challenge in this area is the amount of time necessary to administer neuropsychological testing. The current management of HE requires accurate and prompt diagnosis, elimination of precipitating factors, and administration of pharmacologic therapy tailored to the particular patient. In episodic or mild persistent HE, nonabsorbable disaccharides (lactulose and lactitol) remain the most widely prescribed medications, although this practice is changing toward using rifaximin as the first-line therapy in many cases. The benefits of intestinal decontamination by rifaximin on endotoxemia and gut-derived cytokines may be much more profound than initially imagined, both in the treatment of HE and in other inflammatory issues related to cirrhosis. Ammonia scavengers are useful for patients intolerant to lactulose or antibiotics or as adjunctive treatment in those already on lactulose and rifaximin. Nutritional supplementation with zinc or L-carnitine may be useful. AST-120, LOPA, acarbose, and rivastigmine are still under investigation. Patients with OHE should be considered for liver transplantation. The treatment of HE is currently a burgeoning area of interest. Over the last several years, high-quality studies have been conducted on the various pharmacologic therapies for HE, and as more data emerge, it is hoped that HE will become a much more easily treated complication of decompensated liver disease. In the interim, it is important that physicians continue to screen for MHE and treat patients early in addition to continuing to provide current treatments for OHE.

REFERENCES

1. Voight M, Conn H. Hepatic encephalopathy. In: Robson SC, Trey C, Kirsch RE (editors). Diagnosis and management of liver disease. Chapman & Hall, London, p. 140–147, Chapter 13.
2. Frederick RT. Current concepts in the pathophysiology and management of hepatic encephalopathy. Gastroenterol Hepatol 2011;7(4):222–33.
3. Ferenci P, Lockwood A, Mullen K, et al. Hepatic encephalopathy – definition, nomenclature, diagnosis and quantification: final report of the working party at the 11th World Congresses of Gastroenterology, Vienna 1998. Hepatology 2002;35:716–21.
4. Poordad FF. Review article: the burden of hepatic encephalopathy. Aliment Pharmacol Ther 2007;25(Suppl 1):3–9.
5. Romero-Gomez M, Boza F, Garcia-Valdecasas MS, et al. Subclinical hepatic encephalopathy predicts the development of overt hepatic encephalopathy. Am J Gastroenterol 2001;96:2718–23.
6. Boyer TD, Haskal ZJ. American Association for the Study of Liver Diseases. The role of transjugular intrahepatic portosystemic shunt in the management of portal hypertension. Hepatology 2005;41:386–400.
7. Bajaj JS, Heuman DM, Wade JB, et al. Rifaximin improves driving simulator performance in a randomized trial of patients with minimal hepatic encephalopathy. Gastroenterology 2011;140:478–87.
8. Riordan SM, Williams R. Gut flora and hepatic encephalopathy in patients with cirrhosis. N Engl J Med 2010;362(12):1140–1.
9. Leevy CB, Phillips JA. Hospitalizations during the use of rifaximin versus lactulose for the treatment of hepatic encephalopathy. Dig Dis Sci 2007;52:737–41.
10. Bajaj JS, Wade JB, Gibson DP, et al. The multi-dimensional burden of cirrhosis and hepatic encephalopathy on patients and caregivers. Am J Gastroenterol 2011;106:1646–53.
11. Higginson IJ, Gao W, Jackson D, et al. Short-form Zarit caregiver burden interviews were valid in advanced conditions. J Clin Epidemiol 2010;63:535–42.
12. Bustamante J, Rimola A, Ventura PJ, et al. Prognostic significance of hepatic encephalopathy in patients with cirrhosis. J Hepatol 1999;30:890–5.
13. Stewart CA, Malinchoc M, Kim WR, et al. Hepatic encephalopathy as a predictor of survival in patients with end-stage liver disease. Liver Transpl 2007;13:1366–71.
14. Bajaj JS, Schubert CM, Sanyal AJ, et al. Severity of chronic cognitive impairment in cirrhosis increases with number of episodes of overt hepatic encephalopathy. J Hepatol 2010;52(Suppl 1):S66.
15. Bajaj JS, Schubert CM, Heuman DM, et al. Persistence of cognitive impairment after resolution of overt hepatic encephalopathy. Gastroenterology 2010;138(7):2332–40.
16. Fichet J, Mercier E, Genee O, et al. Prognosis and 1-year mortality of intensive care unit patients with severe hepatic encephalopathy. J Crit Care 2009;24:364–70.
17. Phear EA, Sherlock S. Summer skill WH. Blood-ammonium levels in liver disease and hepatic coma. Lancet 1955;268:836–40.
18. Conn HO, Lieberthal MM. The hepatic coma syndromes and lactulose. Baltimore (MD): Williams & Wilkins; 1979.
19. Olde Damink SW, Jalan R, Redhead DN, et al. Interorgan ammonia and amino acid metabolism in metabolically stable patients with cirrhosis and a TIPSS. Hepatology 2002;36:1163–71.

20. Romero-Gomez M, Ramos-Guerrero R, Grande L, et al. Intestinal glutaminase activity is increased in liver cirrhosis and correlates with minimal hepatic encephalopathy. J Hepatol 2004;41:49–54.
21. Haussinger D, Sies H, Gerok W. Functional hepatocyte heterogeneity in ammonia metabolism. The intercellular glutamine cycle. J Hepatol 1985;1:3–14.
22. Vinay P, Kemieux G, Gougoux A, et al. Regulation of glutamine metabolism in dog kidney in vivo. Kidney Int 1986;29:68–79.
23. Tizianello A, Deferrari G, Garibotto G, et al. Renal ammoniagenesis in an early stage of metabolic acidosis in man. J Clin Invest 1982;69:240–50.
24. Tizianello A, Deferrari G, Garibotto G, et al. Renal ammoniagenesis during the adaptation to metabolic acidosis in man. Contrib Nephrol 1988;63:105–13.
25. Olde Damink SW, Jalan R, Deutz NE, et al. The kidney plays a major role in the hyperammonemia seen after simulated or actual GI bleeding in patients with cirrhosis. Hepatology 2003;37:1277–85.
26. Donovan JP, Schafer DF, Shaw BW Jr, et al. Cerebral edema and increased intracranial pressure in chronic liver disease. Lancet 1998;351:719–21.
27. Kavitt RT, Yang VL, Jensen DM. Cerebral edema and hyperammonemia after transjugular intrahepatic portosystemic shunt placement in a cirrhotic patient. Clin Gastroenterol Hepatol 2008;6:1054–6.
28. Norenberg MD, Itzhak Y, Bender AS. The peripheral benzodiazepine receptor and neurosteroids in hepatic encephalopathy. Adv Exp Med Biol 1997;420: 95–111.
29. Mullen KD, Szauter KM, Kaminsky-Russ K. "Endogenous" benzodiazepine activity in body fluids of patients with hepatic encephalopathy. Lancet 1990; 336:81–3.
30. Garcia-Ayllon MS, Cauli O, Silveyra MX, et al. Brain cholinergic impairment in liver failure. Brain 2008;131:2946–56.
31. Mendez M, Mendez-Lopez M, Lopez L, et al. Acetylcholinesterase activity in an experimental rat model of type C hepatic encephalopathy. Acta Histochem 2011;113:358–62.
32. Basu P, Shah NJ, Krishnaswamy N, et al. Transdermal rivastigmine for treatment of encephalopathy in liver cirrhosis – a randomized placebo controlled trial (TREC TRIAL). J Hepatol 2010;52(Suppl 1):S67–8.
33. Guevara M, Baccaro ME, Torre A, et al. Hyponatremia is a risk factor of hepatic encephalopathy in patients with cirrhosis: a prospective study with time-dependent analysis. Am J Gastroenterol 2009;104:1382–9.
34. Angeli P, Wong F, Watson H, et al. CAPPS investigators. Hyponatremia in cirrhosis: results of a patient population survey. Hepatology 2006;44:1535–42.
35. Vaquero J, Chung C, Blei AT. Brain edema in acute liver failure. A window to the pathogenesis of hepatic encephalopathy. Ann Hepatol 2003;2:12–22.
36. Blei AT. Infection, inflammation, and hepatic encephalopathy, synergism redefined. J Hepatol 2004;40:327–30.
37. Pedersen HR, Ring-Larsen H, Olsen NV, et al. Hyperammonemia acts synergistically with lipopolysaccharide in inducing changes in cerebral hemodynamics in rats anaesthetized with pentobarbital. J Hepatol 2007;47:245–52.
38. Perez del Pulgar S, Pizcueta P, Engel P, et al. Enhanced monocyte activation and hepatotoxicity in response to endotoxin in portal hypertension. J Hepatol 2000;32:25–31.
39. Lumsden AB, Henderson JM, Kutner MH. Endotoxin levels measured by a chromogenic assay in portal, hepatic, and peripheral blood in patients with cirrhosis. Hepatology 1988;8:232–6.

40. Kalambokis GN, Tsianos EV. Rifaximin reduces endotoxemia and improves liver function and disease severity in patients with decompensated cirrhosis. Hepatology 2012;55:655–6.
41. Tilg H, Wilmer A, Vogel W, et al. Serum levels of cytokines in chronic liver diseases. Gastroenterology 1992;103:264–74.
42. Garcia-Tsao G. Gut microflora in the pathogenesis of the complications of cirrhosis. Best Pract Res Clin Gastroenterol 2004;18:353–72.
43. Kalambokis G, Tsianos EV. Endotoxaemia in the pathogenesis of cytopenias in liver cirrhosis. Could simple antibiotics raise blood counts? Med Hypotheses 2011;76:105–9.
44. Kalambokis GN, Mouzaki A, Rodi M, et al. Rifaximin improves thrombocytopenia in patients with alcoholic cirrhosis in association with reduction of endotoxaemia. Liver Int 2012;32:467–75.
45. McGrath KM, Stuart JJ, Richards F II. Correlation between serum IgG, platelet membrane IgG, and platelet function in hypergammaglobulinemic states. Br J Haematol 1979;42:585–91.
46. Kajihara M, Jato S, Okazaki Y, et al. A role of autoantibody-mediated platelet destruction in thrombocytopenia in patients with cirrhosis. Hepatology 2003; 37:1267–76.
47. Violi F, Ferri D, Basili S, et al. Association between low-grade disseminated intravascular coagulation and endotoxemia in patients with liver cirrhosis. Gastroenterology 1995;109:531–9.
48. Schwager I, Jungi TW. Effect of human recombinant cytokines on the induction of macrophages procoagulant activity. Blood 1994;83:152–60.
49. Cordoba J, Blei AT. Hepatic encephalopathy. In: Schiff ER, Sorrell MF, Maddrey WC, editors. Schiff's diseases of the liver, vol. 1, 10th edition. Philadelphia: Lippincott Williams & Wilkins; 2007. p. 569–99.
50. Hassanein T, Blei AT, Perry W, et al. Performance of the hepatic encephalopathy scoring algorithm in a clinical trial of patients with cirrhosis and severe hepatic encephalopathy. Am J Gastroenterol 2009;104:1392–400.
51. Williams R, James OF, Morgan MY. Evaluation of the efficacy and safety of rifaximin in the treatment of hepatic encephalopathy: a double-blind, randomized, dose-finding multi-centre study. Eur J Gastroenterol Hepatol 2000;12: 203–8.
52. Conn HO, Leevy CM, Vlahcevic ZR, et al. Comparison of lactulose and neomycin in the treatment of chronic portal-systemic-encephalopathy: a double blind controlled trial. Gastroenterology 1977;72:573–83.
53. Weissenborn K, Ennen JC, Schomerus H, et al. Neuropsychological characterization of hepatic encephalopathy. J Hepatol 2001;34:768–73.
54. Schomerus H, Hamster W. Quality of life in cirrhotics with minimal hepatic encephalopathy. Metab Brain Dis 2001;16:37–41.
55. Stewart CA, Smith GE. Minimal hepatic encephalopathy. Nat Clin Pract Gastroenterol Hepatol 2007;4(12):677–85.
56. McCrea M, Cordoba J, Vessey M, et al. Neuropsychological characterization and detection of subclinical hepatic encephalopathy. Arch Neurol 1996;53(8): 758–63.
57. Weissenborn K, Scholz M, Hinrichs H, et al. Neurophysiological characterization of hepatic encephalopathy. J Hepatol 2001;34:768–73.
58. Quero JC, Schalm SW. Subclinical hepatic encephalopathy. Semin Liver Dis 1996;16:321–8.
59. Kamath PS. The need for better clinical trials. Hepatology 2008;48:1–3.

60. Bajaj JS, Etemadian A, Hafeezullah M, et al. Testing for minimal hepatic encephalopathy in the United States: an AASLD survey. Hepatology 2007;45:833–4.
61. Blei AT, Cordoba J. Practice Parameters Committee of the American College of Gastroenterology. Hepatic encephalopathy. Am J Gastroenterol 2001;96: 1968–76.
62. Riordan SM, Williams R. Treatment of hepatic encephalopathy. N Engl J Med 1997;337(7):473–9.
63. Munoz SJ. Hepatic encephalopathy. Med Clin North Am 2008;92:795–812.
64. Caruana P, Shah N. Hepatic encephalopathy: are NH_4 levels and protein restriction obsolete? Pract Gastroenterol 2011;95:6–18.
65. Morgan MY, Blei A, Grungreiff K, et al. The treatment of hepatic encephalopathy. Metab Brain Dis 2007;22:389–405.
66. Als-Nielsen B, Gluud LL, Gluud C. Non-absorbable disaccharides for hepatic encephalopathy: systematic review of randomized trials. BMJ 2004;328:1046.
67. Sotil EU, Gottstein J, Ayala E, et al. Impact of preoperative overt hepatic encephalopathy on neurocognitive function after liver transplantation. Liver Transpl 2009;15:184–92.
68. Bass NM. Review article the current pharmacological therapies for hepatic encephalopathy. Aliment Pharmacol Ther 2007;25(Suppl 1):23–31.
69. Watanabe A, Sakai T, Sato S. Clinical efficacy of lactulose in cirrhotic patients with and without subclinical hepatic encephalopathy. Hepatology 1997;26:1410–4.
70. Sidhu SS, Goyal O, Mishra BP, et al. Rifaximin improves psychometric performance and health-related quality of life in patients with minimal hepatic encephalopathy (The RIME Trial). Am J Gastroenterol 2011;106(2):307–16.
71. Mcphail MJ, Leech R, Grover VP, et al. Functional core modulation following treatment of minimal hepatic encephalopathy with l-ornithine l-aspartate: a potential novel mechanism of action. 46th annual meeting of the european-association-for-the-study-of-the-liver (EASL) 2011;54:S74–5.
72. Devrajani BR, Shah SZ, Devrajani T, et al. Precipitating factors of hepatic encephalopathy at a tertiary care hospital Jamshoro, Hyderabad. J Pak Med Assoc 2009;59:683–6.
73. Strauss E, Gomes de Sa Ribeiro Mde F. Bacterial infections associated with hepatic encephalopathy: prevalence and outcome. Ann Hepatol 2003;2: 41–5.
74. Zushi S, Imai Y, Fukuda K, et al. Endoscopic coagulation therapy is successful for improving encephalopathy in cirrhotic patients with gastric antral vascular ectasia. Dig Endosc 2005;17:32–5.
75. Jalan R, Kapoor D. Enhanced renal ammonia excretion following volume expansion in patients with well compensated cirrhosis of the liver. Gut 2003;52: 1041–5.
76. Pockros P, Hassanein T, Vierling J, et al. Phase 2, multicenter, randomized study of AST-120 (spherical carbon adsorbent) vs. lactulose in the treatment of low-grade hepatic encephalopathy. J Hepatol 2009;50(Supp 1):S43–4.
77. Kramer L, Tribl B, Gendo A, et al. Partial pressure of ammonia versus ammonia in hepatic encephalopathy. Hepatology 2000;31:30–4.
78. Ong JP, Aggarwal A, Krieger D, et al. Correlation between ammonia levels and the severity of hepatic encephalopathy. Am J Med 2003;114:188–93.
79. Plauth M, Roske AE, Romaniuk P, et al. Post-feeding hyperammonaemia in patients with transjugular intrahepatic portosystemic shunt and liver cirrhosis: role of small intestinal ammonia release and route of nutrient administration. Gut 2000;46:849–55.

80. Weissenborn K, Tietge UJ, Bokemeyer M, et al. Liver transplantation improves hepatic myelopathy: evidence by three cases. Gastroenterology 2003;124: 346–51.
81. Als-Nielsen B, Gluud LL, Gluud C. Nonabsorbable disaccharides for hepatic encephalopathy. Cochrane Database Syst Rev 2004;2:CD003044.
82. Sharma BC, Sharma P, Agrawal A, et al. Secondary prophylaxis of hepatic encephalopathy: an open label randomized controlled trial of lactulose versus placebo. Gastroenterology 2009;137:885–91.
83. Lukers B, Nierman DM, Schiano TD. Lactulose: how many ways can one drug be prescribed? Am J Gastroenterol 2011;106(9):1726–7.
84. Bass N. Treatment of patients with hepatic encephalopathy: review of the latest data from EASL 2011. Gastroenterol Hepatol 2011;7(Suppl 9):1–15.
85. Malaguarnera M, Gargante MP, Malaguarnera G, et al. Bifidobacterium combined with fructo-oligosaccharide versus lactulose in the treatment of patients with hepatic encephalopathy. Eur J Gastroenterol Hepatol 2010;22:199–206.
86. Iwasa M, Nakao M, Kato Y, et al. Dietary fiber decreases ammonia levels in patients with cirrhosis. Hepatology 2005;41:217–8 [author reply: 219].
87. Liu Q, Duan ZP, Ha DK, et al. Synbiotic modulation of gut flora: effect on minimal hepatic encephalopathy in patients with cirrhosis. Hepatology 2004;39: 1441–9.
88. Seyan AS, Hughes RD, Shawcross DL. Changing face of hepatic encephalopathy: role of inflammation and oxidative stress. World J Gastroenterol 2010;16: 3347–57.
89. Gentile S, Guarino G, Romano M, et al. A randomized controlled trial of acarbose in hepatic encephalopathy. Clin Gastroenterol Hepatol 2005;3:184–91.
90. Gerard L, Garey KW, DuPont HL. Rifaximin: a nonabsorbable rifamycin antibiotic for use in nonsystemic gastrointestinal infections. Expert Rev Anti Infect Ther 2005;3:201–11.
91. Jiang ZD, DuPont HL. Rifaximin: in vitro and in vivo antibacterial activity – a review. Chemotherapy 2005;51(Suppl 1):67–72.
92. Debbia EA, Maioli E, Roveta S, et al. Effects of rifaximin on bacterial virulence mechanisms at supra-and sub-inhibitory concentrations. J Chemother 2008; 20:186–94.
93. Sanyal A, Younossi ZM, Bass NM, et al. Randomised clinical trial: rifaximin improves health-related quality of life in cirrhotic patients with hepatic encephalopathy – a double-blind placebo-controlled study. Aliment Pharmacol Ther 2011;34:853–61.
94. Sanyal A, Bass N, Mullen K, et al. Rifaximin treatment improved quality of life in patients with hepatic encephalopathy: results of a large, randomized, placebo-controlled trial. J Hepatol 2010;52(Suppl 1):S7.
95. Bass NM, Mullen KD, Sanyal A, et al. Rifaximin treatment in hepatic encephalopathy. N Engl J Med 2010;362:1071–81.
96. Mullen KD, Poordad F, Rossaro L, et al. Long term efficacy and survival in patients treated with the gut-selective antibiotic rifaximin (550 mg BID) for the maintenance of remission from overt hepatic encephalopathy. Gastroenterol Hepatol 2011;7(6 Suppl 9):1–15.
97. Vlachogiannakos K, Viazis N, Vasianopoulou P, et al. Long-term administration of rifaximin improves the prognosis of patients with alcohol-related decompensated cirrhosis: a case-control study. Hepatology 2010;52:328A.
98. Leise MD, Pedersen R, Kamath PS, et al. Impact of rifaximin treatment on survival in patients with end-stage liver disease. Hepatology 2010;52:331A.

99. Jiang Q, Jiang G, Welty TE, et al. Naloxone in the management of hepatic encephalopathy. J Clin Pharm Ther 2010;35:333–41.
100. Als-Nielsen B, Gluud LL, Gluud C. Benzodiazepine receptor antagonists for hepatic encephalopathy. Cochrane Database Syst Rev 2004;2:CD002798.
101. Cordoba J, Lopez-Hellin J, Planas M, et al. Normal protein diet for episodic hepatic encephalopathy: results of a randomized study. J Hepatol 2004;41: 38–43.
102. Bajaj JS. Review article: the modern management of hepatic encephalopathy. Aliment Pharmacol Ther 2010;31(5):537–47.
103. Balzola F, Sanna C, Ottobrelli A, et al. Chronic hepatic encephalopathy (HE) in patients with severe liver cirrhosis: efficacy of the wheat and milk protein free diet in the reduction of clinical episodes. Gastroenterol Hepatol 2011; 7(6 Suppl 9):1–15.
104. Takuma Y, Nouso K, Makino Y, et al. Clinical trial: oral zinc in hepatic encephalopathy. Aliment Pharmacol Ther 2010;32:1080–90.
105. Jiang Q, Jiang XH, Zheng MH, et al. L-ornithine-l-aspartate in the management of hepatic encephalopathy: a meta-analysis. J Gastroenterol Hepatol 2009;24:9–14.
106. Ocera therapeutics completes first in human studies with OCR-002 for the treatment of hyperammonemia and hepatic encephalopathy. San Diego, CA: Ocera; 2010.
107. Als-Nielsen B, Koretz RL, Kjaergard L, et al. Branched-chain amino acids for hepatic encephalopathy. Cochrane Database Syst Rev 2003;2:CD001939.
108. Malaguarnera M, Vacante M, Motta M, et al. Acetyl-L-carnitine improves cognitive functions in severe hepatic encephalopathy: a randomized and controlled clinical trial. Metab Brain Dis 2011;26:281–9.
109. Hassanein TI, Tofteng F, Brown RS Jr, et al. Randomized controlled study of extracorporeal albumin dialysis for hepatic encephalopathy in advanced cirrhosis. Hepatology 2007;46:1853–62.
110. Riggio O, Masini A, Efrati C, et al. Pharmacological prophylaxis of hepatic encephalopathy after transjugular intrahepatic portosystemic shunt: a randomized controlled study. J Hepatol 2005;42(5):674–9.
111. Kanematsu T, Koyanagi N, Matsumata T, et al. Lack of preventive effect of branched-chain amino acid solution on postoperative hepatic encephalopathy in patients with cirrhosis: a randomized, prospective trial. Surgery 1988;104(3): 482–8.
112. Rolachon A, Zarski JP, Lutz JM, et al. Is the intestinal lavage with a solution of mannitol effective in the prevention of post-hemorrhagic hepatic encephalopathy in patients with liver cirrhosis? Results of a randomized prospective study. Gastroenterol Clin Biol 1994;18(12):1057–62.
113. Uribe M, Campollo O, Vargas F, et al. Acidifying enemas (lactitol and lactose) vs. nonacidifying enemas (tap water) to treat acute portal-systemic encephalopathy: a double-blind, randomized clinical trial. Hepatology 1987;7(4):639–43.
114. Kircheis G, Nilius R, Held C, et al. Therapeutic efficacy of L-ornithine-L-aspartate infusions in patients with cirrhosis and hepatic encephalopathy: results of a placebo-controlled, double-blind study. Hepatology 1997;25(6):1351–60.
115. Stauch S, Kircheis G, Adler G, et al. Oral L-ornithine-L-aspartate therapy of chronic hepatic encephalopathy: results of a placebo-controlled double-blind study. J Hepatol 1998;28(5):856–64.
116. Sushma S, Dasarathy S, Tandon RK, et al. Sodium benzoate in the treatment of acute hepatic encephalopathy: a double-blind randomized trial. Hepatology 1992;16(1):138–44.

117. Reding P, Duchateau J, Bataille C. Oral zinc supplementation improves hepatic encephalopathy. Results of a randomized controlled trial. Lancet 1984;2(8401): 493–5.
118. Riggio O, Ariosto F, Merli M, et al. Short-term oral zinc supplementation does not improve chronic hepatic encephalopathy. Results of a double-blind crossover trial. Dig Dis Sci 1991;36(9):1204–8.

Shortness of Breath in the Patient with Chronic Liver Disease

Paul Y. Kwo, MD

KEYWORDS

- Dyspnea • Hepatopulmonary syndrome
- Portopulmonary hypertension • Shortness of breath • Cirrhosis
- Hydrothorax

Over the past 40 years, hepatology has grown exponentially with worldwide recognition of the burden of chronic liver disease, including alcoholic liver disease, hepatitis B, hepatitis C, and nonalcoholic fatty liver disease all contributing to a large burden of those with chronic liver disease, end-stage liver disease, and hepatocellular carcinoma.[1,2] Although many new therapeutic options now exist for many of these diseases, patients may present with clinical manifestations of chronic liver disease before detection by routine laboratory testing. Moreover, even in those with known liver disease, extrahepatic complications of chronic liver disease are also common, and clinicians should be familiar with these presentations and develop an approach to evaluate, diagnose, and treat these complications.

One common complaint of patients with chronic liver disease is shortness of breath, or dyspnea. Dyspnea has a broad differential diagnosis, with more than 30 attributable causes involving different organ systems.[3] Moreover, the prevalence of dyspnea is common in both general medicine clinics and emergency clinics. Multiple comorbidities that are common in those with chronic liver disease may also be associated with dyspnea, including older age, smoking, morbid obesity, and female gender.

DIFFERENTIAL DIAGNOSIS

The differential diagnosis of shortness of breath is broad, but in general may be divided into pulmonary and nonpulmonary causes. Besides the classic causes (pneumonia, reactive airway disease, bronchitis, chronic obstructive pulmonary disease), the pulmonary causes commonly seen in those with chronic liver disease include the pulmonary vascular complications portopulmonary hypertension and hepatopulmonary syndrome (hepatopulmonary shunts). Because cirrhosis is also associated

---

Potential conflicts: None.
Gastroenterology/Hepatology Division, Indiana University School of Medicine, 975 West Walnut, IB 327, Indianapolis, IN 46202-5121, USA
E-mail address: pkwo@iupui.edu

Clin Liver Dis 16 (2012) 321–329
doi:10.1016/j.cld.2012.03.007 liver.theclinics.com

with a systemic vasodilated state and high cardiac output, pulmonary edema and volume overload may also be a parenchymal pulmonary cause of shortness of breath in the patient with liver disease.[4] A hepatic hydrothorax or ascites causing abdominal distention is commonly seen in those with chronic liver disease with cirrhosis and decompensation, and ascites is the most common initial presenting sign of decompensated liver disease. Anemia, primarily from portal hypertension-related blood loss in those with chronic liver disease, may be a common cause of shortness of breath in those with cirrhosis.

In a patient with dyspnea, 3 diseases are well known to affect both the lung and liver. Patients with the genetic disorder α1-antitrypsin deficiency may present with end-stage liver disease and/or may develop pulmonary complications, including emphysema and others.[5] Cystic fibrosis is a genetic disorder whereby patients may present with portal hypertension resulting from the classic lesion focal biliary cirrhosis, as well as the more widely recognized pulmonary complications.[6] Lastly, patients with sarcoidosis may present with both pulmonary and hepatic complications.[7]

PHYSICAL EXAMINATION IN A PATIENT WITH LIVER DISEASE AND SHORTNESS OF BREATH

The head examination should include a careful examination for scleral icterus and conjunctival pallor, which may help assess the severity of liver disease as well as determine whether an occult anemia is contributing to the shortness of breath. The presence of xanthelasma over the eyelids and telangiectasias also suggest advanced liver disease, and cyanosis of the lips suggests hypoxemia. The lung examination should assess the quality of breath sounds, looking for the presence of rales, decreased breaths sounds (a hepatic hydrothorax may be found in the right lung greater than two-thirds of the time), or other breath sounds including wheezes and rhonchi, which may be seen in an individual with bronchitis and/or chronic obstructive pulmonary disease. The cardiac examination should carefully assess for the presence of jugular venous distension and hepatojugular reflux. The heart tones should assess for the presence of a gallop or murmur that may be found in anemia, or an increased second heart sound (P_2) that may be recognized in those with portopulmonary hypertension. On abdominal examination, in addition to assessing for the presence or absence of hepatomegaly and splenomegaly or a small liver, one should also assess for ascites and a caput medusa, again providing further evidence of portal hypertension and suggesting more advanced liver disease. The extremity examination may show pedal edema, as well as clubbing and cyanosis of the digits, which may be seen with hepatopulmonary syndrome, portopulmonary hypertension, and other pulmonary complications of liver disease.

LABORATORY TESTS IN A PATIENT WITH DYSPNEA

Laboratory testing should include a complete blood count (CBC) to look for the presence of anemia as well as low platelet and white blood cell count, which may be seen with hypersplenism. Electrolytes, blood urea, nitrogen, and creatinine are important, particularly if diuretic therapy will be a therapeutic option. Thyroid-stimulating hormone is also important, as hypothyroidism may also contribute to dyspnea. Additional studies that are essential in the patient with shortness of breath include a plain chest (posterior/anterior chest) radiograph, looking for evidence of parenchymal pulmonary disease, including pulmonary congestion, pulmonary infiltrates suggestive of pneumonia, or pulmonary nodules in the presence or absence of effusions. If a chest radiograph demonstrates infiltrates in a patient with liver disease, a careful history should be obtained in patients with hepatitis C to see if they have recently received interferon therapy. Particularly at higher doses, interferon has been associated with the development of interstitial lung disease.[8] In addition, certain drugs, including amiodarone, are associated with both liver and pulmonary toxicity.[9] Lastly, an arterial blood gas on room air (typically supine) should be obtained to assess for the presence or absence of hypoxemia.

PULMONARY VASCULAR COMPLICATIONS OF CHRONIC LIVER DISEASE

The 2 primary pulmonary vascular consequences of chronic liver disease include hepatopulmonary syndrome (HPS), which is primarily a gas-exchange disorder characterized by arteriolar hypoxemia, and portopulmonary hypertension (PPH), which is primarily a hemodynamic disorder associated with pulmonary hypertension and right-sided heart failure. The hepatopulmonary syndrome is characterized by a classic triad of chronic liver disease, hypoxemia defined by an alveolar arterial oxygen gradient exceeding 15 mm Hg or PaO_2 on room air of less than 80 mm Hg, and evidence of pulmonary vascular dilation.[10] The prevalence of hepatopulmonary syndrome has been reported to range from 5% to 32% based on data primarily from liver transplant centers, and it has been postulated that the prevalence differences are a function of varying cutoffs for arteriolar-alveolar gradients used to define gas-exchange abnormalities.[11] The clinical presentation of hepatopulmonary syndrome is typically an individual with cirrhosis who presents with dyspnea and is found to have hypoxemia. Individuals may present with cyanosis, finger clubbing, and clinically significant hypoxemia. In addition, the hypoxemia may worsen when the patient moves from a supine to an upright position (orthodeoxia), which produces the clinical symptom of platypnea, or worsening shortness of breath on standing. This condition is a reflection of increased perfusion of the lung bases, where vascular dilation predominates in hepatopulmonary syndrome, leading to worsening oxygen exchange, reduced PaO_2, and the increased subjective feeling of shortness of breath. The diagnostic criteria for hepatopulmonary syndrome are shown in **Box 1**.

Hepatopulmonary syndrome occurs most commonly in those who have established cirrhosis and portal hypertension. The etiology of liver disease does not seem to affect the development of hepatopulmonary syndrome. Moreover, hepatopulmonary syndrome has been reported in those with noncirrhotic portal hypertension, Budd-Chiari syndrome, and acute or chronic liver disease, without evidence of cirrhosis or portal hypertension. The prognosis of hepatopulmonary syndrome is poor, with mortality rates

Box 1
Criteria for the hepatopulmonary syndrome

1. Partial pressure of oxygen <80 mm Hg or alveolar-arterial oxygen gradient $\geq$15 mm Hg
2. Pulmonary vascular dilatation shunting on contrast-enhanced echocardiography or abnormal uptake in the brain (>6%) with radioactive lung-perfusion scanning (rarely done)
3. Portal hypertension (most common) with or without cirrhosis

Degree of Severity:

Mild: partial pressure of oxygen (PaO_2) $\geq$80 mm Hg

Moderate: PaO_2 $\geq$60 to <80 mm Hg

Severe: PaO_2 $\geq$50 to <60 mm Hg

Very severe: PaO_2 <50 mm Hg (<300 mm Hg while the patient is breathing 100% oxygen) of 41% being reported within a mean observation period of 2 to 5 years. The pathogenesis of hepatopulmonary syndrome is related primarily to portal hypertension, which leads to increased production of nitric oxide as a key factor for the development of pulmonary vascular dilation. However, the exact role of nitric oxide remains unclear. The use of nitric oxide inhibitors to treat hepatopulmonary syndrome have had varying outcomes, with inhibitors of nitric oxide both improving and having no effect on arterial oxygenation in the setting of well-documented hepatopulmonary syndrome.[12,13]

The diagnosis of hepatopulmonary syndrome is most commonly obtained through the use of contrast-enhanced transthoracic echocardiography with saline (bubble echo), whereby agitated saline (which produces microbubbles >10 μm in diameter) are administered in a peripheral vein in the arm.[14] The appearance of agitated saline in the left atrium within 3 to 6 beats after right atrial appearance indicates that the agitated saline has passed through the arteriovenous malformations in the pulmonary vasculature without absorption, as under normal circumstances without pulmonary vascular dilation, the microbubbles typically will not pass through a normal pulmonary capillary. An additional method less commonly used is technetium-labeled macroaggregated albumin with quantitative uptake in the brain. Here, tracer activity is demonstrated in both lungs but again, because of the pulmonary vascular dilation, uptake will also be seen in the brain. Typically the normal uptake in the brain is less than 6%, and values greater than this suggest the presence of pulmonary vascular dilation. In rare circumstances, pulmonary angiography may also be used to supplement the diagnosis in those with severe hypoxemia, whereby the possibility of embolizing arteriovenous communications to improve oxygen exchange may be undertaken.

TREATMENT OF HEPATOPULMONARY SYNDROME

There are currently no effective medical therapies for hepatopulmonary syndrome, and orthotopic liver transplant remains the only successful therapy although anecdotal reports have suggested that methylene blue, which inhibits nitric oxide, may be of benefit.[15] Resolution of hypoxemia after transplantation has been shown to be directly related to the severity of hypoxemia before transplantation. Thus, in those with end-stage liver disease and a diagnosis of hepatopulmonary syndrome associated with a PaO_2 of less than 60 mm Hg may be offered an orthotopic liver transplant, and these individuals are given a model for end-stage liver disease (MELD exceptions) score of 22 points, similar to selected patients with hepatocellular carcinoma.[16] Thus, once the diagnosis of hepatopulmonary syndrome is made, referral for orthotopic liver transplant is mandatory because of the poor prognosis.

PORTOPULMONARY HYPERTENSION

Portopulmonary hypertension is defined by the presence of raised pulmonary arterial pressure (mean pulmonary artery pressure >25 mm Hg at rest, >30 mm Hg during exercise), raised pulmonary vascular resistance (240 dyne/s/cm^5) in the presence of a normal pulmonary capillary wedge pressure of less than 15 mm Hg (**Table 1**).[17] Previously, portal pulmonary hypertension was classified as a secondary pulmonary hypertension but now is recognized as a primary pulmonary arterial hypertension associated with chronic liver disease. Before diagnosing portopulmonary hypertension as the cause of shortness of breath, other forms of pulmonary hypertension should be excluded, including thromboembolic disease, interstitial lung disease, untreated obstructive sleep apnea, and volume overload.

The incidence of portopulmonary hypertension is not known but is less than the incidence of hepatopulmonary syndrome.[10] Autopsy studies using various diagnostic

Table 1
Classification of portopulmonary hypertension

	Mild	Moderate	Severe
Mean PAP (mm Hg)	25–34	35–44	>45
Pulmonary vascular resistance (dyne/s/cm^5)	240–500	500–800	>800
Right arterial pressure (mm Hg)	0–5	5–8	>8
Prognosis with OLT	Good	Questionable	Poor
Specific treatment required before OLT[18]	No	Yes	Yes
Reversibility after liver transplantation	Yes	Questionable	No

Abbreviations: OLT, orthotopic liver transplant; PAP, pulmonary artery pressure.

criteria suggest that 2% to 10% of cirrhotic patients have an estimated risk of developing pulmonary hypertension, and in transplant populations the presence of pulmonary hypertension may be seen in up to 16% of those referred for orthotopic liver transplant. Similar to hepatopulmonary syndrome, no clear relationship between the severity of hepatic dysfunction or hepatic venous pressure gradient and the severity of pulmonary hypertension has been demonstrated. The survival rates for portopulmonary hypertension in general are poor, and the development of portopulmonary hypertension is a sign of poor prognosis. However, survival rates have varied markedly in the literature, likely attributable to differing severities of portopulmonary hypertension.

The pathogenesis of portopulmonary hypertension is not known; however, the development of portopulmonary hypertension appears to be independent of the cause of chronic liver disease, though most patients appear to have chronic liver disease with cirrhosis. However, portopulmonary hypertension has also been described in individuals with portal venous thrombosis without chronic liver disease. Thus, the presence of portal hypertension appears to be required. In addition, a hyperdynamic circulation appears to be required, and this physiologic state is present in those with advanced liver disease with portal hypertension. The high cardiac output, in combination with splanchnic vasodilation, leads to increased shear forces in the pulmonary circulation. Unlike hepatopulmonary syndrome, in which this high-output state leads to an abnormally reduced vascular resistance, in portopulmonary hypertension, increased vascular resistance caused by vasoconstriction and pulmonary vascular proliferation of pulmonary arterial endothelial and smooth muscle cells appears to lead to the pulmonary hypertension.[10] A high cardiac output may result in a mild degree of pulmonary hypertension in the presence of normal pulmonary vascular resistance. Portopulmonary hypertension is typically mild to moderate in severity in most patients, with vasoconstriction and medial hypertrophy of the pulmonary arteries being the dominant features in pulmonary hypertension. However, severe portopulmonary hypertension may occur with pulmonary arteriopathy, with obliteration of the vessel lumen by endothelial and smooth muscle cells, and formation of the plexiform lesions indistinguishable from primary pulmonary hypertension. Those with severe disease will present with right-sided heart failure.

The most common presenting symptom in patients with portopulmonary hypertension is shortness of breath or progressive dyspnea on exertion. Other nonspecific symptoms include fatigue, palpitations, syncope, and chest pain, but these are nonspecific. The most common finding on physical examination is an accentuated

P_2 of the second heart sound with a tricuspid regurgitation murmur. In cases of severe portopulmonary hypertension, distended jugular vein, ascites, and hepatojugular reflux may be seen. The diagnosis of portopulmonary hypertension requires demonstration of a raised pulmonary arterial pressure and pulmonary vascular resistance in the absence of volume overload. Transesophageal echocardiography is the initial screening test in the evaluation of patients with suspected portopulmonary hypertension.[18] When performed with contrast, this study can assess cardiac function, assess for the presence of right atrial/right ventricular dilation, and provide an estimate of pulmonary artery pressure if an adequate tricuspid regurgitation jet is available. These findings must be interpreted with caution in the setting of ascites, hepatic hydrothorax, or pericardial effusion. Definitive diagnosis and accurate characterization of pulmonary artery pressures requires right-sided cardiac catheterization, which remains the gold standard. Thus, if transthoracic echocardiography does not provide definitive diagnosis, a right heart catheterization should be obtained.

Therapy for portopulmonary hypertension is similar to that for primary pulmonary hypertension. The vasodilators, including bosentan, sildenafil, and epoprostenol, have all been used to reduce pulmonary artery pressures. Nitric oxide, a potent vasodilator, may reduce pulmonary artery pressures in a select group of patients with portopulmonary hypertension. The only definitive therapy is orthotopic liver transplantation, but patients with portopulmonary hypertension are at high risk for right ventricular decompensation or death during orthotopic liver transplant, as the pulmonary vessels are unable to accommodate the increased preload that occurs during the surgery. This process results in right heart failure with possible myocardial ischemia in the setting of a newly perfused liver, which can increase pulmonary vascular resistance. Besides vasodilators, treatment of mild portopulmonary hypertension includes the use of diuretics and supplemental oxygen for hypoxemia. Those with mean portopulmonary artery pressures <35 mm Hg may undergo orthotopic liver transplantation with outcomes comparable to those without portopulmonary hypertension. Those with mean pulmonary artery pressures of greater than 50 mm Hg should not undergo orthotopic liver transplant, as mortality rates are high. Those with mean pulmonary pressures between 35 and 50 mm Hg have an increased mortality rate, and may benefit from vasodilators before orthotopic liver transplantation. Portopulmonary hypertension may resolve, persist, or even develop de novo after liver transplantation.

HEPATIC HYDROTHORAX

Hepatic hydrothorax is defined as the presence of a significant pleural effusion (>500 mL) in a patient with cirrhosis without underlying pulmonary or cardiac disease. Although those with cirrhosis can generally tolerate substantial volumes of ascitic fluid in the peritoneal cavity, small volumes of fluid within the pleural space can lead to significant shortness of breath/dyspnea. The clinical presentation of hepatic hydrothorax includes shortness of breath with a nonproductive cough, chest discomfort, or fatigue. Physical examination may demonstrate reduced breath sounds at the right base (>80%), though hepatic hydrothorax may be seen as a left-sided effusion less than 15% of the time.[19] Of importance is that the development of cirrhotic ascites is not a prerequisite for the development of hepatic hydrothorax. Large pleural effusions are typically associated with substantial shortness of breath, and patients with large pleural effusions may require rapid intervention, including thoracentesis and/or transjugular intrahepatic portosystemic shunt.

The mechanisms leading to the development of hepatic hydrothorax have not been precisely defined. However, the preponderance of data suggests that direct passage of peritoneal fluid, albeit a diaphragmatic defect, likely explains the majority of cases of hepatic hydrothorax caused by the negative intrathoracic pressure associated with normal respiration. The fluid characteristics of a hepatic hydrothorax are listed in **Table 2**. These values are similar to those of ascitic fluid, though a diagnostic thoracentesis should be performed to exclude infection or an alternative diagnosis. Similar to ascitic fluid, spontaneous bacterial empyema may also occur, and is diagnosed by a polymorphonuclear cell count of greater than 250/mm^3 and a positive fluid culture. For definitive diagnosis, which is rarely required, radionuclide tracers may be used to document migration from the peritoneal to the pleural cavity.

Therapy for hepatic hydrothorax is similar to therapy for ascites, in that generating a negative sodium balance is the primary goal: salt restriction to 2 g per day (88 mEq) as well as the introduction of diuretics (furosemide 40 mg, spironolactone 100 mg) maintaining a 2:5 ratio with maximum doses of 160 mg and 400 mg, respectively. Those who fail to respond to diuretic therapy are candidates for transjugular intrahepatic portosystemic shunt, which leads to symptomatic improvement in most patients with hepatic hydrothorax but does not alter survival in those patients with decompensation. Surgical intervention for hepatic hydrothorax, including pleurodesis, tube thoracostomy, peritoneal venous shunts, AND end-dwelling catheters, have all been reported and should be reserved only as palliative intervention for cases refractory to traditional therapy. Orthotopic liver transplant remains the only intervention that addresses the underlying hepatic dysfunction, in addition to addressing the resolution of portal hypertension.

TENSE ASCITES

The presence of tense ascites may also be associated with dyspnea, although this diagnosis is apparent on examination.[20] An initial large-volume paracentesis of 5 L may typically be performed without postparacentesis colloid infusion, although larger volumes typically require intravenous albumin (8 g/L of fluid removed). Typically a single large-volume paracentesis followed by sodium restriction with diuretic therapy is appropriate therapy, not only to relieve the tense ascites but also to improve the patient's dyspnea.

ANEMIA

The role of anemia in those with chronic liver disease is an often overlooked, yet important etiological factor for shortness of breath in those with liver disease.[21] In the setting of cirrhosis, anemia is common in individuals with chronic liver disease and is likely to have a multifactorial etiology, including hypersplenism, folate deficiency, hemodilution, bone marrow suppression, renal insufficiency, and portal hypertension, with

Table 2
Fluid characteristics of a hepatic hydrothorax

Pleural fluid/serum total protein	<0.5
Pleural fluid/serum LDH	>0.6
Pleural fluid LDH	~200 U/L
Pleural fluid/serum cholesterol	>0.3
Pleural fluid/serum albumin gradient	1.2 g/dL
Pleural fluid/serum bilirubin	<0.6

Abbreviation: LDH, lactate dehydrogenase.

losses from variceal bleeding, portal hypertensive gastropathy, and gastric antral venular ectasia.[22] Anemia can typically be detected on physical examination with conjunctival pallor, and laboratory values can help suggest whether anemia is related to nutritional deficiencies, as is seen in alcoholic liver disease (macrocytosis) or iron deficiency due to portal hypertensive-related blood loss. Treatment is directed toward the underlying cause of anemia.

SUMMARY

The patient with chronic liver disease who complains of shortness of breath should lead to an evaluation that will help determine if primary pulmonary parenchymal or extraparenchymal disease is present, including pulmonary vascular complications, or complications of cirrhosis. The history should vary for a family history of liver disease as well as for signs or symptoms that may lead to a diagnosis of α1-antitrypsin deficiency, cystic fibrosis, or sarcoidosis. Physical examination, CBC, chest radiograph, and arterial blood gas are important initial tests to order. Based on this evaluation, transthoracic echocardiography with agitated saline to look for hepatopulmonary syndrome and to assess for elevated right heart pressures is important. If the origin of the dyspnea is still not clear, a right heart catheterization may be appropriate. Treatment will be directed toward the underlying cause, but most commonly orthotopic liver transplant will provide the best solution for appropriate candidates with shortness of breath, including those with dyspnea related to hepatopulmonary syndrome, portopulmonary hypertension, and hepatic hydrothorax.

REFERENCES

1. Mendez-Sanchez N, Villa AR, Zamora-Valdes D, et al. Worldwide mortality from cirrhosis. Ann Hepatol 2007;6:194–5.
2. Bosetti C, Levi F, Lucchini F, et al. Worldwide mortality from cirrhosis: an update to 2002. J Hepatol 2007;46:827–39.
3. Michelson E, Hollrah S. Evaluation of the patient with shortness of breath: an evidence based approach. Emerg Med Clin North Am 1999;17:221–37, x.
4. Gines P, Cardenas A, Arroyo V, et al. Management of cirrhosis and ascites. N Engl J Med 2004;350:1646–54.
5. Silverman EK, Sandhaus RA. Clinical practice. Alpha1-antitrypsin deficiency. N Engl J Med 2009;360:2749–57.
6. Bhardwaj S, Canlas K, Kahi C, et al. Hepatobiliary abnormalities and disease in cystic fibrosis: epidemiology and outcomes through adulthood. J Clin Gastroenterol 2009;43:858–64.
7. Kahi CJ, Saxena R, Temkit M, et al. Hepatobiliary disease in sarcoidosis. Sarcoidosis Vasc Diffuse Lung Dis 2006;23:117–23.
8. Kumar KS, Russo MW, Borczuk AC, et al. Significant pulmonary toxicity associated with interferon and ribavirin therapy for hepatitis C. Am J Gastroenterol 2002;97:2432–40.
9. Mattar W, Juliar B, Gradus-Pizlo I, et al. Amiodarone hepatotoxicity in the context of the metabolic syndrome and right-sided heart failure. J Gastrointestin Liver Dis 2009;18:419–23.
10. Hoeper MM, Krowka MJ, Strassburg CP. Portopulmonary hypertension and hepatopulmonary syndrome. Lancet 2004;363:1461–8.
11. Swanson KL, Wiesner RH, Krowka MJ. Natural history of hepatopulmonary syndrome: impact of liver transplantation. Hepatology 2005;41:1122–9.

12. Alexander J, Greenough A, Baker A, et al. Nitric oxide treatment of severe hypoxemia after liver transplantation in hepatopulmonary syndrome: case report. Liver Transpl Surg 1997;3:54–5.
13. Brussino L, Bucca C, Morello M, et al. Effect on dyspnoea and hypoxaemia of inhaled N(G)-nitro-L-arginine methyl ester in hepatopulmonary syndrome. Lancet 2003;362:43–4.
14. Rodriguez-Roisin R, Krowka MJ. Hepatopulmonary syndrome—a liver-induced lung vascular disorder. N Engl J Med 2008;358:2378–87.
15. Groneberg DA, Fischer A. Methylene blue improves the hepatopulmonary syndrome. Ann Intern Med 2001;135:380–1.
16. Fallon MB, Mulligan DC, Gish RG, et al. Model for end-stage liver disease (MELD) exception for hepatopulmonary syndrome. Liver Transpl 2006;12:S105–7.
17. Fallon MB. Portopulmonary hypertension: new clinical insights and more questions on pathogenesis. Hepatology 2003;37:253–5.
18. Krowka MJ, Fallon MB, Mulligan DC, et al. Model for end-stage liver disease (MELD) exception for portopulmonary hypertension. Liver Transpl 2006;12: S114–6.
19. Garcia N Jr, Mihas AA. Hepatic hydrothorax: pathophysiology, diagnosis, and management. J Clin Gastroenterol 2004;38:52–8.
20. Runyon BA. Management of adult patients with ascites due to cirrhosis: an update. Hepatology 2009;49:2087–107.
21. Lisman T, Caldwell SH, Porte RJ. Anemia as a potential contributor to bleeding in patients with liver disease – Neglected but not forgotten. J Hepatol 2011;54: 594–5.
22. Sharara AI, Rockey DC. Gastroesophageal variceal hemorrhage. N Engl J Med 2001;345:669–81.

Pruritus in Chronic Cholestatic Liver Disease

Chalermrat Bunchorntavakul, MD[a,b], K. Rajender Reddy, MD[a,*]

KEYWORDS

• Pruritus • Itching • Cholestasis • Liver disease • Pathogenesis
• Management • Opioid antagonist • Cholestyramine

Pruritus is a troublesome complication of chronic liver disease and often occurs in those with cholestasis. It is commonly encountered and well recognized in chronic cholestatic conditions, such as primary biliary cirrhosis (PBC); primary sclerosing cholangitis (PSC); prolonged drug-induced cholestasis, with or without ductopenia; intrahepatic cholestasis of pregnancy (ICP); and cholestasis syndromes associated with genetic mutations, such as progressive familial intrahepatic cholestasis (PFIC) and benign recurrent intrahepatic cholestasis (BRIC). Further, it is also observed in other types of liver disease, such as intrahepatic or extrahepatic biliary obstruction and chronic viral hepatitis.[1,2] This clinical manifestation can significantly negatively affect patients' quality of life, resulting in sleep deprivation, emotional/psychological disturbance, and even suicidal ideation. At an extreme, severe refractory pruritus in patients with chronic cholestasis, and without overt liver failure, has been accepted as an indication for liver transplantation (LT) so that quality of life can be improved.[3]

In the past few decades, some progress has been made in elucidating the pathogenesis of cholestasis-related pruritus. As a result, several potential therapeutic targets have been proposed and treatments directed at them have been investigated. However, there is currently no single established pathogenetic explanation and all available antipruritic treatment options are empiric and are not consistently effective. Thus, the management of pruritus in cholestasis continues to be a challenge and it remains a cause of considerable distress among patients. Based on recent experimental and clinical data, this article outlines the clinical manifestations, pathogenesis, and management of pruritus in cholestasis. The current recommended approach is emphasized, and the experimental interventions are discussed. In addition, the management of pruritus in certain conditions including ICP and BRIC are briefly reviewed.

Conflict of interest: The authors have nothing to disclose.
[a] Division of Gastroenterology and Hepatology, Department of Medicine, University of Pennsylvania, Philadelphia, PA, USA; [b] Department of Medicine, Rajavithi Hospital, College of Medicine, Rangsit University, Rajavithi Road, Rajthewi, Bangkok 10400, Thailand
* Corresponding author. Hospital of the University of Pennsylvania, 2 Dulles, 3400 Spruce Street, Philadelphia, PA 19104.
E-mail address: rajender.reddy@uphs.upenn.edu

Clin Liver Dis 16 (2012) 331–346
doi:10.1016/j.cld.2012.03.010 liver.theclinics.com

MANIFESTATION AND NATURAL HISTORY

PBC has traditionally been the model for the study of pruritus in chronic cholestasis. Pruritus is a common presenting symptom of PBC and is reported in up to 70% to 80% of patients by 10 years after diagnosis; 75% of these patients reported this symptom preceding the diagnosis of PBC.[4,5] Similarly, in PSC, pruritus is a presenting symptom in 20% to 40% of patients and the frequency tends to increase during the course of the disease.[6,7] Pruritus is a prerequisite for the diagnosis of ICP. In patients with biliary tract obstruction, pruritus occurred in 17% of cases of nonmalignant obstruction and in 45% of patients with a malignant obstruction.[8] It has also been reported in 20% of patients with viral hepatitis and in 7% of patients with cirrhosis.[8]

Pruritus associated with cholestasis is often worse at night and can be transiently exacerbated by premenstrual state and psychological stress, whereas it often is relieved by cool temperatures.[4,5] It may be generalized or localized, particularly over the palms and soles, and often without any definable primary skin lesion. However, several cutaneous complications, such as folliculitis, excoriations, prurigo nodularis, and lichenification, can result from long-standing, vigorous scratching activity.[5,9] The intensity of pruritus varies and does not correlate with the severity of underlying liver disease. Once pruritus evolves in PBC, the severity may diminish over time. However, it is unlikely to disappear completely without treatment until a patient develops cirrhosis.[10]

PATHOGENESIS OF PRURITUS OF CHOLESTASIS

Itch-related nerve endings are found throughout the body surface and are inducible by many physical and chemical stimuli, either acting directly on the nerve endings or indirectly via histamine release.[4] The pruritus pathway involves the dorsal horn, the contralateral spinothalamic tract, and the thalamus. Apart from peripheral stimuli, central mediators, such as endogenous opioids, serotonin, and steroids, have also been postulated in the pathogenesis of pruritus.[9] The classic example is when a central phenomenon is invoked after the intrathecal injection of morphine, which then inhibits pain but is associated with pruritus.[11]

The pathogenesis of pruritus in cholestasis has not been clearly elucidated. It is assumed that cholestasis-related pruritus is induced by pruritogenic substance(s) that accumulate as a result of impaired secretion of bile, which either directly or indirectly affect signaling of the pruritus pathway.[4,9,12] This conventional wisdom is supported by an observation that pruritus generally disappears following resolution of bile duct obstruction, the use of procedures that remove substances from circulation, and LT. However, the causative factor(s) have not been conclusively identified. In the past, bile acids (BAs), which interact with peripheral nerve endings and induce an itching sensation, had been implicated as potential pruritogens. More recent attention has been drawn to the pathophysiologic alterations in cholestasis that induce pruritus, mediating mainly via the central pathways, and that include endogenous opioids, serotonin, and, most recently, lysophosphatidic acid (LPA).[4,9,12] Further, several genetic mutations have been shown to increase susceptibility for cholestatic liver disease; however, no genetic susceptibility specific for the occurrence of pruritus has been yet identified.

The Role of BAs

BAs accumulate in the tissue of patients with cholestasis, and they correlate linearly with the serum levels.[13] They are thought to be important pruritogens in patients with cholestasis, presumably by interacting with peripheral nerve endings. This notion is supported by the observations that intradermal injection of BA caused pruritus in healthy volunteers,[14] feeding of BAs aggravated pruritus in PBC,[15] and cholestyramine, an anion exchange resin that enhances luminal clearance of BA, continues to ameliorate pruritus in various cholestatic conditions.[4] However, several arguments question the role of BA as a key mediator of cholestasis-related pruritus. BA levels, in serum, urine, and in tissue, and severity of pruritus have not correlated and their levels have not been able to differentiate between patients with and without pruritus.[9,13] Further, pruritus does not often occur in acute liver failure and extrahepatic bile duct obstruction, and it tends to improve spontaneously in those with progression to advanced-stage cholestatic liver disease; these conditions are associated with highly increased BA levels.[9,12] A recent double-blind, randomized controlled study noted that colesevelam, a newer anion exchange resin with 7-fold higher BA-binding capacity than cholestyramine, significantly decreased serum BA levels, but was unable to show superiority in alleviating the severity of pruritus compared with placebo.[16] Taken together, BAs may be necessary, or at least play some role, as mediators of cholestasis-related pruritus, but it is likely that cofactor(s) and other pathogenetic mechanisms are involved.

Endogenous Opioids

Endogenous opioids, such as met-enkephalins and leu-enkephalins have been implicated in the pathogenesis of cholestasis-related pruritus.[17] Several experimental studies suggest that the central opioidergic tone is increased in patients with cholestasis.[12,17] In a rat model of cholestasis, total opioid activity in plasma was increased,[18,19] central μ opioid receptors were downregulated[20] and a stereospecific naloxone reversible state of analgesia was observed.[18] In cholestatic patients, but not in healthy individuals, oral administration of a potent opioid antagonist induces a constellation of adverse symptoms mimicking an opiate withdrawal reaction.[21] The pruritus activation pathway mediated by opioids remains unclear. It has been explained by a central mode of action[17]; however, a recent study in mice suggested that cholestasis is associated with antinociception caused by local effects of endogenous opioids (ie, met-enkephalins) at the level of sensory nerve endings.[22] Nevertheless, some evidence disputes endogenous opioids as a direct pruritogen in cholestasis.[23,24] A significant correlation between endogenous opioid concentrations and the presence or intensity of pruritus has never been shown.[23,24] Thus, many opioid antagonists have been used to treated cholestatic pruritus with moderate success.[4]

Serotonin

The serotonin neurotransmitter system has also been implicated in the pathogenesis of cholestasis-related pruritus. Following an intradermal injection, serotonin induced scratching behavior in mice[25] and itching sensation in humans.[26] It has also been reported to modulate nociception in rats and, in analogy with the opioid system, may modulate the perception of pruritus.[4] Through unclear mechanisms, a serotonin 5-HT3 receptor antagonist, ondansetron, has been effective in preventing intrathecal morphine-induced pruritus.[27] However, data supporting changes in the serotonin neurotransmitter system in cholestatic patients in lacking.

Autotaxin and Lysophosphatidic Acid Axis

Lysophosphatidic acid, a small but potent bioactive phospholipid with a wide variety of effects in many cell types (ie, cytoskeletal organization, cell migration, cytokine production, platelet and neuronal activation) is formed from lysophosphatidylcholine by the enzyme autotaxin (ATX).[23,28] It has recently been proposed to be a potential pruritogen in cholestasis.[23] Intradermal injection of lysophosphatidic acid (LPA) induces itch-scratch responses in mice in a dose-dependent manner.[23,29] A recent study in a large number of pruritic and nonpruritic cholestatic patients (mainly ICP and PBC) showed that serum LPA levels and ATX activities were increased only in those patients who suffered from pruritus.[23] Further, ATX activity significantly correlated with the intensity of pruritus, and markedly decreased after temporary nasobiliary drainage that then ameliorated pruritus[23] Therefore, the ATX-LPA axis seems to play a critical role in cholestasis-related pruritus. Currently, there is no LPA antagonist or ATX inhibitor available for clinical use and the question of whether or not a treatment targeted at the ATX-LPA axis effectively reduces pruritus is unanswered.

MANAGEMENT OF PRURITUS IN CHRONIC CHOLESTATIC LIVER DISEASE

Apart from treatment directed at cholestatic liver disease, the management of pruritus is largely empiric and several therapeutic targets have been evaluated in clinical studies, including (1) interventions to remove the pruritogens from the body either by preventing absorption and interrupting enterohepatic circulation or directly from the blood; (2) interventions to alter metabolism of the presumed pruritogens in the liver and/or the gut; and (3) interventions to modify central and/or peripheral pruritus signaling pathways (**Table 1**). Pruritus is a sensation that cannot be directly measured, and therefore a reliable assessment method is needed for clinicians and researchers. In clinical trials, pruritus sensation is measured by either a subjective methodology (ie, visual analog scale, descriptive grade scale, questionnaires, log books) or instruments that record the direct behavioral consequences of pruritus (ie, scratching behavior).[4] In the past decade, a scratch activity monitoring system that permits the portable recording of vibrations produced by the act of scratching has been introduced to allow objective quantification of pruritus and has been used in recent clinical studies.[12] However, the interpretation of data obtained from either subjective or objective methodology has been challenging because there is variability in the perception of pruritus and thus in the response as well. Therefore, it is important to carefully examine placebo response rates in pruritus studies before making judgments on the efficacy of any therapeutic intervention. Management strategies for pruritus in chronic cholestatic conditions are categorized according to a rationale based on pathophysiologic mechanisms as well as targets.

Interventions Directing at the Underlying Cholestatic Conditions

Pruritus associated with extrahepatic bile duct obstruction generally disappears with the relief of obstruction. Some cholestatic conditions such as drug-induced cholestasis and ICP spontaneously resolve with the withdrawal of the causative drug, and delivery of the infant and concurrently there is eventual resolution of pruritus. However, some cholestatic conditions such as PBC and PSC are chronic and incurable. Ursodeoxycholic acid (UDCA) is a hydrophilic, tertiary BA with choleretic and hepatoprotective effects and has been used for the treatment of a variety of chronic cholestatic conditions.[30] Although it has been reported to ameliorate pruritus in ICP and some of the pediatric cholestatic conditions,[9,31] in randomized controlled trials for treatment of PBC and PSC, UDCA has been associated with an improvement in liver biochemical tests, but not pruritus.[32,33] Paradoxic worsening of pruritus has been reported anecdotally following introduction of UDCA.[34] Prednisolone, cyclosporin, and methotrexate have also been reported to improve itching in clinical studies of the treatment of PBC.[35–37] A nonsignificant trend toward lower on-treatment pruritus scores was observed in a long-tern follow-up study of low-dose methotrexate.[38] The assessment of pruritus in these studies was not a primary outcome and was done by subjective methodology.

Table 1
Therapeutic options for pruritus in chronic cholestatic liver disease

Cause and Mechanisms of Pruritus	Potential Therapeutic Agents/Interventions	Efficacy and Comments
Underlying cholestasis disease	UDCA	Generally ineffective (except in PBC and ICP)
	MTX, CSA, prednisolone	Limited data
	LT	Effective(II/C1[a]) ;for intractable cases
Increase in BAs	Cholestyramine	Effective (II-2/B1[a]); unpalatable
	Colestipol	Limited data
	Colesevalam	Ineffective
Presumed pruritogens in the circulation and/or tissue	Rifampicin	Effective (I/A1[a]), hepatotoxicity 7%–12%
	Phenobarbital	Borderline effective; heavily sedative
	Flumecinol	Limited data
	Plasmapheresis	Effective; for intractable cases
	MARS	Effective (III/C2[a]); for intractable cases
Increase in endogenous opioids	Naloxone (intravenous)	Effective; opioid withdrawal reaction
	Naltrexone	Effective (I/B1[a]); opioid withdrawal reaction
	Nalmefene	Effective; opioid withdrawal reaction
	Butorphanol	Limited data; addiction potential
Serotonin pathway	Sertraline	Moderately effective (II-2/C2[a])
	Ondansetron	Inconclusive
Modulate nociceptive threshold	Gabapentin	Ineffective
	Propofol	May be effective
	Lidocaine	Limited data
	Dronabinol	Limited data
ATX and LPA axis	LPA antagonist	Not yet available
	ATX inhibitor	Not yet available

Abbreviations: CSA, cyclosporin A; MARS, molecular adsorbent recirculating system; MTX, methotrexate; UDCA, ursodeoxycholic acid.

[a] Categories of evidence according to the EASL Practice Guideline 2009: I, randomized controlled trials; II-1, controlled trials without randomization; II-2, cohort or case-control analytical studies; II-3, multiple time series and/or dramatic uncontrolled experiments; III, opinions of respected authorities and/or descriptive epidemiology. Evidence grading: A, high quality; B, moderate quality; C, low quality. 1, strong recommendation; 2, weak recommendation.

LT is the most effective treatment of end-stage cholestatic liver disease. It is also an accepted option for cholestatic patients with preserved liver function while suffering from intractable and disabling pruritus despite medical therapy.[3] Pruritus generally resolves soon after LT. However, primary cholestatic disease (ie, PBC, PSC) and pruritus can recur in LT recipients and this must be differentiated from chronic graft rejection and biliary and vascular complications.

Interventions Directed at the Removal of the Presumed Pruritogens

BA sequestrants

The nonabsorbable anion exchange resins (ie, cholestyramine, colestipol, and colesevalem) have been widely used to treat cholestasis-associated pruritus, as well as other conditions such as polycythemia vera and uremia.[4] In the intestine, these agents bind the potential pruritogens, particularly BA, and then enhance excretion by preventing their absorption by the terminal ileum and interrupting enterohepatic circulation. There have been no good randomized controlled trials evaluating the efficacy of anion exchange resins for pruritus, and perhaps this is largely because the agents entered widespread use before the era of evidence-based medicine. However, small clinical studies, as well as most expert opinions, support the use of cholestyramine for pruritus in a variety of both intrahepatic and extrahepatic cholestatic conditions in which the improvement is often noticed within a few weeks after initiation of treatment.[4,9,34,39–42] According to earlier studies, 80% to 85% of patients completely or partially responded to cholestyramine in 4 to 11 days, and this response was maintained for up to 6 to 32 months.[41,42] Apart from BA sequestration, cholestyramine may also have an antipruritic effect by inducing the release of cholecystokinin, an endogenous antiopiate.[12,43] This antiopiate effect may explain the tachyphylaxis phenomenon that is reported by some patients.[12] Taken together, particularly when considering its safety and extensive clinical experience, cholestyramine should be used as the first-line therapy for the management of cholestasis-related pruritus.[10,34]

Cholestyramine should be adequately diluted in water or juice and given in escalating and divided doses starting at 4 g/d and titrated up to 16 g/d. The timing of cholestyramine administration in relation to meals is important. The greatest amount of BA for binding by the resin is present in the gallbladder before breakfast, whereas less may be present before lunch and even less before dinner.[4,44] Accordingly, cholestyramine should be taken 30 to 60 minutes before and after breakfast. When up-titrating, a third and fourth dose can be administered following lunch and dinner, respectively.[4,44] Poor compliance is a concerning issue because cholestyramine is unpalatable and often associated with side effects, such as constipation, bloating, and abdominal discomfort. Long-term treatment with cholestyramine is associated with fat malabsorption and vitamin K deficiency, which should be properly monitored. Cholestyramine can interfere with absorption of several drugs (eg, UDCA, thyroid replacement, oral contraceptives) and therefore should ideally be spaced a minimum of 4 hours apart from other medications.[45] Colestipol hydrochloride is another BA-binding resin that was initially developed for the treatment of hypercholesterolemia. Compared with cholestyramine, colestipol seems to be better tolerated, but clinical experience for the treatment of pruritus in cholestasis is limited and controlled studies have not been done. Colesevalem hydrochloride is a potent BA-binding polymer and is probably the most favored agent by patients, because it is formulated as a tablet and associated with minimal gastrointestinal side effects, compared with cholestyramine and colestipol.[4,46] However, colesevalem failed to alleviate the severity of pruritus of cholestasis in a recent randomized placebo-controlled trial.[16]

Plasmapheresis and extracorporeal albumin dialysis

Invasive procedures, including plasmapheresis and extracorporeal albumin dialysis, are intended to remove pruritogens that presumably accumulate in tissues and plasma of patients with cholestasis. Although no controlled studies have been done to date, several case series have suggested that plasmapheresis[47,48] and, more recently, molecular adsorbent recirculating system (MARS) therapy[49–53] are effective in the management of severe and refractory pruritus in various chronic cholestatic conditions. Limitations of these interventions include their invasive nature, cost, and the need for repeated sessions (approximately every 2–4 weeks in most reports) to maintain the response.[47–52] Therefore, these procedures should be reserved as an option for cholestatic patients with severe pruritus who fail noninvasive interventions.

Interventions to Alter the Metabolism of the Presumed Pruritogens

Rifampicin and phenobarbital are pregnane X receptor (also known as steroid and xenobiotic sensing nuclear receptor) agonists that strongly induce hepatic microsomal oxidizing enzymes and biotransformation transporters (ie, CYP3A4, UGT1A1, and MRP2), and these may promote the metabolism and/or the secretion of the potential endogenous pruritogens.[54,55] Phenobarbital has been used to manage patients with cholestasis-related pruritus; however, it has considerable sedative effects and was less effective than rifampicin in a comparative trial.[56,57] Thus more attention has been given to rifampicin, which, in addition to its pregnane X receptor agonist property, competes with BA uptake by hepatocyte and, through its antimicrobial property, modifies secondary BA synthesis in the gut lumen, which then ultimately reduces the level of hepatotoxic lithocholic acid.[4] Further, it may have antiopiate activity.[58] Several small randomized controlled trials have shown that rifampicin (300–600 mg/d) was safe and effective in the treatment of pruritus; these included 1 open labeled trial with up to 2 years' follow-up.[56,59–61] This beneficial effect is supported by 2 meta-analyses; 1 that observed a significant higher proportion of patients with relief of pruritus than control (odds ratio 15.2; 95% confidence interval [CI] 5.2–45.6)[62] and another that concluded that there was a significant reduction in pruritus score (standardized mean change -1.62; 95% CI -3.05 to -0.18).[63]

Rifampicin has been associated with a severe idiosyncratic hypersensitivity reaction (ie, rash, hepatitis, hemolysis, renal failure), opiate withdrawal reaction, and presents drug-drug interactions with concomitant medication(s).[58,61,64] Rifampicin-induced hepatotoxicity has been reported in up to 7% to 12% of cholestatic patients following several weeks or months of rifampicin treatment, and this hepatotoxicity often resolved with treatment discontinuation.[61,64] Several severe cases of rifampicin-induced hepatotoxicity, with some evolving to liver failure and requiring LT, have been reported in the setting of tuberculosis (used in combination with other potentially hepatotoxic antituberculosis agents).[65] Although there is limited experience with the use of rifampicin as monotherapy for pruritus, severe hepatotoxicity seems to be less frequent, but such cases have been reported.[64] Therefore, the use of rifampicin in this context requires regular monitoring of serum alanine aminotransferase (ALT) levels. Rifampicin use may obviate the antidepressive effects of serotonin reuptake inhibition (SSRI), and these should not be used together.[10] More recently, a new inducer of cytochrome P450, flumecinol, was evaluated for pruritus. In a prospective controlled study of 50 patients (46 had PBC), short-term treatment with flumecinol (300 mg/d) was safe and significantly ameliorated pruritus.[66] However, these data have not yet been replicated.

Interventions to Modify Central and/or Peripheral Pruritus Signaling Pathways

Opioid antagonists

In the past decades, opioid antagonists (ie, naloxone, naltrexone, and nalmefene) have been extensively evaluated as treatment of cholestasis-associated pruritus. Convincing results from several controlled clinical studies applying both subjective and behavioral methodology,[67–73] as well as a meta-analysis that included 5 randomized controlled trials with a total of 84 participants (standardized mean change in pruritus score: -0.68, 95% CI -1.19 to -0.17) showed benefit from these opioid antagonists.[63] Intravenous infusion of naloxone (0.2 μg/kg/min) is associated with a significant decrease in pruritus[67,68]; however, the parenteral mode of administration is not practical for chronic use, and should be reserved as temporary treatment of selected patients with intractable and severe exacerbation of pruritus.[12] To manage pruritus in the long term, orally administered opioid antagonists have been evaluated. A significant improvement in pruritus in most patients has been reported in controlled clinical studies of oral naltrexone (25–50 mg/d)[69,72–74] and nalmefene (2 mg orally twice daily, and with increasing doses until a satisfactory clinical response was achieved; most patients required up to 30 to 80 mg/d, with 2 patients tolerating a dose of 240 mg/d).[70,71]

A reaction like opiate withdrawal, which is characterized by anorexia, nausea, pallor, colicky abdominal pain, tachycardia, and increase in blood pressure, is a common complication of opioid antagonists in patients with cholestasis. This reaction may begin within 1 hour after administration of treatment and is generally alleviated after 2 or 3 days while continuing therapy.[4,12,68–72,75] Although most patients experience a mild reaction, it is difficult to predict the severity of withdrawal-like reaction, thus limiting the broader acceptance of this type of intervention. To prevent or minimize the development of this reaction, 3 approaches have been recommended: (1) starting oral naltrexone (12.5–25 mg twice daily) or nalmefene (2 mg twice daily) at the lowest possible dose, with gradual stepwise increases until the subjective reduction of pruritus is achieved[4,12,70]; (2) initiating therapy with continuously infused naloxone at a low dose (0.002 μg/kg/min), gradually increasing the dose to 0.2 to 0.8 μg/kg/min and then switching to small doses of orally bioavailable opioid antagonists[76]; and (3) coadministering clonidine during the first week of treatment.[75] A sustained exacerbation of pruritus (so-called breakthrough phenomenon) in the early weeks of treatment, after an initial response, may be encountered in up to one-third of patients during naltrexone and nalmefene therapy.[69,70] This phenomenon is explained by a reversal of downregulated central opioid receptors during the treatment, leading to a transiently increased sensitivity to endogenous opioids.[4] It may be preventable by interrupting treatment for 2 days every week[74] and is then managed by increments in the doses.[70] In addition, tolerance and severe exacerbation of pruritus have also been reported in a study of nalmefene.[70] Compared with naltrexone, nalmefene has longer half-life, higher oral bioavailability, and higher receptor affinity; however, it seemed to be associated with more treatment-adverse events in a long-term clinical study,[70] which limits the use of nalmefene in patients with pruritus.

An activation of κ opioid receptor inhibits pruritus evoked by morphine in an animal model.[77] The spray form of butorphanol, a κ receptor agonist and μ opioid receptor antagonist, resulted in marked reduction of severe pruritus associated with chronic hepatitis C.[12] The addiction potential of butorphanol may limit wide acceptance of this agent.[12]

Serotonin modulators

Ondansetron is a serotonin 5-HT3 receptor antagonist used mainly as an antiemetic but it has also been used to prevent morphine-induced pruritus.[27] Earlier placebo-controlled studies (1 per oral 24 mg/d[78] and 1 intravenous 4–8 mg[79]) supported the use of ondansetron to treat cholestasis-associated pruritus. However, the considerable limitations of these studies are that they are small, have heterogeneous sample populations, and outcomes had subjective assessments. These results were not confirmed by subsequent studies that applied behavioral methodology.[80,81]

More recently, sertraline, an antidepressant of the SSRI class, has been evaluated in pruritus. In a retrospective study of 32 patients with pruritus caused by PBC, 6 of 7 subjects who had been given sertraline for another indication improved considerably, and pruritus completely subsided in 3 of those individuals.[82] Subsequently, in a small, double-blinded, randomized placebo-controlled crossover study, treatment with sertraline (75–100 mg/d) was noted to be safe and effective in reducing pruritus (33% improvement in pruritus score), but complete resolution of pruritus was not observed.[83]

Patients with depression at baseline improved their depression score after sertraline therapy, and this improvement was independent of a decrease in pruritus score.[83] The investigators proposed that sertraline mediated its effect through serotonergic signals in the central nervous system that provide inhibitory signals to the itch pathways, which involves both a physical sensation and an emotional response, culminating in the desire to scratch.

Agents that modulate the threshold of nociception

The notion of altered neurotransmission in the mediation of the pruritus of cholestasis has led to the study of drugs with neuropsychiatric effects as treatment of pruritus.[84] Because pruritus is a nociceptive stimulus, gabapentin, a drug that increases the threshold of nociception and is used mainly for neuropathic pain and epilepsy, has been evaluated in patients with pruritus from various conditions, such as uremia, burns, and induced by morphine, with variable success.[85–87] In cholestatic patients, gabapentin (300–2400 mg/d) did not provide a significant therapeutic advantage compared with placebo in a randomized controlled study.[84] It was associated with an increase in the perception of pruritus and in scratch activity in some patients.[84]

A cannabinoid agonist, dronabinol, increased nociception threshold in cholestatic rats.[88] Preliminary observation reported that dronabinol (5 mg at bedtime) was associated with symptom improvement in those with intractable pruritus and who failed conventional treatment.[89] Anesthetic agents have also been used for cholestasis-related pruritus. In a small, double-blind, randomized controlled, crossover study, subhypnotic doses of propofol (2 doses of 15 mg) have been shown to be effective for the short-term symptomatic relief of liver disease–associated pruritus (treatment success was achieved in 85% and 10% of patients receiving propofol and placebo respectively; $P<.01$).[90] Minor adverse events were observed; 15% discomfort at injection site and 10% dizziness. Lidocaine has also been reported to improve cholestasis-related pruritus.[91,92]

Antihistamines

Antihistamines have been commonly prescribed empirically for itching in allergic and dermatologic conditions. They may have nonspecific antipruritic effects in patients with cholestasis; however, no systematic study to evaluate their efficacy has been reported. Antihistamine-mediated sedation may help insomnia, a problematic and disabling symptom in patients with pruritus.[10]

ALGORITHM FOR THE MANAGEMENT OF PRURITUS IN CHOLESTATIC LIVER DISEASE

A thorough medical history and careful physical examination are necessary in cholestatic patients who experience pruritus. Concomitant dermatologic conditions must be sorted out, because the management in those cases may be different. Disease-specific management for primary chronic cholestatic disease, such as UDCA or immunosuppressive agents, should be adequately provided because this may relieve pruritus. Extrahepatic bile duct obstruction should be excluded by appropriate imaging and, if necessary, cholangiographic studies and corrected, if possible. Patients with end-stage liver disease should be listed for LT. Taking into consideration all available evidence of efficacy and risk/benefit ratio for the several interventions, guidelines for the management of pruritus in cholestatic liver disease were developed in 2009 by the European Association for the Study of the Liver (EASL)[34] and the American Association for the Study of Liver Diseases (AASLD),[10] and are summarized in **Fig. 1**. Both guidelines recommend cholestyramine as first-line treatment, and rifampicin, naltrexone, and sertraline respectively as second-line, third-line, and fourth-line

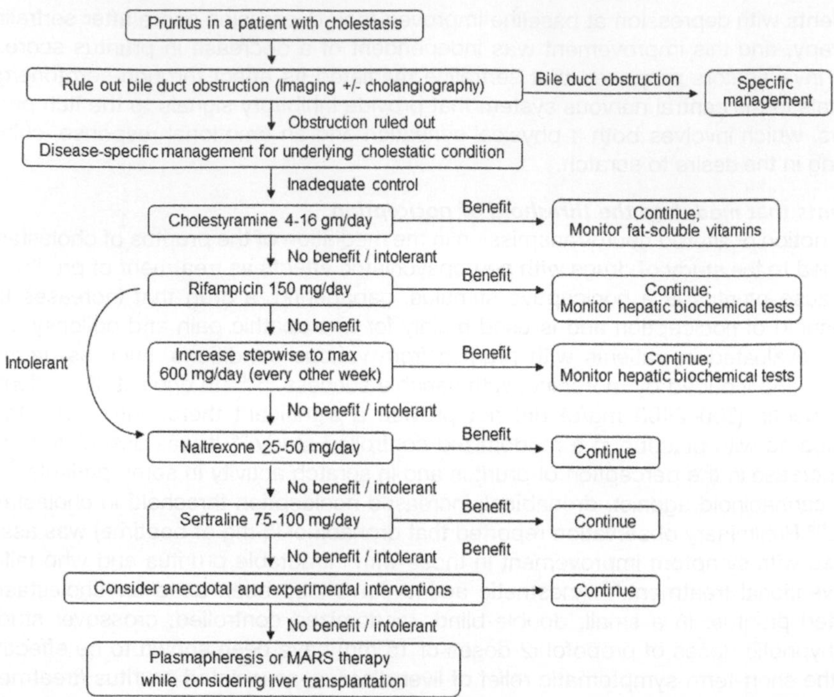

Fig. 1. Algorithm for the management of pruritus in the patients with cholestatic liver disease. (*Adapted from* European Association for the Study of the Liver (EASL). Clinical practice guidelines: management of cholestatic liver disease. J Hepatol 2009;51(2):237–67; with permission.)

line treatments.[10,34] Sertraline may be an interesting option for patients with pruritus who also have depression. If patients have sleep disturbance, sedative antihistamines or short-acting benzodiazepines may be helpful.

The management for patients who fail the described agents may be problematic. A trial of experimental agents, such as propofol,[90] dronabinol,[89] ondansetron,[78,79] gabapentin,[84] butorphanol,[9,12] flumecinol,[66] cimetidine,[34] metronidazole,[1] lidocaine,[91,92] and stanozolol,[93] may be pursued and these may have variable success. The supporting evidence for the use of these agents comes from small clinical trials and anecdotal observations. Patients with severe pruritus are at risk of depression and suicide. These patients may require hospitalization for parenteral administration of medications such as naloxone.[10] Invasive interventions of MARS and plasmapheresis can be used as well and are often reserved for those who fail interventions with medications and have a poor quality of life. LT is reserved for patients with intractable pruritus who have failed all options.[10,34]

PRURITUS IN SPECIAL CHOLESTASIS POPULATIONS

ICP

Unlike other cholestatic conditions, the management of pruritus in ICP is unique. Pruritus is generally the only disturbing symptom and any risk to the mother and fetus from treatment of this symptom needs to be taken into consideration. The diagnosis of ICP is based on (1) pruritus in pregnancy, often in the third trimester; and (2) increased serum ALT activity and fasting BA levels.[34] Pruritus often becomes progressively more severe as the pregnancy advances and typically resolves spontaneously within 48 hours after delivery.[31] ICP is not associated with significant or ongoing hepatic impairment, but it affects maternal well-being and carries a high risk of adverse fetal outcomes (ie, fetal distress, intrauterine fetal death, preterm delivery).[31,34] Pruritus associated with ICP has been treated with cholestyramine and antihistamines, but they are often ineffective and not well tolerated.[31,34] UDCA is safe (pregnancy risk category B) and well tolerated in pregnancy.[34,59,94,95] It is recommended as the first-line treatment of ICP[34] because several clinical studies reported that UDCA (10–20 mg/kg/d) was associated with relief of pruritus, decrease in levels of endogenous BAs, restoration of ALT levels, and improvement in fetal outcomes.[59,94–97] *S*-Adenosylmethionine (SAMe) is a physiologic compound formed from the metabolism of methionine, and is involved in the BA detoxification process in the hepatocyte. Randomized controlled studies of SAMe for the treatment of pruritus in ICP have shown conflicting results.[96–99] Although SAMe is less effective than UDCA, they may have an additive effect.[96,97] In theory, rifampicin (pregnancy risk category C) may enhance BA export induced by UDCA.[31] Because several ICP cases do not adequately respond to UDCA monotherapy, SAMe and rifampicin as adjunctive treatments have been recommended to treat pruritus.[31,34] Dexamethasone (12 mg/d for 7 days) promotes fetal lung maturity, but is ineffective in reducing pruritus and ALT levels in patients with ICP.[100]

BRIC

BRIC is characterized by acute episodes of cholestasis, jaundice and severe pruritus that, after weeks or months, completely resolve to start again following an asymptomatic period of months to years.[34] It is caused by mutations in the coding sequence of the FIC1 gene (ATP8B1 and ABCB11) located on chromosome 18q21.[101] BRIC presents during adolescence and adulthood, and represents the benign form of PFIC. No effective evidence-based therapy is known. However, UDCA and rifampicin, as well as nasobiliary drainage, have been anecdotally reported to favorably affect the course of BRIC.[34,102]

REFERENCES

1. Bergasa NV. Update on the treatment of the pruritus of cholestasis. Clin Liver Dis 2008;12(1):219–34, x.
2. Lebovics E, Seif F, Kim D, et al. Pruritus in chronic hepatitis C: association with high serum bile acids, advanced pathology, and bile duct abnormalities. Dig Dis Sci 1997;42(5):1094–9.
3. Murray KF, Carithers RL Jr. AASLD practice guidelines: evaluation of the patient for liver transplantation. Hepatology 2005;41(6):1407–32.
4. Mela M, Mancuso A, Burroughs AK. Review article: pruritus in cholestatic and other liver diseases. Aliment Pharmacol Ther 2003;17(7):857–70.
5. Rishe E, Azarm A, Bergasa NV. Itch in primary biliary cirrhosis: a patients' perspective. Acta Derm Venereol 2008;88(1):34–7.
6. Broome U, Olsson R, Loof L, et al. Natural history and prognostic factors in 305 Swedish patients with primary sclerosing cholangitis. Gut 1996;38(4):610–5.
7. Tischendorf JJ, Hecker H, Kruger M, et al. Characterization, outcome, and prognosis in 273 patients with primary sclerosing cholangitis: a single center study. Am J Gastroenterol 2007;102(1):107–14.
8. McPhedran NT, Henderson RD. Pruritus and jaundice. Can Med Assoc J 1965; 92:1258–60.

9. Kremer AE, Oude Elferink RP, Beuers U. Pathophysiology and current management of pruritus in liver disease. Clin Res Hepatol Gastroenterol 2011;35(2):89–97.
10. Lindor KD, Gershwin ME, Poupon R, et al. Primary biliary cirrhosis. Hepatology 2009;50(1):291–308.
11. Slappendel R, Weber EW, Benraad B, et al. Itching after intrathecal morphine. Incidence and treatment. Eur J Anaesthesiol 2000;17(10):616–21.
12. Bergasa NV. The pruritus of cholestasis. J Hepatol 2005;43(6):1078–88.
13. Ghent CN, Bloomer JR, Klatskin G. Elevations in skin tissue levels of bile acids in human cholestasis: relation to serum levels and to pruritus. Gastroenterology 1977;73(5):1125–30.
14. Varadi DP. Pruritus induced by crude bile and purified bile acids. Experimental production of pruritus in human skin. Arch Dermatol 1974;109(5):678–81.
15. Ricci P, Hofmann AF, Hagey LR, et al. Adjuvant cholylsarcosine during ursodeoxycholic acid treatment of primary biliary cirrhosis. Dig Dis Sci 1998;43(6):1292–5.
16. Kuiper EM, van Erpecum KJ, Beuers U, et al. The potent bile acid sequestrant colesevelam is not effective in cholestatic pruritus: results of a double-blind, randomized, placebo-controlled trial. Hepatology 2010;52(4):1334–40.
17. Jones EA, Bergasa NV. The pruritus of cholestasis: from bile acids to opiate agonists. Hepatology 1990;11(5):884–7.
18. Bergasa NV, Alling DW, Vergalla J, et al. Cholestasis in the male rat is associated with naloxone-reversible antinociception. J Hepatol 1994;20(1):85–90.
19. Swain MG, Rothman RB, Xu H, et al. Endogenous opioids accumulate in plasma in a rat model of acute cholestasis. Gastroenterology 1992;103(2):630–5.
20. Bergasa NV, Rothman RB, Vergalla J, et al. Central mu-opioid receptors are down-regulated in a rat model of cholestasis. J Hepatol 1992;15(1–2):220–4.
21. Thornton JR, Losowsky MS. Plasma methionine enkephalin concentration and prognosis in primary biliary cirrhosis. BMJ 1988;297(6658):1241–2.
22. Nelson L, Vergnolle N, D'Mello C, et al. Endogenous opioid-mediated antinociception in cholestatic mice is peripherally, not centrally, mediated. J Hepatol 2006;44(6):1141–9.
23. Kremer AE, Martens JJ, Kulik W, et al. Lysophosphatidic acid is a potential mediator of cholestatic pruritus. Gastroenterology 2010;139(3):1008–18, 1018 e1001.
24. Spivey JR, Jorgensen RA, Gores GJ, et al. Methionine-enkephalin concentrations correlate with stage of disease but not pruritus in patients with primary biliary cirrhosis. Am J Gastroenterol 1994;89(11):2028–32.
25. Inagaki N, Nagao M, Igeta K, et al. Scratching behavior in various strains of mice. Skin Pharmacol Appl Skin Physiol 2001;14(2):87–96.
26. Hagermark O. Peripheral and central mediators of itch. Skin Pharmacol 1992;5(1):1–8.
27. George RB, Allen TK, Habib AS. Serotonin receptor antagonists for the prevention and treatment of pruritus, nausea, and vomiting in women undergoing cesarean delivery with intrathecal morphine: a systematic review and meta-analysis. Anesth Analg 2009;109(1):174–82.
28. van Meeteren LA, Moolenaar WH. Regulation and biological activities of the autotaxin-LPA axis. Prog Lipid Res 2007;46(2):145–60.
29. Hashimoto T, Ohata H, Momose K. Itch-scratch responses induced by lysophosphatidic acid in mice. Pharmacology 2004;72(1):51–6.
30. Paumgartner G, Beuers U. Mechanisms of action and therapeutic efficacy of ursodeoxycholic acid in cholestatic liver disease. Clin Liver Dis 2004;8(1):67–81, vi.

31. Geenes V, Williamson C. Intrahepatic cholestasis of pregnancy. World J Gastroenterol 2009;15(17):2049–66.
32. Lindor KD. Ursodiol for primary sclerosing cholangitis. Mayo Primary Sclerosing Cholangitis-Ursodeoxycholic Acid Study Group. N Engl J Med 1997;336(10):691–5.
33. Talwalkar JA, Souto E, Jorgensen RA, et al. Natural history of pruritus in primary biliary cirrhosis. Clin Gastroenterol Hepatol 2003;1(4):297–302.
34. EASL Clinical Practice Guidelines: management of cholestatic liver diseases. J Hepatol 2009;51(2):237–67.
35. Kaplan MM, Schmid C, Provenzale D, et al. A prospective trial of colchicine and methotrexate in the treatment of primary biliary cirrhosis. Gastroenterology 1999;117(5):1173–80.
36. Mitchison HC, Palmer JM, Bassendine MF, et al. A controlled trial of prednisolone treatment in primary biliary cirrhosis. Three-year results. J Hepatol 1992;15(3):336–44.
37. Wiesner RH, Ludwig J, Lindor KD, et al. A controlled trial of cyclosporine in the treatment of primary biliary cirrhosis. N Engl J Med 1990;322(20):1419–24.
38. Hendrickse MT, Rigney E, Giaffer MH, et al. Low-dose methotrexate is ineffective in primary biliary cirrhosis: long-term results of a placebo-controlled trial. Gastroenterology 1999;117(2):400–7.
39. Carey JB Jr, Williams G. Relief of the pruritus of jaundice with a bile-acid sequestering resin. JAMA 1961;176:432–5.
40. Van Itallie TB, Hashim SA, Crampton RS, et al. The treatment of pruritus and hypercholesteremia of primary biliary cirrhosis with cholestyramine. N Engl J Med 1961;265:469–74.
41. Datta DV, Sherlock S. Treatment of pruritus of obstructive jaundice with cholestyramine. Br Med J 1963;1(5325):216–9.
42. Datta DV, Sherlock S. Cholestyramine for long term relief of the pruritus complicating intrahepatic cholestasis. Gastroenterology 1966;50(3):323–32.
43. Wiertelak EP, Maier SF, Watkins LR. Cholecystokinin antianalgesia: safety cues abolish morphine analgesia. Science 1992;256(5058):830–3.
44. Javitt NB. Letter: timing of cholestyramine doses in cholestatic liver disease. N Engl J Med 1974;290(23):1328–9.
45. Rust C, Sauter GH, Oswald M, et al. Effect of cholestyramine on bile acid pattern and synthesis during administration of ursodeoxycholic acid in man. Eur J Clin Invest 2000;30(2):135–9.
46. Aldridge MA, Ito MK. Colesevelam hydrochloride: a novel bile acid-binding resin. Ann Pharmacother 2001;35(7-8):898–907.
47. Cohen LB, Ambinder EP, Wolke AM, et al. Role of plasmapheresis in primary biliary cirrhosis. Gut 1985;26(3):291–4.
48. Omokawa S, Yamashita M, Malchesky PS, et al. Therapeutic plasmapheresis for cholestatic liver diseases: study of 9 cases. Prog Clin Biol Res 1990;337:233–6.
49. Montero JL, Pozo JC, Barrera P, et al. Treatment of refractory cholestatic pruritus with molecular adsorbent recirculating system (MARS). Transplant Proc 2006;38(8):2511–3.
50. Pares A, Cisneros L, Salmeron JM, et al. Extracorporeal albumin dialysis: a procedure for prolonged relief of intractable pruritus in patients with primary biliary cirrhosis. Am J Gastroenterol 2004;99(6):1105–10.
51. Pares A, Herrera M, Aviles J, et al. Treatment of resistant pruritus from cholestasis with albumin dialysis: combined analysis of patients from three centers. J Hepatol 2010;53(2):307–12.

52. Ambinder EP, Cohen LB, Wolke AM, et al. The clinical effectiveness and safety of chronic plasmapheresis in patients with primary biliary cirrhosis. J Clin Apher 1985;2(3):219–23.
53. Bellmann R, Graziadei IW, Feistritzer C, et al. Treatment of refractory cholestatic pruritus after liver transplantation with albumin dialysis. Liver Transpl 2004;10(1): 107–14.
54. Chen J, Raymond K. Roles of rifampicin in drug-drug interactions: underlying molecular mechanisms involving the nuclear pregnane X receptor. Ann Clin Microbiol Antimicrob 2006;5:3.
55. Marschall HU, Wagner M, Zollner G, et al. Complementary stimulation of hepatobiliary transport and detoxification systems by rifampicin and ursodeoxycholic acid in humans. Gastroenterology 2005;129(2):476–85.
56. Bachs L, Pares A, Elena M, et al. Comparison of rifampicin with phenobarbitone for treatment of pruritus in biliary cirrhosis. Lancet 1989;1(8638):574–6.
57. Bloomer JR, Boyer JL. Phenobarbital effects in cholestatic liver diseases. Ann Intern Med 1975;82(3):310–7.
58. Kreek MJ, Garfield JW, Gutjahr CL, et al. Rifampin-induced methadone withdrawal. N Engl J Med 1976;294(20):1104–6.
59. Glantz A, Reilly SJ, Benthin L, et al. Intrahepatic cholestasis of pregnancy: amelioration of pruritus by UDCA is associated with decreased progesterone disulphates in urine. Hepatology 2008;47(2):544–51.
60. Podesta A, Lopez P, Terg R, et al. Treatment of pruritus of primary biliary cirrhosis with rifampin. Dig Dis Sci 1991;36(2):216–20.
61. Bachs L, Pares A, Elena M, et al. Effects of long-term rifampicin administration in primary biliary cirrhosis. Gastroenterology 1992;102(6):2077–80.
62. Khurana S, Singh P. Rifampin is safe for treatment of pruritus due to chronic cholestasis: a meta-analysis of prospective randomized-controlled trials. Liver Int 2006;26(8):943–8.
63. Tandon P, Rowe BH, Vandermeer B, et al. The efficacy and safety of bile acid binding agents, opioid antagonists, or rifampin in the treatment of cholestasis-associated pruritus. Am J Gastroenterol 2007;102(7):1528–36.
64. Prince MI, Burt AD, Jones DE. Hepatitis and liver dysfunction with rifampicin therapy for pruritus in primary biliary cirrhosis. Gut 2002;50(3):436–9.
65. Kumar R, Bhatia V, Khanal S, et al. Antituberculosis therapy-induced acute liver failure: magnitude, profile, prognosis, and predictors of outcome. Hepatology 2010;51(5):1665–74.
66. Turner IB, Rawlins MD, Wood P, et al. Flumecinol for the treatment of pruritus associated with primary biliary cirrhosis. Aliment Pharmacol Ther 1994;8(3):337–42.
67. Bergasa NV, Talbot TL, Alling DW, et al. A controlled trial of naloxone infusions for the pruritus of chronic cholestasis. Gastroenterology 1992;102(2):544–9.
68. Bergasa NV, Alling DW, Talbot TL, et al. Effects of naloxone infusions in patients with the pruritus of cholestasis. A double-blind, randomized, controlled trial. Ann Intern Med 1995;123(3):161–7.
69. Wolfhagen FH, Sternieri E, Hop WC, et al. Oral naltrexone treatment for cholestatic pruritus: a double-blind, placebo-controlled study. Gastroenterology 1997;113(4):1264–9.
70. Bergasa NV, Schmitt JM, Talbot TL, et al. Open-label trial of oral nalmefene therapy for the pruritus of cholestasis. Hepatology 1998;27(3):679–84.
71. Bergasa NV, Alling DW, Talbot TL, et al. Oral nalmefene therapy reduces scratching activity due to the pruritus of cholestasis: a controlled study. J Am Acad Dermatol 1999;41(3 Pt 1):431–4.

72. Terg R, Coronel E, Sorda J, et al. Efficacy and safety of oral naltrexone treatment for pruritus of cholestasis, a crossover, double blind, placebo-controlled study. J Hepatol 2002;37(6):717–22.
73. Mansour-Ghanaei F, Taheri A, Froutan H, et al. Effect of oral naltrexone on pruritus in cholestatic patients. World J Gastroenterol 2006;12(7):1125–8.
74. Carson KL, Tran TT, Cotton P, et al. Pilot study of the use of naltrexone to treat the severe pruritus of cholestatic liver disease. Am J Gastroenterol 1996;91(5): 1022–3.
75. Thornton JR, Losowsky MS. Opioid peptides and primary biliary cirrhosis. BMJ 1988;297(6662):1501–4.
76. Jones EA, Dekker LR. Florid opioid withdrawal-like reaction precipitated by naltrexone in a patient with chronic cholestasis. Gastroenterology 2000;118(2): 431–2.
77. Ko MC, Lee H, Song MS, et al. Activation of kappa-opioid receptors inhibits pruritus evoked by subcutaneous or intrathecal administration of morphine in monkeys. J Pharmacol Exp Ther 2003;305(1):173–9.
78. Muller C, Pongratz S, Pidlich J, et al. Treatment of pruritus in chronic liver disease with the 5-hydroxytryptamine receptor type 3 antagonist ondansetron: a randomized, placebo-controlled, double-blind cross-over trial. Eur J Gastroenterol Hepatol 1998;10(10):865–70.
79. Schworer H, Hartmann H, Ramadori G. Relief of cholestatic pruritus by a novel class of drugs: 5-hydroxytryptamine type 3 (5-HT3) receptor antagonists: effectiveness of ondansetron. Pain 1995;61(1):33–7.
80. Jones EA, Molenaar HA, Oosting J. Ondansetron and pruritus in chronic liver disease: a controlled study. Hepatogastroenterology 2007;54(76):1196–9.
81. O'Donohue JW, Pereira SP, Ashdown AC, et al. A controlled trial of ondansetron in the pruritus of cholestasis. Aliment Pharmacol Ther 2005;21(8):1041–5.
82. Browning J, Combes B, Mayo MJ. Long-term efficacy of sertraline as a treatment for cholestatic pruritus in patients with primary biliary cirrhosis. Am J Gastroenterol 2003;98(12):2736–41.
83. Mayo MJ, Handem I, Saldana S, et al. Sertraline as a first-line treatment for cholestatic pruritus. Hepatology 2007;45(3):666–74.
84. Bergasa NV, McGee M, Ginsburg IH, et al. Gabapentin in patients with the pruritus of cholestasis: a double-blind, randomized, placebo-controlled trial. Hepatology 2006;44(5):1317–23.
85. Sheen MJ, Ho ST, Lee CH, et al. Preoperative gabapentin prevents intrathecal morphine-induced pruritus after orthopedic surgery. Anesth Analg 2008; 106(6):1868–72.
86. Vila T, Gommer J, Scates AC. Role of gabapentin in the treatment of uremic pruritus. Ann Pharmacother 2008;42(7):1080–4.
87. Ahuja RB, Gupta R, Gupta G, et al. A comparative analysis of cetirizine, gabapentin and their combination in the relief of post-burn pruritus. Burns 2011;37(2): 203–7.
88. Gingold AR, Bergasa NV. The cannabinoid agonist WIN 55, 212-2 increases nociception threshold in cholestatic rats: implications for the treatment of the pruritus of cholestasis. Life Sci 2003;73(21):2741–7.
89. Neff GW, O'Brien CB, Reddy KR, et al. Preliminary observation with dronabinol in patients with intractable pruritus secondary to cholestatic liver disease. Am J Gastroenterol 2002;97(8):2117–9.
90. Borgeat A, Wilder-Smith OH, Mentha G. Subhypnotic doses of propofol relieve pruritus associated with liver disease. Gastroenterology 1993;104(1):244–7.

91. Villamil AG, Bandi JC, Galdame OA, et al. Efficacy of lidocaine in the treatment of pruritus in patients with chronic cholestatic liver diseases. Am J Med 2005; 118(10):1160–3.
92. Watson WC. Intravenous lignocaine for relief of intractable itch. Lancet 1973; 1(7796):211.
93. Seymour CA, Summerton CB. Effect of stanozolol on itching in primary biliary cirrhosis. Br Med J (Clin Res Ed) 1988;296(6628):1066–7.
94. Kondrackiene J, Beuers U, Kupcinskas L. Efficacy and safety of ursodeoxycholic acid versus cholestyramine in intrahepatic cholestasis of pregnancy. Gastroenterology 2005;129(3):894–901.
95. Palma J, Reyes H, Ribalta J, et al. Ursodeoxycholic acid in the treatment of cholestasis of pregnancy: a randomized, double-blind study controlled with placebo. J Hepatol 1997;27(6):1022–8.
96. Binder T, Salaj P, Zima T, et al. Randomized prospective comparative study of ursodeoxycholic acid and S-adenosyl-L-methionine in the treatment of intrahepatic cholestasis of pregnancy. J Perinat Med 2006;34(5):383–91.
97. Roncaglia N, Locatelli A, Arreghini A, et al. A randomised controlled trial of ursodeoxycholic acid and S-adenosyl-L-methionine in the treatment of gestational cholestasis. BJOG 2004;111(1):17–21.
98. Frezza M, Surrenti C, Manzillo G, et al. Oral S-adenosylmethionine in the symptomatic treatment of intrahepatic cholestasis. A double-blind, placebo-controlled study. Gastroenterology 1990;99(1):211–5.
99. Ribalta J, Reyes H, Gonzalez MC, et al. S-adenosyl-L-methionine in the treatment of patients with intrahepatic cholestasis of pregnancy: a randomized, double-blind, placebo-controlled study with negative results. Hepatology 1991;13(6): 1084–9.
100. Glantz A, Marschall HU, Lammert F, et al. Intrahepatic cholestasis of pregnancy: a randomized controlled trial comparing dexamethasone and ursodeoxycholic acid. Hepatology 2005;42(6):1399–405.
101. van der Woerd WL, van Mil SW, Stapelbroek JM, et al. Familial cholestasis: progressive familial intrahepatic cholestasis, benign recurrent intrahepatic cholestasis and intrahepatic cholestasis of pregnancy. Best Pract Res Clin Gastroenterol 2010;24(5):541–53.
102. Stapelbroek JM, van Erpecum KJ, Klomp LW, et al. Nasobiliary drainage induces long-lasting remission in benign recurrent intrahepatic cholestasis. Hepatology 2006;43(1):51–3.

Chronic Hepatitis B Infection

Alexander Kuo, MD*, Robert Gish, MD

KEYWORDS

• Hepatitis B virus • HBV genotype • HBsAg quantification
• Mother-to-child transmission • Liver transplantation

An estimated 350 to 400 million people worldwide are chronically infected with hepatitis B virus (HBV). The greatest burden of disease lies in Asia, where 75% of infected persons reside, and Africa, which is home to 12% of infected persons.[1] In China, certain islands in the Pacific, and regions of sub-Saharan Africa, up to 60% to 90% of the population have some serologic marker of HBV infection.[2] An estimated 2 million infected persons live in the United States, with a significant proportion being immigrants from endemic regions, especially Asia.[3–5] Although most patients with HBV do not suffer serious sequelae of infection, 15% to 40% can develop cirrhosis or hepatocellular carcinoma (HCC).[6]

In many endemic regions throughout Asia, HBV is largely vertically transmitted (**Table 1**).[7–9] Persons infected in this manner usually experience a prolonged period with normal alanine aminotransferase (ALT) levels and high HBV DNA levels. Liver histology shows minimal or no necroinflammation. This immune tolerant phase of infection can last for decades without progression of disease.[13,14] Throughout sub-Saharan Africa, the Mediterranean region, and Alaska, HBV transmission commonly occurs through close person-to-person contact during childhood.[10,15,16] Infected children usually are hepatitis B e antigen positive (HBeAg[+]), and have high HBV DNA levels and increased ALT, with HBeAg seroconversion occurring around the onset of puberty. In Western countries, HBV is largely transmitted in adulthood through blood exposure, including via sexual exposure or injection drug use, and immediately enters the immune active/clearance phase.[11,12]

Financial disclosures: Alexander Kuo has nothing to disclose.
Robert Gish has relevant consulting relationships with Roche/Genentech, Gilead, BMS. All research, consulting, and promotional fees are placed in a UCSD fund for research and education.
Division of Gastroenterology, University of California, San Diego, 200 West Arbor Drive M/C 8413, San Diego, CA 92103, USA
* Corresponding author.
E-mail address: alkuo@ucsd.edu

Clin Liver Dis 16 (2012) 347–369
doi:10.1016/j.cld.2012.03.003
1089-3261/12/$ – see front matter

Table 1
Risk of developing chronic HBV infection varies by age and method of exposure

Acute HBV Exposure	Risk of Developing Chronic HBV Infection (%)
Newborns of HBeAg(+) mothers[7]	90
Infants and children less than age 5 years[8,9]	25–30
Adults[10–12]	5

PHASES OF HBV INFECTION

The immune response against acute HBV infection and the subsequent natural history of chronic infection largely depend on the age of infection (**Figs. 1** and **2**). Chronic HBV can be divided into 4 states: immune tolerant, HBeAg(+) chronic hepatitis, HBeAg(–) chronic hepatitis, and the inactive carrier state.

The immune tolerant phase is most common after perinatal infection with wild-type HBV. After decades of quiescence, it can evolve into HBeAg(+) chronic hepatitis characterized by persistent or episodic increases in ALT level (flares). In persons with increased ALT levels (>20 IU/mL for women and >30 IU/mL for men), the rate of spontaneous HBeAg seroconversion ranges from 8% to 12% per year, with up to 80% of those achieving HBeAg seroconversion transitioning to the inactive carrier state characterized by normal ALT level and low or undetectable HBV DNA.[14,15,17–19] However, after HBeAg seroconversion, some persons can show persistently increased ALT and

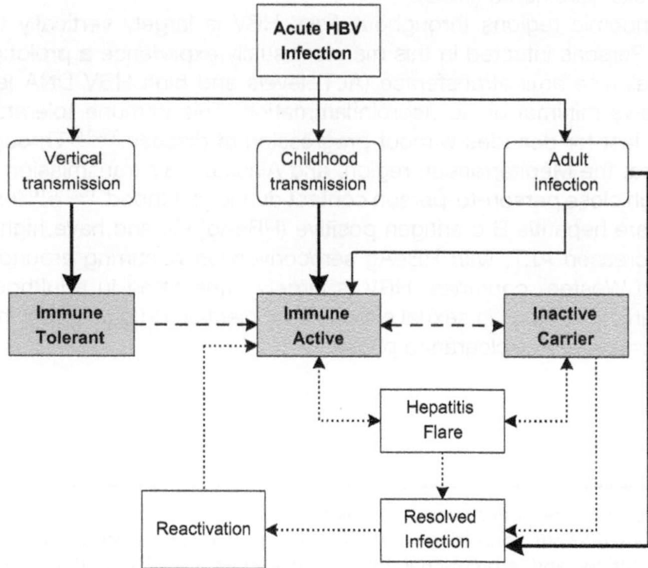

Fig. 1. Natural history of acute hepatitis B infection. Vertical transmission usually results in immune tolerant infection; childhood transmission commonly leads to immune active infection; and adult exposure generally leads to resolved infection, although some develop chronic infection. Transition between the immune tolerant, immune active, and inactive carrier phases of chronic infection is dynamic. Immune active chronic hepatitis leads to necroinflammation and fibrosis progression, and increases the risk of developing cirrhosis and HCC. (*Adapted from* Hepatitis Web Study, University of Washington. Available at: http://depts.washington.edu/hepstudy/hepB/history/chronic/discussion.html; with permission.)

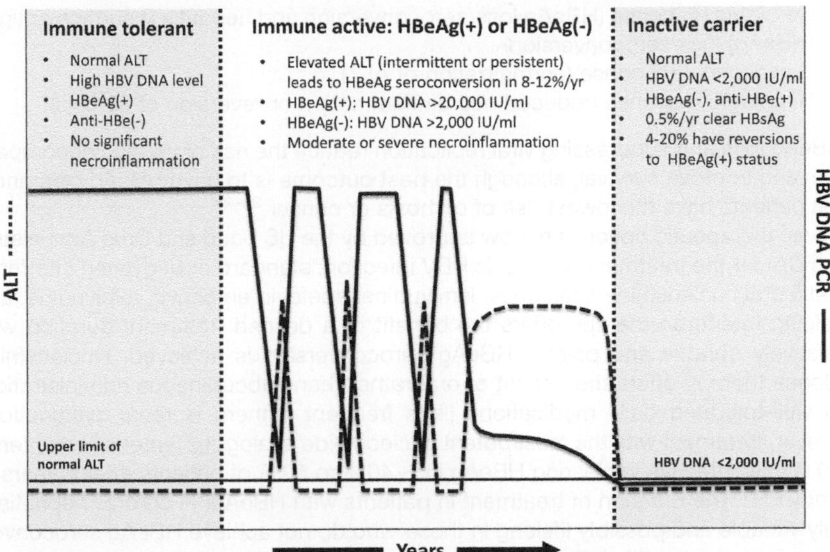

Fig. 2. Major phases of chronic hepatitis B infection. The natural history of HBV infection can be divided into 4 major phases: the immune tolerant phase, HBeAg(+) chronic hepatitis, HBeAg(–) chronic hepatitis, and the inactive carrier state. These states do not occur in all patients and transitions between states are dynamic and can be nonconsecutive.

high HBV DNA levels, and have evidence of necroinflammation on biopsy when the attempts at immune clearance are ineffective[20]: a fourth state termed HBeAg(–) chronic hepatitis. This HBeAg(–) phase is marked by the emergence of core or precore mutations that decrease eAg production yet viral replication and virion production continue in the liver. HBeAg(–) chronic hepatitis is usually associated with a fluctuating course of hepatitis and 1 to 2 $\log_{10}$ lower average HBV DNA levels compared with persons with HBeAg(+) chronic hepatitis. The longer a person remains in the immune active phase of infection, either HBeAg(+) or (–), the greater the degree of necroinflammation, fibrosis, and the greater the risk of developing cirrhosis or HCC.

Each of these major phases is associated with characteristic patterns of ALT, HBV DNA levels, HBeAg, liver histology, and response to antiviral therapy. Transition between phases is dynamic and patients do not always cycle through all phases during the course of their infection. For example, up to 20% of those in the inactive carrier state can revert back to HBeAg positivity and experience reactivation with flares of hepatitis, and a subgroup of patients move directly from HBeAg(+) to HBeAg(–) chronic hepatitis disease.[19,21,22] Many patients who are HBeAg(+) are coinfected with core or precore mutations and thus have a mixed infection.

TREATMENT OPTIONS FOR CHRONIC HBV

Because HBV is a DNA virus that integrates into the host genome and persists in the form of an intracellular replicative intermediary, covalently closed circular DNA, complete elimination of the virus from an infected person is not attainable. Long-term goals of antiviral therapy for HBV are to prevent progression to cirrhosis, liver decompensation, and development of HCC. Various treatment end points include:

- Virologic response (suppression of viral replication to undetectability by polymerase chain reaction)

- Serologic response (HBeAg loss/seroconversion and hepatitis B surface antigen [HBsAg] loss/seroconversion)
- Biochemical response (normalization of ALT)
- Histologic response (reduced necroinflammation or reversion of fibrosis).

HBeAg loss and suppressing viral replication reduce the risk of hepatic decompensation and improve survival, although the best outcome is to have HBsAg clearance, when patients have the lowest risk of cirrhosis or cancer.[23–25]

Seven therapeutic options are now approved by the US Food and Drug Administration (FDA) for the treatment of chronic HBV infection: standard or pegylated interferon α and 5 oral nucleos(t)ide analogues: lamivudine, adefovir, entecavir, telbivudine, and tenofovir. Interferon therapy offers the benefit of a defined treatment duration with a relatively durable end point if HBeAg seroconversion is achieved. Nucleos(t)ide analogue therapy offers the benefit of oral rather than subcutaneous administration, with well-tolerated daily medications (less frequent if there is renal dysfunction). However, treatment with the most potent nucleos(t)ide analogues (entecavir and tenofovir) is only effective in clearing HBeAg in ~40% to 50% of patients after 5 years of therapy.[26,27] The duration of treatment in patients with HBeAg(+) chronic hepatitis is highly variable and possibly lifelong in those who do not achieve HBeAg seroconversion or in patients with HBeAg(–) chronic hepatitis in whom HBeAg serologic end points do not apply. Prolonged therapy increases the risk of viral breakthrough by selecting for antiviral resistance mutants. When choosing first-line oral therapeutic options, one must remember the axiom "There is no resistance without replication." The best therapies should therefore be highly potent, well tolerated, and have a high genetic barrier to resistance.[28]

In order of potency, the oral nucleos(t)ide analogues can be ranked in the following order: entecavir and tenofovir > telbivudine > lamivudine > adefovir (**Table 2**). In addition to being the most potent inhibitors of HBV DNA replication, entecavir and tenofovir also have the highest genetic barriers to resistance. With no well-defined resistance mutation to tenofovir, the term pharmacologic barrier has been used to define this outcome.[28] In treatment-naive HBeAg(+) patients, entecavir resistance was seen in ~1% after 5 years of therapy.[38,39] No tenofovir resistance mutations have been clearly identified to date through up to 240 weeks of treatment.[37,40,41] In contrast, lamivudine resistance develops after a single point mutation, M204V/I, and is seen in 23% of patients after 1 year and up to 80% at 5 years.[42–45] Telbivudine resistance is seen in 5% at 1 year and 25% at 2 years in HBeAg(+) patients.[36] Adefovir resistance is seen in 20% to 29% at 5 years in HBeAg(–) patients and 42% in HBeAg(+) patients.[33,46] Given the greater potency and low rates of antiviral resistance, entecavir and tenofovir should be considered as first-line therapy in patients starting oral nucleos(t)ide analogues for chronic HBV.

The efficacy of each drug in both HBeAg(+) and HBeAg(–) chronic HBV is reviewed in **Tables 2** and **3**. Rates of antiviral resistance as well as the commonly associated resistance mutations are reviewed in **Table 4**.

Immune Tolerant and Inactive Carrier Phases of Infection

For patients in the immune tolerant or inactive carrier phases of infection, there is no clear role for antiviral therapy given the low efficacy of interferon or nucleos(t)ide analogues in the setting of normal ALT level. In studies of lamivudine in HBeAg(+) patients, HBeAg seroconversion occurred in only 2% of patients with normal ALT level compared with 21% of patients with ALT level 2 to 5 times normal, and 47% of patients with ALT level more than 5 times normal.[58] In making the decision as to

Table 2
Responses to antiviral therapy in patients with HBeAg(+) chronic HBV

	PegIFN 180 μg Every Week, 48 Weeks[29] (%)	Lamivudine 100 mg Every Day, 48–52 Weeks[30–32] (%)	Adefovir 10 mg Every Day, 48 Weeks[33,34] (%)	Entecavir 0.5 mg Every Day, 48 Weeks[35] (%)	Telbivudine 600 mg Every Day, 52 Weeks[36] (%)	Tenofovir 300 mg Every Day, 48 Weeks[37] (%)
Loss of HBV DNA	25	40–44	21	67	60	76
Loss of HBeAg	30	17–32	24	22	26	—
HBeAg seroconversion	27	16–21	12/48[a]	21	22	21
Loss of HBsAg	3	1	0	2	0	3
Normalization of ALT	39	41–75	48	68	77	68
Durability of response	—	50–80	~90	69	~80	—

[a] 12% HBeAg seroconversion after 1 year and 50% after 5 years.

Table 3
Responses to antiviral therapy in patients with HBeAg(−) chronic HBV

	PegIFN 180 µg Every Week, 48 Weeks[29] (%)	Lamivudine 100 mg Every Day, 48–52 Weeks[47–50] (%)	Adefovir 10 mg Every Day, 48 Weeks[51] (%)	Entecavir 0.5 mg Every Day, 48 Weeks[52,53] (%)	Telbivudine 600 mg Every Day, 52 Weeks[36] (%)	Tenofovir 300 mg Every Day, 48 Weeks[37] (%)
Loss of HBV DNA	63	60–73	51	90	88	93
Loss of HBsAg	—	—	—	—	—	0
Normalization of ALT	38	60–79	72	78	74	76
Durability of response	~20	<10	~5	3	—	—

Table 4
Rates of drug resistance at year of antiviral therapy for HBV

Drug	Rates of Drug Resistance at Year of Treatment (% Patients)					Resistance Mutations
	Year 1	Year 2	Year 3	Year 4	Year 5	
Lamivudine[42–45]	23	46	55	71	80	M204V/I
Entecavir (naïve)[38,39]	0.1	0.4	1.1	1.1	1.2	M204V/I, T184, S202, M250
Entecavir (lamivudine-resistant)[38,39]	6–7	15–16	35	43	51[54]	—
Telbivudine (naïve)[36,55]	—	—	—	—	—	M204I
HBeAg(+)	5	25	—	—	—	—
HBeAg(–)	2	11	—	—	—	—
Adefovir (naïve)	—	—	—	—	—	N236T, A181V/T
HBeAg(+)[33]	0	—	—	—	20	—
HBeAg(–)[46]	0	3	11	18	29	—
Adefovir (lamivudine-resistant)[56,57]	18[a]	22[b]	—	—	—	—
Tenofovir[37]	0	0[c]	0[40]	—	0[41]	No confirmed reports

[a] 18% adefovir resistance mutations were seen in patients with lamivudine resistance who were switched to adefovir.
[b] 79% of patients in this study had previous lamivudine exposure.
[c] Emtricitabine was added to patients who remained viremic at week 72.

whether to start antiviral therapy, one needs to consider the long-term risk of developing resistance to oral nucleos(t)ide analogues if the likelihood of achieving a serologic end point is low.[29,58–60] These patients should be closely monitored with serial ALT and HBV DNA measurements every 3 to 6 months to confirm that they remain in either the immune tolerant or inactive carrier stages of infection and have not progressed or reverted to chronic hepatitis.[61]

HBeAg(+) Chronic Hepatitis B

For patients with HBeAg(+) chronic hepatitis, the goals of therapy are to suppress viral replication, normalize ALT level, and achieve the serologic end points of HBeAg loss, HBeAg seroconversion, and HBsAg loss and HBsAg seroconversion. For patients with predictors of response to interferon (increased ALT level, low HBV DNA level, and HBV genotypes A and B vs C or D), treatment with interferon offers the advantage of a finite 12-month course of therapy.[62,63] With oral nucleos(t)ide analogues, treatment duration is generally greater than 12 months and treatment discontinuation can be considered if HBV DNA is undetectable and HBeAg loss (and possibly seroconversion) is achieved with at least 6 to 12 months of consolidation therapy, although this serologic end point is not universally durable. It has been proposed that the durability of HBeAg seroconversion can be increased by extending this so-called consolidation therapy, beyond 6 to 12 months after HBeAg seroconversion is achieved.

HBeAg(–) Chronic Hepatitis B

For patients with HBeAg(–) chronic hepatitis, HBeAg seroconversion is not possible and HBsAg seroconversion is a rare event. Therefore, the short-term and long-term goals of therapy are normalization of ALT and complete suppression of viral replication. Contrary to patients with HBeAg(+) chronic hepatitis, there are no clear predictors of interferon responsiveness in patients with HBeAg(–) chronic hepatitis. Treatment with nucleos(t)ide analogues results in a greater percentage of undetectable HBV DNA compared with HBeAg(+) patients, because of the 1 to 2 log_{10} lower average baseline HBV DNA levels found in HBeAg(–) patients. The optimal duration of therapy with nucleos(t)ide analogues is generally recommended to be lifelong given the high risk of relapse (90%–97%) after treatment is stopped in patients who achieve a sustained response (normalization of ALT level with undetectable HBV DNA).[36,37,47,51–53]

VIRAL FACTORS ASSOCIATED WITH DISEASE PROGRESSION AND RESPONSE TO ANTIVIRAL THERAPY

Role of HBV Genotype

Ten distinct genotypes of HBV (A to J) with several subtypes have been identified, each with predominant patterns of geographic distribution.[64] Genotypes Ae and D are more common in Europe and North America. Genotypes B and C are more common in the Asia-Pacific region. More specifically, genotype Aa is found in sub-Saharan Africa, West Africa, and the Philippines, as well as in immigrant populations in Europe. Genotype B is most common in Southeast Asia, Southern China, Alaska, Canada, and Greenland. Genotype C is found in East Asia, Northern China, Korea, Taiwan, and in immigrant populations in Australia, although genotype D is predominant in Africa, southern and eastern Europe, certain islands in the South Pacific, the Mediterranean, and India. In the United States the most common genotypes are A (35%), B (22%), C (31%), and D (10%), with E to G comprising only 2% of chronic infections.[65] In Asia, where genotypes B and C predominate, patients with genotype B have been shown to have higher rates of spontaneous HBeAg seroconversion compared with genotype C (47% vs 27% at 52 months) with an annual incidence of 15.5% versus 7.9%, respectively.[66] In a Spanish study of 258 patients with chronic HBV, there was no difference in the rate of spontaneous HBeAg seroconversion between genotypes A and D, although the durability of HBeAg seroconversion was higher in genotype A than in genotype D (55% vs 32%).[67]

HBV genotype C has been linked to a higher risk of cirrhosis and HCC in several East Asian studies.[68,69] In a study of 2762 Taiwanese patients with chronic HBV, genotype C was associated with an increased risk of developing HCC compared with genotype B, with a hazard ratio of 2.35 (1.68–3.30, 95% confidence interval [CI]; *P*<.001).[70] Given the lower rate of spontaneous HBeAg seroconversion in patients with genotype C compared with genotype B, it is possible that patients with genotype C chronic HBV have longer periods of HBeAg(+) chronic hepatitis, with frequent hepatitis flares that lead to fibrosis progression and cirrhosis. The higher viral replication seen in genotype C may also play a role in disease severity.[71]

Although testing for HBV genotype is not specifically recommended in current practice guidelines, there is a review of the usefulness of genotyping in each guideline and a delineation of usefulness in cases in which interferon is used by the American Association for the Study of Liver Diseases (AASLD), the European Association for the Study of the Liver, and the Asian Pacific Association for the Study of the Liver (**Fig. 3**). In a randomized study of pegylated interferon monotherapy versus combination therapy with pegylated interferon and lamivudine in a largely White cohort with HBeAg(+) chronic HBV in whom the mode of transmission was vertical in only 23%, HBeAg seroconversion was more common in genotypes A (47%) and B (44%) compared with genotypes C (28%) and D (25%).[63] In a randomized study of pegylated interferon, lamivudine, or the combination in a largely East Asian cohort with HBeAg(+)

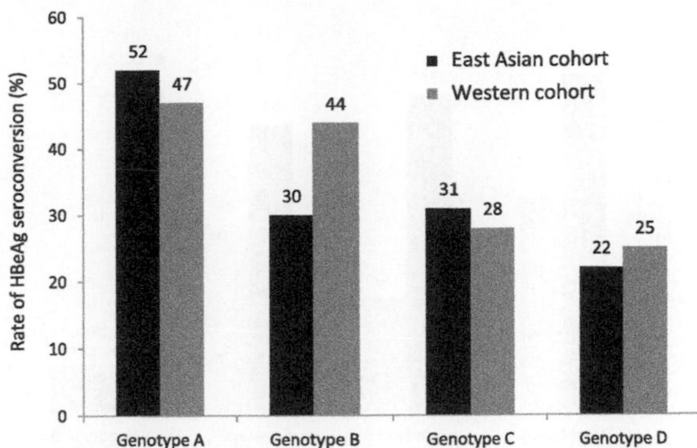

Fig. 3. Rates of HBeAg seroconversion 6 months after a 1-year course of pegylated interferon therapy by HBV genotype in East Asian and Western patients with HBeAg(+) chronic HBV. (*Data from* Lau GK, Piratvisuth T, Luo KX, et al. Peginterferon Alfa-2a, lamivudine, and the combination for HBeAg-positive chronic hepatitis B. N Engl J Med 2005;352(26):2682–95; and Janssen HL, van Zonneveld M, Senturk H, et al. Pegylated interferon alfa-2b alone or in combination with lamivudine for HBeAg-positive chronic hepatitis B: a randomised trial. Lancet 2005;365(9454):123–9.)

chronic HBV, HBeAg seroconversion in the pegylated interferon monotherapy arm was more common in genotype A (52%, 12/23) than in genotypes B (30%, 23/76), C (31%, 50/162), or D (22%, 2/9), although these results should be viewed with some caution given the small number of patients in this study with genotypes A or D.[29] HBsAg seroconversion was uncommon in this study but the rates appeared to differ by genotype in the pegylated interferon monotherapy arm: A (22%, 5/23), B (0%, 0/76), C (10%, 3/31), and D (0%, 0/9).

These studies suggest that HBeAg and possibly HBsAg seroconversion rates are higher in patients with genotype A infection treated with interferon therapy, although the findings require further confirmation. Further research into the role of HBV genotype in predicting response to interferon is needed before its use can be recommended in making treatment decisions. Although data are mounting that HBV genotype predicts response to interferon-based therapy, there is no clear evidence that HBV genotype is a predictor of response with nucleos(t)ide analogue therapy.[72]

Role of IL28B Genetic Polymorphisms

Recent studies have also suggested an association between IL28B polymorphisms and serologic response with pegylated interferon therapy. In a study of 205 patients with HBeAg(+) chronic HBV in European and Asian centers treated with pegylated interferon ± lamivudine, IL28B AA at rs12980275 was associated with HBeAg seroconversion with odds ratio of 3.16 (1.26–8.52, 95% CI; P = .013) after adjusting for HBV genotype, HBV DNA level, ALT level, and combination therapy.[73] The adjusted odds ratio for seroconversion for IL28B CC at rs12979860 was 2.86 (1.15–7.80, 95% CI; P = .024). The prevalence of IL28B CC at rs12979860 by genotype in this study was A 39%, B 88%, C 91%, and D 52%, highlighting the high prevalence of this favorable allele in Asian populations, who are largely genotypes B and C. Both IL28B AA and CC were associated with higher rates of HBeAg seroconversion in patients with genotypes A, B, and C, but not in patients with genotype D (**Fig. 4**), highlighting that clinicians must take a comprehensive approach to assessing treatment recommendations for patients and need to include both viral and host factors in the treatment decisions.

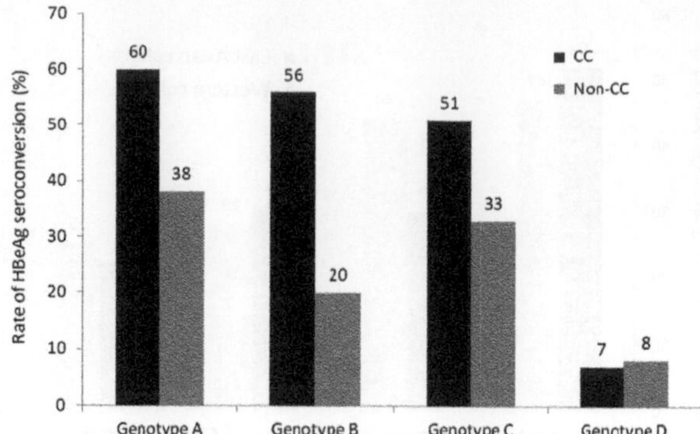

Fig. 4. HBeAg seroconversion rates by genotype and IL28B rs12979860 polymorphism. (*Adapted from* Sonneveld MJ, Wong VW, Woltman AM, et al. Polymorphisms near IL28B and serologic response to peginterferon in HBeAg-positive patients with chronic hepatitis B. Gastroenterology 2012;142(3):513–20; with permission.)

Role of HBsAg Quantification

Recent data have emerged describing the potential value of HBsAg quantification in understanding the natural history of chronic HBV infection as well as in predicting response to interferon therapy in a manner analogous to the response-guided therapy paradigm used in the treatment of chronic hepatitis C infection. HBsAg and HBV DNA levels vary during the natural history of chronic HBV infection as patients transition between phases. During the immune tolerant phase, HBsAg and HBV DNA levels are at their highest. Both levels decline during the chronic hepatitis phase, especially in patients who undergo natural HBeAg seroconversion, and reach their lowest levels during the inactive carrier state.[74–76]

Current definitions of the 4 major phases of HBV infection lack a well-defined consensus on biochemical, serologic, or virologic criteria, which opens the door for misclassification of patients, especially in distinguishing between cases of true inactive carriers and those with HBeAg(−) chronic hepatitis with normal or minimally increased ALT and low HBV DNA levels, as well as HBeAg(+) patients with mixed infection with precore or core mutations. Numerous reports have shown that patients with HBeAg(−) chronic hepatitis generally have higher HBsAg and HBV DNA levels than inactive carriers and that the ratio of HBsAg to HBV DNA is highest in the inactive carrier state compared with other phases of infection.[74–77] These data raise the possibility of more clearly defining the various phases of infection through use of threshold values for HBsAg and HBV DNA combined with HBsAg/HBV DNA ratios, although the optimal cutoff values for disease definition have not been defined.

Rates of sustained response with a 12-month course of pegylated interferon therapy range from 20% to 30% depending on HBeAg status. Because only a few patients achieve a sustained response, efforts to predict ultimate response to therapy could allow some patients to discontinue futile interventions or encourage others to continue based on favorable on-treatment predictors. The recent development of commercially available HBsAg quantification assays has allowed providers to follow HBsAg levels during the course of antiviral therapy. A small study from Hong Kong of HBeAg(+) patients showed that HBsAg levels less than 1500 IU/mL at week 12 of treatment with pegylated interferon monotherapy or combination therapy with lamivudine was associated with a 46% HBeAg seroconversion rate after completing 12 months of therapy. In patients who sustained an HBsAg level less than 300 IU/mL at 24 weeks, the rate of HBeAg seroconversion was 62%. In comparison, only 14% of patients with week 12 HBsAg levels greater than 1500 IU/mL in this study achieved HBeAg seroconversion.[74] Another retrospective analysis of HBeAg(+) patients treated with 48 weeks of pegylated interferon with or without lamivudine showed that week 12 HBsAg levels less than 1500 IU/mL or 1500 to 20,000 IU/mL were associated with HBeAg seroconversion rates of 57% and 32%, respectively.[78]

In HBeAg(−) patients, on-treatment declines in HBsAg level also seem to correlate with end of treatment response. In a study from France, 48 patients with HBeAg(−) HBV were treated with 48 weeks of pegylated interferon and 25% achieved a sustained virologic response (SVR), defined as HBV DNA less than 70 IU/mL 6 months after treatment completion. Eight of the 9 patients who showed $\geq$0.5 $\log_{10}$ decline of HBsAg levels at week 12 achieved SVR (89%). In contrast, only 4 of the 39 patients who had less than 0.5 $\log_{10}$ decline at week 12 were able to achieve SVR (10%). Patients who showed $\geq$0.5 $\log_{10}$ decline of HBsAg levels at week 24 achieved SVR at a rate of 92%.[79]

For patients with HBeAg(+) HBV treated with nucleos(t)ide analogues, current practice guidelines suggest stopping treatment 12 months after HBeAg seroconversion is achieved. However, the durability of response ranges from 50% to 90% (see **Table 2**). In patients with HBeAg(−) HBV, treatment is recommended to be continued indefinitely unless HBsAg loss is achieved. Data on the predictive role of HBsAg decline with nucleos(t)ide analogue treatment are accumulating. In a small study of 17 patients who achieved HBeAg seroconversion with telbivudine, on-treatment week 104 HBsAg level less than 100 IU/mL was associated with sustained response in 93%. No patients with week 104 HBsAg level greater than 100 IU/mL achieved a sustained response.[80] In a separate study of entecavir therapy in HBeAg(+) patients, greater than 1 log IU/ml decline in HBsAg levels on treatment was associated with HBeAg loss in 80% compared with 30% after 1 year of treatment.[81]

These data suggest that week 12 and 24 on-treatment HBsAg thresholds can be useful in predicting response to interferon-based therapy, with the negative predictive values appearing to be more robust than the positive predictive values. Data for on-treatment HBsAg decline with nucleos(t)ide analogue therapy are beginning to reach critical mass, with more than 150 articles on HBsAg quantification. HBsAg quantification is used broadly in Europe and Asia, although there seems to be a requirement for more work to be done before these data can be incorporated into AASLD practice guidelines.

HBV TREATMENT IN SPECIAL POPULATIONS

Mother-to-Child Transmission

Globally, mother-to-child transmission (MTCT) is the predominant mode of transmission, especially throughout the Asia-Pacific region. The risk of transmission can reach as high as 90% in the absence of prophylaxis.[7,82] The combination of passive and active immune prophylaxis consisting of hepatitis B immunoglobulin (HBIG) given to the infant within 12 hours of birth and recombinant HBV immunization given at birth, 1 month, and 6 months can reduce the risk of MTCT to as low as ~5%.[82,83] Despite prophylaxis, MTCT rates remain high at approximately 10% to 30% in HBeAg(+) mothers with high HBV DNA levels (>10^6 copies/mL $\approx$ 200,000 IU/mL), possibly because of intrauterine transmission as well as the higher infectivity associated with high levels of viremia.[84–87] HBeAg may play an immune modulating role by inducing tolerance in the infant and increasing the rate of chronic infection, although the data are not conclusive.[88,89] MTCT is rare in HBeAg(−) mothers, although this is more likely to be caused by the lack of infectivity of the HBeAg(–) viral disease. If disease transmission occurs, the child develops HBeAg(+) disease. Rather than changes in immune modulation in the absence of HBeAg, it may be the lower HBV DNA levels seen in these mothers that influence infection transmission.[90,91] In an Australian study of 313 HBsAg(+) pregnant women whose infants received HBIG and HBV immunization, transmission rates were 7% (4/61) in HBeAg(+) mothers, 0% (0/252) in HBeAg(–) mothers, 9% (20/222) in mothers with HBV DNA levels greater than 10^8 copies/mL (≈20,000,000 IU/mL), and 0% (0/91) in mothers with HBV DNA levels less than 10^8 copies/mL.[85]

Although the use of nucleos(t)ide analogues in patients during the immune tolerant phase of infection is generally not warranted, using antiviral therapies during pregnancy to lower HBV DNA levels in pregnant mothers before delivery to minimize the risk of MTCT has been investigated. Because organogenesis is largely completed during the first trimester, initiation of nucleos(t)ide analogue therapy has focused on the second and most commonly the third trimester. Data on the lack of risk of birth defects are most robust with lamivudine despite its classification as FDA pregnancy class C (**Table 5**). In data including 10,530 pregnancies from the Antiretroviral

Table 5
FDA pregnancy categories for HBV therapies

Category	Description	Drug(s)
A	Adequate and well-controlled (AWC) studies in pregnant women have failed to show a risk to the fetus in the first trimester of pregnancy (and there is no evidence of a risk in later trimesters)	None
B	Animal reproduction studies have failed to show a risk to the fetus and there are no AWC studies in pregnant women, or animal studies show a risk and AWC studies in pregnant women have not shown a risk during the first trimester (and there is no evidence of risk in later trimesters)	Telbivudine Tenofovir
C	Animal reproduction studies have shown an adverse effect on the fetus, there are no AWC studies in humans, and the benefits from the use of the drug in pregnant women may be acceptable despite its potential risks, or animal studies have not been conducted and there are no AWC studies in humans	Adefovir Entecavir Lamivudine Interferon α2b Peginterferon α2a
D	There is positive evidence of human fetal risk based on adverse reaction data from investigational or marketing experience or studies in humans, but the potential benefits from the use of the drug in pregnant women may be acceptable despite its potential risks (eg, if the drug is needed in a life-threatening situation or serious disease for which safer drugs cannot be used or are ineffective)	None
X	Studies in animals or humans have shown fetal abnormalities or there is positive evidence of fetal risk based on adverse reaction reports from investigational or marketing experience, or both, and the risk of the use of the drug in a pregnant woman clearly outweighs any possible benefit (eg, safer drugs or other forms of therapy are available)	None

Pregnancy Registry, the rate of birth defects was found to be no different in infants born from mothers (mostly human immunodeficiency virus [HIV] monoinfected and HIV/HBV coinfected) who were exposed to lamivudine during the first or second trimesters (3.1% and 2.7%, respectively), compared with the baseline rates of birth defects. The rate of birth defects was similarly low among 1921 pregnancies with tenofovir exposure during the first or second trimesters (2.4% and 2.0%, respectively). The registry included few mothers with exposure to adefovir (n = 59), entecavir (n = 40), or telbivudine (n = 22), so conclusions regarding these therapies could not be drawn from this dataset.[92] The data supporting a pregnancy risk category B classification for telbivudine are from animal research only; there are no adequate and well-controlled studies of telbivudine in pregnant women.

In a multicenter, double-blind, randomized controlled trial of 150 HBsAg(+) mothers with high levels of viremia (HBV DNA levels >1000 meq/mL ≈250,000,000 IU/mL), the addition of lamivudine started at week 32 of pregnancy and continued 4 weeks post partum; the combination of this with immune prophylaxis (vaccine plus HBIG) given to the infant at birth was more effective at preventing MTCT than the combination of HBIG and HBV immunization alone, with transmission rates of 18% and 39%, respectively.[93] In a recent Chinese study of 229 HBeAg(+) pregnant women between weeks 20 and 32 of gestation and with HBV DNA levels greater than 1.0×10^7 copies/mL, 135 women were initiated on telbivudine 600 mg daily, with treatment stopped 4 weeks post partum in immune tolerant mothers and continued forward in those with chronic HBV; 94 women who refused telbivudine served as controls. At delivery, 33% of the women who received telbivudine had undetectable HBV DNA (<500 copies/mL). The MTCT rate was 0% in the telbivudine group compared with 8% in the control group (P = .002). No congenital abnormalities in the infants were observed.[94]

For HBsAg(+) pregnant women, the addition of a nucleos(t)ide analogue during the third trimester can significantly lower the risk of MTCT. Given the cumulative experience in pregnancy, lamivudine and telbivudine should be considered first-line options. Tenofovir, given its pregnancy risk category B classification, may also be considered. However, no prospective trials with tenofovir in pregnancy are available. There is no consensus on the precise threshold levels for HBV DNA at which antiviral therapy should be initiated, although the risk of MTCT seems to be increased more than 10^6 copies/mL or 200,000 IU/mL.

After Liver Transplantation

In the current era of numerous potent, well-tolerated, oral nucleos(t)ide analogues, hepatic decompensation in patients with HBV-related cirrhosis is becoming a less common event. Treatment with lamivudine has been shown to delay HBV disease progression and reduce the risk of developing HCC, thereby theoretically delaying or eliminating the need for liver transplantation in some instances.[95,96] Consequently, HBV-related cirrhosis as an indication for transplantation in the United States is also becoming less common, with only 4.2% of registrants on waiting lists for liver transplant in the United States from 1985 to 2006 listed for HBV-related liver disease.[97]

Recurrent HBV infection after liver transplantation can occur in patients with a history of acute or chronic HBV before transplantation or in HBsAg(−) recipients of an anti-HBc(+) donor allograft. Before the routine use of HBIG to prevent recurrence, HBV was a poor indication for liver transplantation because of the high rate of recurrent HBV and rapid progression to cirrhosis, a pattern being replicated with recurrent hepatitis C. The use of HBIG in the posttransplant period reduced the risk of recurrent

HBV from 80% to 90% down to 15% to 36%.[98] The addition of oral nucleos(t)ide analogues to HBIG has further reduced the risk of recurrent HBV and patients transplanted for HBV-related liver disease now have one of the best long-term outcomes of any indication for liver transplantation, with 5-year survival rates of more than 85%.[99]

For liver transplant recipients who are HBsAg(+) before transplant, nucleos(t)ide analogue treatment is usually started before transplant, if possible, to reduce the viral load and possibly stabilize or improve hepatic function. Posttransplant prophylaxis, most commonly consisting of intravenous HBIG and lamivudine, has been shown to reduce the risk of recurrent HBV to 0% to 10%.[98,100,101] Conversion of long-term intravenous HBIG to intramuscular HBIG has been shown to be similarly effective at preventing recurrent HBV at a lower cost.[102] Withdrawal of long-term HBIG has been shown to be safe, with low risk of recurrent HBV in patients adherent to nucleos(t)ide analogue therapy. In a study of 21 patients who were maintained on nucleos(t)ide analogue monotherapy after HBIG was withdrawn a median of 26 months after transplant, HBV recurrence was seen in 0% at 2 years and 9% at 4 years, but all cases became HBV DNA undetectable on follow-up testing.[103] In a separate single-center retrospective study, HBV immunization was attempted and long-term HBIG was withdrawn in 12 patients a median of 63 months after transplant, with nucleos(t)ide analogue monotherapy continued forward. Although no patients developed protective levels of anti-HBs, HBV recurrence in this group was 0%.[104] An Italian study of HBIG withdrawal reported HBV recurrence in 4 of 29 patients, although noncompliance was a factor in 3 of the 4 patients who recurred on lamivudine monotherapy.[105] These studies suggest that HBIG withdrawal is safe and does not lead to high rates of HBV recurrence, especially in patients who are adherent to their oral antiviral therapy. The recurrence rate may be even lower with more potent antivirals with high genetic barriers to resistance such as entecavir and tenofovir. In a case series from Hong Kong, 80 patients transplanted for HBV-related disease received entecavir monotherapy for prophylaxis against HBV recurrence. After a median follow-up of 26 months, 91% lost HBsAg and 98.8% had undetectable HBV DNA levels, with no entecavir resistance mutations seen.[106]

For recipients of anti-HBc(+) donor livers, posttransplant management has varied from center to center, with many using a combination of HBIG and a nucleos(t)ide analogue (usually lamivudine) and others using nucleos(t)ide analogue monotherapy. However, the logic behind the use of HBIG in the setting of donors with serologic evidence of previous HBV exposure was unclear. Given the low or absent level of HBV replication in these recipients it was argued that oral antiviral therapy should be sufficient to prevent recurrence. A recent systematic review that included 13 studies reported a risk of HBV recurrence of 3.6% in the HBIG + lamivudine group and 2.7% in the lamivudine monotherapy group. The investigators concluded that the use of HBIG + lamivudine is not more effective than lamivudine alone at preventing recurrence.[107] As with the prevention of recurrent HBV in patients transplanted for HBV-related liver disease, the risk of recurrence in recipients of anti-HBc(+) donor livers may be further reduced with the use of more potent antivirals.

Patients Receiving Chemotherapy or Immunosuppressive Therapy

HBV reactivation in patients receiving chemotherapy or immunosuppressive therapy related to organ transplantation or rheumatologic or gastroenterologic disorders is well documented and associated with significant morbidity and mortality.[108,109] Because of the increasing use of potent immunomodulating agents in the treatment of these disorders, prevention of HBV reactivation in these populations is an important public health concern.[110] The reported incidence of HBV reactivation in HBsAg(+) patients receiving chemotherapy without prophylaxis is between 14% and 85%, with mortality as high as 60% to 70%, depending on the type of malignancy and the chemotherapeutic agent used,[109,111–113] with reactivation rates highest in regimens containing corticosteroids or rituximab.[114,115] Patients who are anti-HBc(+) but HBsAg(–) and either anti-HBs(+) or (–) are also susceptible to HBV reactivation, although the risk is lower, at an estimated 3% to 6%.

HBV reactivation can be largely prevented with prophylactic use of oral nucleos(t)ide analogues. Lamivudine has been shown to reduce the risk of HBV reactivation by 79% to 100%, thus avoiding any interruption or discontinuation of chemotherapy.[110,111,116–118] Prophylactic antiviral therapy is preferred to starting treatment after reactivation has occurred because treatment in this setting is often ineffective in attenuating the course of hepatic injury or preventing fulminant hepatic failure. AASLD guidelines suggest that lamivudine or telbivudine can be used if the anticipated treatment duration is ≤12 months and the baseline HBV DNA level is undetectable. Tenofovir or entecavir is recommended for longer treatment durations.[61] Antiviral therapy should be started at least 1 week before chemotherapy or immunosuppressive therapy is begun and should be continued 6 months after immunomodulating therapy is completed. Although lamivudine has been recommended in guidelines from numerous liver disease societies, entecavir or tenofovir may be preferable in all patients (at least those with an initial viral load >2000 IU/mL), because these agents offer high genetic barriers to resistance compared with lamivudine, in which resistance has been documented in as little as 12 weeks.

At our institution, all patients scheduled to receive chemotherapy or immunosuppressive therapy are screened for HBsAg, anti-HBs, and anti-HBc. Patients testing positive for either HBsAg or anti-HBc are reflexively tested for quantitative HBV DNA. All patients who test positive for HBsAg or have detectable HBV DNA are started on prophylactic antiviral therapy with tenofovir 300 mg daily or entecavir 0.5 mg daily if they have a glomerular filtration rate more than 70 (with dose adjustments made for renal failure), with therapy continued throughout their treatment course. Patients who are isolated anti-HBc(+) are not started on prophylactic antiviral therapy. Instead, liver enzymes are monitored monthly with HBsAg and quantitative HBV DNA every 3 months during chemotherapy/immunomodulating therapy, or if liver enzymes increase. Given the higher rate of HBV reactivation in patients undergoing bone marrow transplantation or treatment with rituximab therapy, these patients are recommended to receive prophylactic treatment with entecavir or tenofovir.

SUMMARY

The appropriate management of patients with HBV infection requires a clear understanding of the natural history of this complex disease. Knowing when to start antiviral therapy is just as important as knowing which therapy to choose. Recent advances suggest that using HBsAg quantification or HBsAg/HBV DNA ratios can help to better define phases of infection, and is especially helpful for distinguishing true inactive carriers from patients with HBeAg(–) chronic hepatitis. Host and viral factors such as HBV genotype and IL28B genotype seem to be useful predictors of interferon responsiveness and may be able to help physicians decide whom to treat. On-treatment HBsAg kinetics could potentially be useful in creating interferon-specific response-guided therapy algorithms analogous to those that exist for hepatitis V virus therapy. As for therapy, pegylated interferon remains a viable option for patients who prefer a finite 12-month course of treatment. However, oral nucleos(t)ide analogues

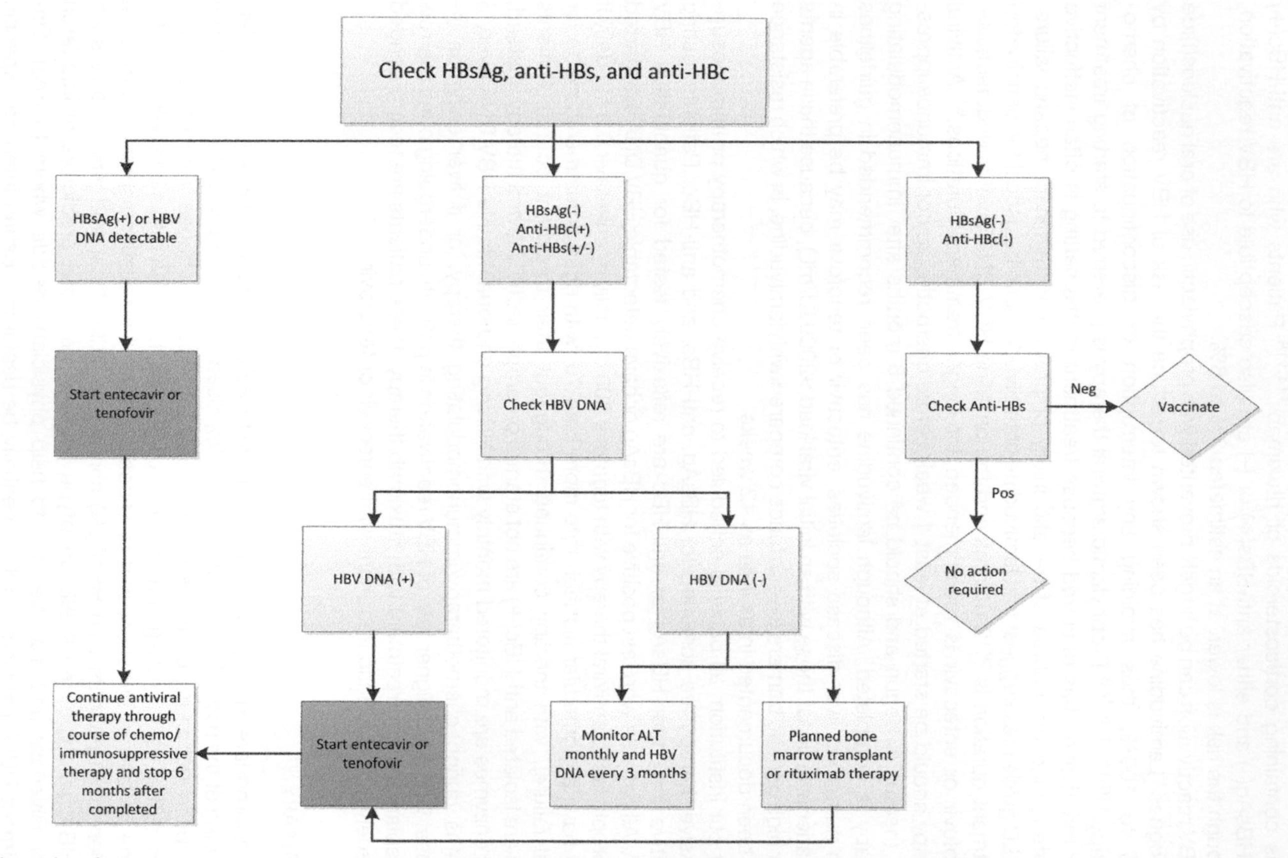

Fig. 5. Algorithm for preventing HBV reactivation in patients receiving chemotherapy or immunosuppressive therapy.

can offer similar rates of HBeAg seroconversion, albeit with longer durations of treatment. For HBeAg(–)patients, treatment duration is likely lifelong in the absence of HBsAg seroconversion.

The optimal management of HBV in special populations is becoming clearer. For women in the third trimester of pregnancy who have high HBV DNA levels (>10^6 copies/mL or 200,000 IU/mL), treatment with lamivudine, telbivudine, or tenofovir, combined with passive and active immune prophylaxis of the newborn, can decrease the risk of MTCT. In the postliver transplant population, the availability of potent nucleos(t)ide analogues with high genetic barriers to resistance such as entecavir and tenofovir makes long-term HBIG unnecessary; this costly drug can be safely discontinued with no additional risk of HBV recurrence. We propose a simple algorithm for preventing HBV reactivation in patients who plan to receive chemotherapy or immunomodulatory drugs and suggest that entecavir or tenofovir should supplant lamivudine as first-line agents in this setting **Fig. 5**.

REFERENCES

1. Gust ID. Epidemiology of hepatitis B infection in the Western Pacific and South East Asia. Gut 1996;38(Suppl 2):S18–23.
2. Lin X, Robinson NJ, Thursz M, et al. Chronic hepatitis B virus infection in the Asia-Pacific region and Africa: review of disease progression. J Gastroenterol Hepatol 2005;20(6):833–43.
3. Mast EE, Weinbaum CM, Fiore AE, et al. A comprehensive immunization strategy to eliminate transmission of hepatitis B virus infection in the United States: recommendations of the Advisory Committee on Immunization Practices (ACIP) Part II: immunization of adults. MMWR Recomm Rep 2006;55(RR-16): 1–33 [quiz: CE31-34].
4. Lavanchy D. Hepatitis B virus epidemiology, disease burden, treatment, and current and emerging prevention and control measures. J Viral Hepat 2004; 11(2):97–107.
5. Gish RG, Gadano AC. Chronic hepatitis B: current epidemiology in the Americas and implications for management. J Viral Hepat 2006;13(12):787–98.
6. Bosch FX, Ribes J, Cleries R, et al. Epidemiology of hepatocellular carcinoma. Clin Liver Dis 2005;9(2):191–211, v.
7. Beasley RP, Hwang LY, Lee GC, et al. Prevention of perinatally transmitted hepatitis B virus infections with hepatitis B virus infections with hepatitis B immune globulin and hepatitis B vaccine. Lancet 1983;2(8359):1099–102.
8. Beasley RP, Hwang LY, Lin CC, et al. Incidence of hepatitis B virus infections in preschool children in Taiwan. J Infect Dis 1982;146(2):198–204.
9. Coursaget P, Yvonnet B, Chotard J, et al. Age- and sex-related study of hepatitis B virus chronic carrier state in infants from an endemic area (Senegal). J Med Virol 1987;22(1):1–5.
10. McMahon BJ, Alward WL, Hall DB, et al. Acute hepatitis B virus infection: relation of age to the clinical expression of disease and subsequent development of the carrier state. J Infect Dis 1985;151(4):599–603.
11. Stroffolini T, Mele A, Tosti ME, et al. The impact of the hepatitis B mass immunisation campaign on the incidence and risk factors of acute hepatitis B in Italy. J Hepatol 2000;33(6):980–5.
12. McQuillan GM, Coleman PJ, Kruszon-Moran D, et al. Prevalence of hepatitis B virus infection in the United States: the National Health and Nutrition Examination Surveys, 1976 through 1994. Am J Public Health 1999;89(1):14–8.

13. McMahon BJ. Epidemiology and natural history of hepatitis B. Semin Liver Dis 2005;25(Suppl 1):3–8.
14. Lok AS, Lai CL, Wu PC, et al. Spontaneous hepatitis B e antigen to antibody seroconversion and reversion in Chinese patients with chronic hepatitis B virus infection. Gastroenterology 1987;92(6):1839–43.
15. Bortolotti F, Guido M, Bartolacci S, et al. Chronic hepatitis B in children after e antigen seroclearance: final report of a 29-year longitudinal study. Hepatology 2006;43(3):556–62.
16. Dusheiko GM, Brink BA, Conradie JD, et al. Regional prevalence of hepatitis B, delta, and human immunodeficiency virus infection in southern Africa: a large population survey. Am J Epidemiol 1989;129(1):138–45.
17. Hoofnagle JH, Dusheiko GM, Seeff LB, et al. Seroconversion from hepatitis B e antigen to antibody in chronic type B hepatitis. Ann Intern Med 1981;94(6):744–8.
18. Fattovich G, Rugge M, Brollo L, et al. Clinical, virologic and histologic outcome following seroconversion from HBeAg to anti-HBe in chronic hepatitis type B. Hepatology 1986;6(2):167–72.
19. Hsu YS, Chien RN, Yeh CT, et al. Long-term outcome after spontaneous HBeAg seroconversion in patients with chronic hepatitis B. Hepatology 2002;35(6):1522–7.
20. Hadziyannis SJ, Vassilopoulos D. Hepatitis B e antigen-negative chronic hepatitis B. Hepatology 2001;34(4 Pt 1):617–24.
21. McMahon BJ, Holck P, Bulkow L, et al. Serologic and clinical outcomes of 1536 Alaska Natives chronically infected with hepatitis B virus. Ann Intern Med 2001;135(9):759–68.
22. Davis GL, Hoofnagle JH, Waggoner JG. Spontaneous reactivation of chronic hepatitis B virus infection. Gastroenterology 1984;86(2):230–5.
23. Fattovich G, Giustina G, Realdi G, et al. Long-term outcome of hepatitis B e antigen-positive patients with compensated cirrhosis treated with interferon alfa. European Concerted Action on Viral Hepatitis (EUROHEP). Hepatology 1997;26(5):1338–42.
24. Lin SM, Sheen IS, Chien RN, et al. Long-term beneficial effect of interferon therapy in patients with chronic hepatitis B virus infection. Hepatology 1999;29(3):971–5.
25. Lau DT, Everhart J, Kleiner DE, et al. Long-term follow-up of patients with chronic hepatitis B treated with interferon alfa. Gastroenterology 1997;113(5):1660–7.
26. Chang TT, Lai CL, Kew Yoon S, et al. Entecavir treatment for up to 5 years in patients with hepatitis B e antigen-positive chronic hepatitis B. Hepatology 2010;51(2):422–30.
27. Marcellin P, Muti M, Gane E, et al. Five years of treatment with tenofovir DF for chronic hepatitis B infection is associated with sustained virologic suppression and significant regression of histological fibrosis and cirrhosis. Hepatology 2011;54(4 Suppl):1011a [abstract: 1375].
28. Gish R, Jia J, Locarnini S, et al. Selection of chronic hepatitis B therapy with high barrier to resistance. Lancet Infect Dis 2012. [Epub ahead of print].
29. Lau GK, Piratvisuth T, Luo KX, et al. Peginterferon Alfa-2a, lamivudine, and the combination for HBeAg-positive chronic hepatitis B. N Engl J Med 2005;352(26):2682–95.
30. Dienstag JL, Schiff ER, Wright TL, et al. Lamivudine as initial treatment for chronic hepatitis B in the United States. N Engl J Med 1999;341(17):1256–63.

31. Lai CL, Chien RN, Leung NW, et al. A one-year trial of lamivudine for chronic hepatitis B. Asia Hepatitis Lamivudine Study Group. N Engl J Med 1998;339(2):61–8.
32. Schalm SW, Heathcote J, Cianciara J, et al. Lamivudine and alpha interferon combination treatment of patients with chronic hepatitis B infection: a randomised trial. Gut 2000;46(4):562–8.
33. Marcellin P, Chang TT, Lim SG, et al. Long-term efficacy and safety of adefovir dipivoxil for the treatment of hepatitis B e antigen-positive chronic hepatitis B. Hepatology 2008;48(3):750–8.
34. Marcellin P, Chang TT, Lim SG, et al. Adefovir dipivoxil for the treatment of hepatitis B e antigen-positive chronic hepatitis B. N Engl J Med 2003;348(9): 808–16.
35. Chang TT, Gish RG, de Man R, et al. A comparison of entecavir and lamivudine for HBeAg-positive chronic hepatitis B. N Engl J Med 2006;354(10):1001–10.
36. Lai CL, Gane E, Liaw YF, et al. Telbivudine versus lamivudine in patients with chronic hepatitis B. N Engl J Med 2007;357(25):2576–88.
37. Marcellin P, Heathcote EJ, Buti M, et al. Tenofovir disoproxil fumarate versus adefovir dipivoxil for chronic hepatitis B. N Engl J Med 2008;359(23):2442–55.
38. Colonno RJ, Rose R, Baldick CJ, et al. Entecavir resistance is rare in nucleoside naive patients with hepatitis B. Hepatology 2006;44(6):1656–65.
39. Perrillo RP. Current treatment of chronic hepatitis B: benefits and limitations. Semin Liver Dis 2005;25(Suppl 1):20–8.
40. Snow-Lampart A, Chappell B, Curtis M, et al. No resistance to tenofovir disoproxil fumarate detected after up to 144 weeks of therapy in patients monoinfected with chronic hepatitis B virus. Hepatology 2011;53(3):763–73.
41. Marcellin P, Heathcote E, Corsa A, et al. No detectable resistance to tenofovir disoproxil fumarate (TDF) following up to 240 weeks of treatment in patients with HBeAg+ and HBeAg- chronic hepatitis B virus infection [abstract 238]. 62nd Annual Meeting for the American Association for the Study of Liver Diseases, San Francsico (CA), November 4–8, 2011.
42. Lai CL, Ratziu V, Yuen MF, et al. Viral hepatitis B. Lancet 2003;362(9401): 2089–94.
43. Leung NW, Lai CL, Chang TT, et al. Extended lamivudine treatment in patients with chronic hepatitis B enhances hepatitis B e antigen seroconversion rates: results after 3 years of therapy. Hepatology 2001;33(6):1527–32.
44. Benhamou Y, Bochet M, Thibault V, et al. Long-term incidence of hepatitis B virus resistance to lamivudine in human immunodeficiency virus-infected patients. Hepatology 1999;30(5):1302–6.
45. Lok AS, Lai CL, Leung N, et al. Long-term safety of lamivudine treatment in patients with chronic hepatitis B. Gastroenterology 2003;125(6):1714–22.
46. Hadziyannis SJ, Tassopoulos NC, Heathcote EJ, et al. Long-term therapy with adefovir dipivoxil for HBeAg-negative chronic hepatitis B for up to 5 years. Gastroenterology 2006;131(6):1743–51.
47. Santantonio T, Mazzola M, Iacovazzi T, et al. Long-term follow-up of patients with anti-HBe/HBV DNA-positive chronic hepatitis B treated for 12 months with lamivudine. J Hepatol 2000;32(2):300–6.
48. Lok AS, Hussain M, Cursano C, et al. Evolution of hepatitis B virus polymerase gene mutations in hepatitis B e antigen-negative patients receiving lamivudine therapy. Hepatology 2000;32(5):1145–53.
49. Hadziyannis SJ, Papatheodoridis GV, Dimou E, et al. Efficacy of long-term lamivudine monotherapy in patients with hepatitis B e antigen-negative chronic hepatitis B. Hepatology 2000;32(4 Pt 1):847–51.

50. Lau DT, Khokhar MF, Doo E, et al. Long-term therapy of chronic hepatitis B with lamivudine. Hepatology 2000;32(4 Pt 1):828–34.
51. Hadziyannis SJ, Tassopoulos NC, Heathcote EJ, et al. Adefovir dipivoxil for the treatment of hepatitis B e antigen-negative chronic hepatitis B. N Engl J Med 2003;348(9):800–7.
52. Lai CL, Shouval D, Lok AS, et al. Entecavir versus lamivudine for patients with HBeAg-negative chronic hepatitis B. N Engl J Med 2006;354(10):1011–20.
53. Shouval D, Lai CL, Chang TT, et al. Relapse of hepatitis B in HBeAg-negative chronic hepatitis B patients who discontinued successful entecavir treatment: the case for continuous antiviral therapy. J Hepatol 2009;50(2):289–95.
54. Tenney DJ, Rose RE, Baldick CJ, et al. Long-term monitoring shows hepatitis B virus resistance to entecavir in nucleoside-naive patients is rare through 5 years of therapy. Hepatology 2009;49(5):1503–14.
55. Liaw YF, Gane E, Leung N, et al. 2-Year GLOBE trial results: telbivudine is superior to lamivudine in patients with chronic hepatitis B. Gastroenterology 2009; 136(2):486–95.
56. Lee YS, Suh DJ, Lim YS, et al. Increased risk of adefovir resistance in patients with lamivudine-resistant chronic hepatitis B after 48 weeks of adefovir dipivoxil monotherapy. Hepatology 2006;43(6):1385–91.
57. Fung SK, Chae HB, Fontana RJ, et al. Virologic response and resistance to adefovir in patients with chronic hepatitis B. J Hepatol 2006;44(2):283–90.
58. Perrillo RP, Lai CL, Liaw YF, et al. Predictors of HBeAg loss after lamivudine treatment for chronic hepatitis B. Hepatology 2002;36(1):186–94.
59. Chien RN, Liaw YF, Atkins M. Pretherapy alanine transaminase level as a determinant for hepatitis B e antigen seroconversion during lamivudine therapy in patients with chronic hepatitis B. Asian Hepatitis Lamivudine Trial Group. Hepatology 1999;30(3):770–4.
60. Marcellin P, Lau GK, Bonino F, et al. Peginterferon alfa-2a alone, lamivudine alone, and the two in combination in patients with HBeAg-negative chronic hepatitis B. N Engl J Med 2004;351(12):1206–17.
61. Lok AS, McMahon BJ. Chronic hepatitis B: update 2009. Hepatology 2009; 50(3):661–2.
62. Erhardt A, Blondin D, Hauck K, et al. Response to interferon alfa is hepatitis B virus genotype dependent: genotype A is more sensitive to interferon than genotype D. Gut 2005;54(7):1009–13.
63. Janssen HL, van Zonneveld M, Senturk H, et al. Pegylated interferon alfa-2b alone or in combination with lamivudine for HBeAg-positive chronic hepatitis B: a randomised trial. Lancet 2005;365(9454):123–9.
64. Lin CL, Kao JH. The clinical implications of hepatitis B virus genotype: recent advances. J Gastroenterol Hepatol 2011;26(Suppl 1):123–30.
65. Chu CJ, Keeffe EB, Han SH, et al. Hepatitis B virus genotypes in the United States: results of a nationwide study. Gastroenterology 2003;125(2):444–51.
66. Kao JH, Chen PJ, Lai MY, et al. Hepatitis B virus genotypes and spontaneous hepatitis B e antigen seroconversion in Taiwanese hepatitis B carriers. J Med Virol 2004;72(3):363–9.
67. Sanchez-Tapias JM, Costa J, Mas A, et al. Influence of hepatitis B virus genotype on the long-term outcome of chronic hepatitis B in western patients. Gastroenterology 2002;123(6):1848–56.
68. Kao JH, Chen PJ, Lai MY, et al. Hepatitis B genotypes correlate with clinical outcomes in patients with chronic hepatitis B. Gastroenterology 2000;118(3): 554–9.

69. Chan HL, Hui AY, Wong ML, et al. Genotype C hepatitis B virus infection is associated with an increased risk of hepatocellular carcinoma. Gut 2004;53(10):1494–8.
70. Yang HI, Yeh SH, Chen PJ, et al. Associations between hepatitis B virus genotype and mutants and the risk of hepatocellular carcinoma. J Natl Cancer Inst 2008;100(16):1134–43.
71. Sugiyama M, Tanaka Y, Kato T, et al. Influence of hepatitis B virus genotypes on the intra- and extracellular expression of viral DNA and antigens. Hepatology 2006;44(4):915–24.
72. Wiegand J, Hasenclever D, Tillmann HL. Should treatment of hepatitis B depend on hepatitis B virus genotypes? A hypothesis generated from an explorative analysis of published evidence. Antivir Ther 2008;13(2):211–20.
73. Sonneveld MJ, Wong VW, Woltman AM, et al. Polymorphisms near IL28B and serological response to peginterferon in HBeAg-positive patients with chronic hepatitis B. Gastroenterol 2012;142(3):513–520.e1.
74. Chan HL, Wong VW, Chim AM, et al. Serum HBsAg quantification to predict response to peginterferon therapy of e antigen positive chronic hepatitis B. Aliment Pharmacol Ther 2010;32(11–12):1323–31.
75. Jaroszewicz J, Calle Serrano B, Wursthorn K, et al. Hepatitis B surface antigen (HBsAg) levels in the natural history of hepatitis B virus (HBV)-infection: a European perspective. J Hepatol 2010;52(4):514–22.
76. Nguyen T, Thompson AJ, Bowden S, et al. Hepatitis B surface antigen levels during the natural history of chronic hepatitis B: a perspective on Asia. J Hepatol 2010;52(4):508–13.
77. Brunetto MR, Oliveri F, Colombatto P, et al. Hepatitis B surface antigen serum levels help to distinguish active from inactive hepatitis B virus genotype D carriers. Gastroenterology 2010;139(2):483–90.
78. Piratvisuth T, Marcellin P, Popescu M, et al. Hepatitis B surface antigen: association with sustained response to peginterferon alfa-2a in hepatitis B e antigen-positive patients. Hepatol Int 2011. [Epub ahead of print].
79. Moucari R, Mackiewicz V, Lada O, et al. Early serum HBsAg drop: a strong predictor of sustained virological response to pegylated interferon alfa-2a in HBeAg-negative patients. Hepatology 2009;49(4):1151–7.
80. Cai W, Xie Q, An B, et al. On-treatment serum HBsAg level is predictive of sustained off-treatment virologic response to telbivudine in HBeAg-positive chronic hepatitis B patients. J Clin Virol 2010;48(1):22–6.
81. Jung YK, Kim JH, Lee YS, et al. Change in serum hepatitis B surface antigen level and its clinical significance in treatment-naive, hepatitis B e antigen-positive patients receiving entecavir. J Clin Gastroenterol 2010;44(9):653–7.
82. Wong VC, Ip HM, Reesink HW, et al. Prevention of the HBsAg carrier state in newborn infants of mothers who are chronic carriers of HBsAg and HBeAg by administration of hepatitis-B vaccine and hepatitis-B immunoglobulin. Double-blind randomised placebo-controlled study. Lancet 1984;1(8383):921–6.
83. Lee C, Gong Y, Brok J, et al. Effect of hepatitis B immunisation in newborn infants of mothers positive for hepatitis B surface antigen: systematic review and meta-analysis. BMJ 2006;332(7537):328–36.
84. Farmer K, Gunn T, Woodfield DG. A combination of hepatitis B vaccine and immunoglobulin does not protect all infants born to hepatitis B e antigen positive mothers. N Z Med J 1987;100(827):412–4.
85. Wiseman E, Fraser MA, Holden S, et al. Perinatal transmission of hepatitis B virus: an Australian experience. Med J Aust 2009;190(9):489–92.

86. del Canho R, Grosheide PM, Schalm SW, et al. Failure of neonatal hepatitis B vaccination: the role of HBV-DNA levels in hepatitis B carrier mothers and HLA antigens in neonates. J Hepatol 1994;20(4):483–6.
87. van Zonneveld M, van Nunen AB, Niesters HG, et al. Lamivudine treatment during pregnancy to prevent perinatal transmission of hepatitis B virus infection. J Viral Hepat 2003;10(4):294–7.
88. Milich DR, Jones JE, Hughes JL, et al. Is a function of the secreted hepatitis B e antigen to induce immunologic tolerance in utero? Proc Natl Acad Sci U S A 1990;87(17):6599–603.
89. Xu DZ, Yan YP, Choi BC, et al. Risk factors and mechanism of transplacental transmission of hepatitis B virus: a case-control study. J Med Virol 2002;67(1): 20–6.
90. Burk RD, Hwang LY, Ho GY, et al. Outcome of perinatal hepatitis B virus exposure is dependent on maternal virus load. J Infect Dis 1994;170(6):1418–23.
91. Yang YJ, Liu CC, Chen TJ, et al. Role of hepatitis B immunoglobulin in infants born to hepatitis B e antigen-negative carrier mothers in Taiwan. Pediatr Infect Dis J 2003;22(7):584–8.
92. Antiretroviral Pregnancy Registry. Interim report: 1 January 1989 through 31 July 2011. Available at: http://www.apregistry.com/forms/interim_report.pdf. Accessed November 12, 2011.
93. Xu WM, Cui YT, Wang L, et al. Lamivudine in late pregnancy to prevent perinatal transmission of hepatitis B virus infection: a multicentre, randomized, double-blind, placebo-controlled study. J Viral Hepat 2009;16(2):94–103.
94. Han GR, Cao MK, Zhao W, et al. A prospective and open-label study for the efficacy and safety of telbivudine in pregnancy for the prevention of perinatal transmission of hepatitis B virus infection. J Hepatol 2011;55(6):1215–21.
95. Fontana RJ, Keeffe EB, Carey W, et al. Effect of lamivudine treatment on survival of 309 North American patients awaiting liver transplantation for chronic hepatitis B. Liver Transpl 2002;8(5):433–9.
96. Liaw YF, Sung JJ, Chow WC, et al. Lamivudine for patients with chronic hepatitis B and advanced liver disease. N Engl J Med 2004;351(15):1521–31.
97. Kim WR, Terrault NA, Pedersen RA, et al. Trends in waiting list registration for liver transplantation for viral hepatitis in the United States. Gastroenterology 2009;137(5):1680–6.
98. Han SH, Ofman J, Holt C, et al. An efficacy and cost-effectiveness analysis of combination hepatitis B immune globulin and lamivudine to prevent recurrent hepatitis B after orthotopic liver transplantation compared with hepatitis B immune globulin monotherapy. Liver Transpl 2000;6(6):741–8.
99. Bzowej N, Han S, Degertekin B, et al. Liver transplantation outcomes among Caucasians, Asian Americans, and African Americans with hepatitis B. Liver Transpl 2009;15(9):1010–20.
100. Dumortier J, Chevallier P, Scoazec JY, et al. Combined lamivudine and hepatitis B immunoglobulin for the prevention of hepatitis B recurrence after liver transplantation: long-term results. Am J Transplant 2003;3(8):999–1002.
101. Markowitz JS, Martin P, Conrad AJ, et al. Prophylaxis against hepatitis B recurrence following liver transplantation using combination lamivudine and hepatitis B immune globulin. Hepatology 1998;28(2):585–9.
102. Anderson RD, Chinnakotla S, Guo L, et al. Intramuscular hepatitis B immunoglobulin (HBIG) and nucleosides for prevention of recurrent hepatitis B following liver transplantation: comparison with other HBIG regimens. Clin Transplant 2007;21(4):510–7.

103. Wong SN, Chu CJ, Wai CT, et al. Low risk of hepatitis B virus recurrence after withdrawal of long-term hepatitis B immunoglobulin in patients receiving maintenance nucleos(t)ide analogue therapy. Liver Transpl 2007;13(3):374–81.
104. Weber NK, Forman LM, Trotter JF. HBIg discontinuation with maintenance oral anti-viral therapy and HBV vaccination in liver transplant recipients. Dig Dis Sci 2010;55(2):505–9.
105. Buti M, Mas A, Prieto M, et al. Adherence to Lamivudine after an early withdrawal of hepatitis B immune globulin plays an important role in the long-term prevention of hepatitis B virus recurrence. Transplantation 2007;84(5):650–4.
106. Fung J, Cheung C, Chan SC, et al. Entecavir monotherapy is effective in suppressing hepatitis B virus after liver transplantation. Gastroenterology 2011;141(4):1212–9.
107. Saab S, Waterman B, Chi AC, et al. Comparison of different immunoprophylaxis regimens after liver transplantation with hepatitis B core antibody-positive donors: a systematic review. Liver Transpl 2010;16(3):300–7.
108. Aomatsu T, Komatsu H, Yoden A, et al. Fulminant hepatitis B and acute hepatitis B due to intrafamilial transmission of HBV after chemotherapy for non-Hodgkin's lymphoma in an HBV carrier. Eur J Pediatr 2010;169(2):167–71.
109. Hou JK, Velayos F, Terrault N, et al. Viral hepatitis and inflammatory bowel disease. Inflamm Bowel Dis 2010;16(6):925–32.
110. Loomba R, Rowley A, Wesley R, et al. Systematic review: the effect of preventive lamivudine on hepatitis B reactivation during chemotherapy. Ann Intern Med 2008;148(7):519–28.
111. Lubel JS, Angus PW. Hepatitis B reactivation in patients receiving cytotoxic chemotherapy: diagnosis and management. J Gastroenterol Hepatol 2010;25(5):864–71.
112. Evens AM, Jovanovic BD, Su YC, et al. Rituximab-associated hepatitis B virus (HBV) reactivation in lymphoproliferative diseases: meta-analysis and examination of FDA safety reports. Ann Oncol 2011;22(5):1170–80.
113. Alexopoulou A, Theodorou M, Dourakis SP, et al. Hepatitis B virus reactivation in patients receiving chemotherapy for malignancies: role of precore stop-codon and basic core promoter mutations. J Viral Hepat 2006;13(9):591–6.
114. Cheng AL, Hsiung CA, Su IJ, et al. Steroid-free chemotherapy decreases risk of hepatitis B virus (HBV) reactivation in HBV-carriers with lymphoma. Hepatology 2003;37(6):1320–8.
115. Yeo W, Chan TC, Leung NW, et al. Hepatitis B virus reactivation in lymphoma patients with prior resolved hepatitis B undergoing anticancer therapy with or without rituximab. J Clin Oncol 2009;27(4):605–11.
116. Dai MS, Wu PF, Shyu RY, et al. Hepatitis B virus reactivation in breast cancer patients undergoing cytotoxic chemotherapy and the role of preemptive lamivudine administration. Liver Int 2004;24(6):540–6.
117. Martyak LA, Taqavi E, Saab S. Lamivudine prophylaxis is effective in reducing hepatitis B reactivation and reactivation-related mortality in chemotherapy patients: a meta-analysis. Liver Int 2008;28(1):28–38.
118. Hsu C, Hsiung CA, Su IJ, et al. A revisit of prophylactic lamivudine for chemotherapy-associated hepatitis B reactivation in non-Hodgkin's lymphoma: a randomized trial. Hepatology 2008;47(3):844–53.

Alcoholic Hepatitis: A Clinician's Guide

Gina Choi, MD[a], Bruce Allen Runyon, MD[b,*]

KEYWORDS

• Alcoholic liver disease • Pentoxifylline • Corticosteroids
• Discriminant function

Although physical examination and laboratory test results are characteristic in alcoholic hepatitis (AH), the diagnosis may be missed with time-wasting evaluations for fever and leukocytosis and associated with potentially harmful, invasive procedures, such as endoscopic retrograde cholangiopancreatography (ERCP) in pursuit of jaundice.

When severe, AH is life-threatening. Early detection and initiation of appropriate treatment are imperative. Treatment includes abstinence, nutritional supplementation, and specific medical therapy. Although corticosteroids have been used most frequently, the superiority and lower incidence of side effects of pentoxifylline (PTX) in a randomized trial have led to increased use of this drug. The side effects and duration of appropriate treatment with steroids (abrupt discontinuation vs taper) make the steroid option less appealing. In 2009, a study investigating physician preferences in treating severe AH observed that more physicians in the United States preferred PTX to steroids.[1] Finally, baclofen can be started towards the end of hospitalization to reduce alcohol craving and recidivism.

INTRODUCTION

Dr Gordon Beckett and colleagues first used the term, *acute alcoholic hepatitis*, in 1961: "Severe jaundice may occur in alcoholics at an earlier stage, and before cirrhosis is established, when it is accompanied by marked constitutional disturbances—fever, anorexia, abdominal pain, nausea, and vomiting…the illness tends to run a protracted course, often ends fatally, but is potentially recoverable with suitable treatment."[2] Beckett's description of this clinical syndrome remains incredibly accurate 50 years later. Alcoholic liver disease and its complications, including AH, continue to have an impact on society and represent a challenging clinical entity. Thus, it remains important for clinicians to be able to recognize and treat this complex disease.

The authors have nothing to disclose relative to this subject matter.

[a] Department of Medicine, David Geffen School of Medicine at UCLA, 11301 Wilshire Boulevard, Building 115, Room 215, Los Angeles, CA 90043, USA; [b] Department of Medicine, Santa Monica/UCLA Medical Center, 1223 16th Street, Santa Monica, CA 90404, USA

* Corresponding author.

E-mail address: BARunyon@mednet.ucla.edu

Clin Liver Dis 16 (2012) 371–385
doi:10.1016/j.cld.2012.03.015 **liver.theclinics.com**
1089-3261/12/$ – see front matter

EPIDEMIOLOGY

Alcohol consumption is ubiquitous in the United States and represents a large burden on society. The literature estimates that 67.3% of the adult population drinks alcohol each year and 7.4% (11% in men and 4% in women) meet *Diagnostic and Statistical Manual of Mental Disorders* (Fourth Edition) criteria for alcohol abuse or dependence.[3] In 1998, the total estimated cost of alcohol abuse was $185 billion with health care costs accounting for 14%.[4] The net effect of alcohol consumption on health is detrimental, with an estimated 3.8% of all global deaths and 4.6% of global disability-adjusted life-years attributable to alcohol.[5] More recent data published by the National Institute on Alcohol Abuse and Alcoholism revealed that cirrhosis was the 12th leading cause of death in the United States, with a total of 29,925 deaths in 2007, 48.1% of which were alcohol related. The proportion of alcohol-related cirrhosis was highest (70.6%) among decedents aged 25 to 34.[6] When expanded diagnosis codes (liver failure, viral hepatitis, and hepatobiliary cancer) were used, liver disease was the 8th leading cause of death in 2006, with 60,810 deaths.[7]

RISK FACTORS

The volume of alcohol ingested is the most important risk factor for the development of alcoholic liver disease. The risk of developing cirrhosis increases with the ingestion of greater than 60 g per day to 80 g per day of alcohol for more than 10 years in men and greater than 20 g per day in women.[8] Only 6% to 41% of those drinking at this level, however, develop cirrhosis.[9] Bellentani and colleagues[10] showed that even in patients with an extremely high daily alcohol intake (>120 g/d), only 13.5% developed alcohol-induced liver damage. They also found that the risk of cirrhosis or noncirrhotic chronic liver disease increased with a daily alcohol intake of greater than 30 g. The odds of developing either cirrhosis or noncirrhotic liver disease with a daily alcohol intake greater than 30 g per day were 13.7 and 23.6, respectively, when compared with nondrinkers.

In addition to the amount and duration of alcohol intake, a variety of genetic and gender-related factors influence the development of alcoholic liver disease. For example, women have a significantly higher relative risk of developing alcohol-related liver disease than men for any given level of alcohol intake.[8] In addition, excess body weight (body mass index [BMI] >27 kg/m^2 in men and BMI >25 kg/m^2 in women) has been identified as an independent risk factor. A population-based study has shown that being overweight worsens survival specifically in AH. Also, liver steatosis/steatohepatitis related to being overweight may be synergistic in worsening alcohol-related liver injury.[11] Recently, BMI has come to the forefront in light of increasing numbers of gastric bypass patients presenting with AH. Removal or exclusion of a portion of the gastric mucosa leads to lack of metabolism and detoxification of the alcohol.[12]

Furthermore, several polymorphisms of genes encoding alcohol-metabolizing enzymes have been reported in their association with alcoholism and liver damage induced by alcohol in different populations. A higher frequency of the allele ADH1B*1 is associated with increased risk of developing alcoholic liver disease in a group of Mexican mestizos.[13] Epidemiologically, compared with nonhispanic whites, all hispanic subgroups except Cubans have much higher cirrhosis mortality.[14]

DIAGNOSIS

Diagnosis of AH requires a high index of suspicion followed by a detailed clinical history. Questions to ask patients with suspected AH are detailed in **Box 1**. Obtaining such a history can be difficult if patients feel ashamed about their drinking habits and

Box 1
Questions pertinent to suspected alcohol history

Do you drink alcohol?

Have you ever drunk alcohol?

When did you have your very first alcoholic drink?

What is your preference of alcoholic beverage?

Do you drink at home? Alone? Or with others?

How many days of the week are drinking days for you? Every day?

Have you been drinking all of your adult life or were there periods of abstinence?

How many drinks do you drink on an average day? In an average week? (One drink = 12 oz of beer [360 mL], 4 oz of wine [120 mL], or 1.5 oz of hard liquor [45 mL]).[15]

Have you ever gotten into financial difficulties because of your drinking?

Any arrests for public intoxication or legal difficulties?

Have you been through an alcohol education or detoxification program? How many?

Do you attend Alcoholics Anonymous? How often?

When was your last drink?

minimize the duration and volume of alcohol intake. Lengthy discussions, including interviews with family members and friends, are often required to confirm a diagnosis. Alcoholism and alcohol-related health problems are common in patients seen in county hospitals. Patients in private health systems, however, are questioned less rigorously or may be asked only a few cursory questions that are easily evaded. Thus, the diagnosis is often missed.

CLINICAL FEATURES

The clinical presentation of AH is reflective of the inflammatory features characteristic of this disorder. Classically, AH presents with fever, jaundice, hepatomegaly, and, occasionally, signs of decompensated liver disease, such as ascites and hepatic encephalopathy.[16]

History

Heavy drinkers who dramatically increase their alcohol intake in response to recent life crises are most at risk for AH. These triggers include divorce, death of a (alcoholic) parent, and loss of employment. Patients who drink only part time in the evenings and on weekends may drink full time once they have no structure to their schedule. After months of this pattern, they may become ill and jaundiced and seek medical attention. Usually they stop drinking spontaneously a few weeks before accessing the health care system. At this point, drinking alcohol worsens their condition and they realize that the alcohol has caused their illness. Occasionally, they refuse medical attention until they collapse or are too confused to resist an ambulance to the emergency room.

Jaundice and increasing abdominal girth are the most common symptoms that bring them to medical attention. Patients can also have nonspecific complaints, such as anorexia, nausea, vomiting, abdominal pain, and weight loss. Many complain that their muscles disappeared as their abdomen began to swell. Malnutrition is seen in approximately 90% of patients with AH.[17]

Physical Examination

Fever ranging from 100.4° to 104° due to AH and not attributable to infection can be seen in more than half of patients diagnosed with severe AH.[18] Patients with AH often undergo extensive fever work-ups. Mild to elevated leukocytosis (up to 40,000/μL) can be seen with AH.[19] Various reports in the literature correlate a severe leukomoid reaction with a poor prognosis.[20,21] Clinicians can be led astray by the presence of both fever and leukocytosis, leading to concern for sepsis that overshadows the possibility of AH, particularly if a patient's history is unclear. Nonetheless, because these patients are often profoundly nutrient deficient and have comorbidities, such as cirrhosis, they are at increased risk of infection and warrant a full infectious evaluation.[18] They should undergo a chest radiograph, blood cultures, abdominal paracentesis (if ascites is present), and urinalysis with urine culture. Clinicians must keep in mind, however, that a concomitant leukocytosis can be present without an infection due to AH alone and discontinue antibiotics if they are not warranted. The presence of jaundice in this context can raise the question of biliary obstruction. ERCP, too often with resulting pancreatitis, may be inappropriately performed and should be avoided.

On physical examination, the presence of a hepatic bruit strongly supports a diagnosis of AH. In one series of 101 patients with AH, 58% of patients with severe AH had a hepatic bruit.[22]

Laboratory Values

Serum aspartate aminotransferase (AST) levels are typically elevated 2 to 6 times the upper limits of normal in severe AH. Levels of AST greater than 500 IU/L or alanine transaminase (ALT) greater than 200 IU/L are rarely seen with AH (other than alcoholic foamy degeneration, in which case AST can rise as high as 730 IU/L, or concomitant acetominophen overdose) and suggest another cause.[23,24] A serum AST/ALT ratio greater than or equal to 2 differentiates alcoholic liver disease from other liver diseases, such as chronic hepatitis C without cirrhosis, with ratios less than 2, or nonalcoholic steatohepatitis, with ratios less than 1.[25] Other nonspecific but established markers of alcohol intake include γ-glutamyltransferase (GGT) activity and erythrocyte mean corpuscular volume.[26] As the severity of alcohol-related liver injury increases, the bilirubin can increase with a concomitant decrease in GGT.[27]

Testing for iron overload should be avoided. Ferritin ng/ml may be in the thousands in AH but normalizes after a few months of abstinence and improvement in the inflammatory state.[28] Hemochromatosis does not present with deep jaundice and inflammatory features.

Nuclear Medicine Scan

A technetium sulfur colloid liver spleen scan can augment a diagnosis of AH noninvasively.[29] A reincarnation of this scan, known as the *perfused hepatic mass*, can be estimated by the colloid shift. It uses single-photon emission CT of the sulfur colloid distribution between the liver, spleen, and bone marrow.[30] In AH, there is a characteristic pattern of colloid shift where the liver is barely visible and the colloid is preferentially taken up by the spleen and bone marrow. Currently, this is not a widely applied technique. It is becoming more relevant, however, as evidenced by a recent study using data from the Hepatitis C Antiviral Long-Term Treatment against Cirrhosis trial. Disease severity was measured by quantitative liver function tests, including the perfused hepatic mass, to predict risk for future clinical outcomes. This perfused hepatic mass showed utility in assessing prognosis in liver disease.[31] Given that no new equipment is needed to perform this study, a liver scan represents an existing technology that has the ability to aid in diagnosis of AH.

Liver Biopsy

Clinical and laboratory features are often enough to diagnose AH with a high degree of certainty. A liver biopsy, however, can confirm a diagnosis. This becomes particularly useful during a pretransplant evaluation when there is concern for AH. Occasionally, patients and families may deny alcohol intake or overestimate periods of abstinence. Biopsy for AH is rare, especially given its potential complications and the availability of noninvasive options, such as the colloid liver spleen scan.

On the rare occasion when a biopsy is performed, it is usually done transjugularly due to ascites and/or coagulopathy. The major pathologic manifestations of alcoholic liver injury include steatosis, steatohepatitis, and cirrhosis.[32] The most common characteristic finding on pathology is macrovesicular steatosis, which can also be seen in nonalcoholic fatty liver disease. Mallory bodies can be seen in up to 65% of patients with AH but can also be found in other causes of hepatocyte injury and are not pathognomonic of AH.[33] Intrahepatic cholestasis is also seen and requires clinicians to evaluate for other causes of cholestasis, such as drug toxicity or viral hepatitis.

PROGNOSIS IN AH

Various scoring systems have been created to quantify the severity of AH (**Table 1**). The Maddrey discriminant function (MDF) was first introduced in 1978 to predict mortality and to identify patients who may benefit from prednisolone treatment.[34] A value of 32 was used to identify patients with a mortality rate above 50% at 1 month. The drawbacks of the MDF were outlined by Dunn and colleagues,[35] the most notable being the lack of standardized PT measurements, and by O'Shea and colleagues,[24]

Table 1
Prognosis in alcoholic hepatitis

Scoring System	Calculation	Treatment Threshold
MDF	MDF = 4.6 × [PT in seconds − control PT] + serum bilirubin in mg/dL	MDF ≥32
MELD	MELD = 3.78 [Ln serum bilirubin (mg/dL)] + 11.2 [Ln INR] + 9.57 [Ln serum creatinine (mg/dL)] + 6.43 http://www.mayoclinic.org/meld/[a]	MELD >20
GAHS	1 Points: age <50, WBC <15, BUN <5, PT ratio <1.5, bilirubin <7.3 2 Points: age ≥50, WBC ≥15, BUN ≥5, PT ratio 1.5–2, bilirubin 7.3–14.6 3 Points: PT ratio ≥2, bilirubin >14.6 • Calculate on hospital days 1 and 7 http://www.mdcalc.com/glasgow-alcoholic-hepatitis-score[a]	GAHS ≥9
Lille model	Bilirubin on days 0 and day 7, creatinine day 0, albumin day 0, PT day 0 http://www.lillemodel.com/score.asp?score=lillept[a]	Lille >0.45

Abbreviations: BUN, blood urea nitrogen; GAHS, glasgow alcoholic hepaitits score; LN, natural logarithm; MDF, Maddrey discriminant function; MELD, mayo end-stage liver disease; PT, prothrombin time; WBC, white blood cell count.

[a] Web links included for on-line calculators.

who observed that "although it is a continuous measure, its interpretation (using a threshold of 32) has converted it into an essentially categorical method of classification."

In response, other scoring systems, including the model for end-stage liver disease (MELD), the Glasgow alcoholic hepatitis score (GAHS),[36] and the Lille model, have been proposed to predict mortality. A retrospective cohort study showed that the MELD was comparable to MDF in predicting 30-day and 90-day mortality.[35] A MELD score greater than or equal to 20 at the time of admission has the highest sensitivity and specificity for predicting in-hospital mortality and outperformed both the MDF and the Child-Turcotte-Pugh score.[37] The GAHS was less sensitive for predicting 30-day and 90-day mortality compared with the MDF and the MELD score. Among patients with an MDF greater than or equal to 32, however, there was no appreciable benefit from treatment with corticosteroids in patients with a GAHS less than 9. GAHS greater than or equal to 9 has an extremely poor prognosis without pharmacotherapy.[38] The Lille model was highly predictive of death at 6 months. A Lille score greater than 0.45, or a nonresponder, corresponds to 40% of cases that do not respond to steroid therapy.[39]

In summary, based on a Scandinavian study, the MELD and the Lille model for predicting the mortality of patients with AH performed similarly with areas under the receiver operating characteristic curve for 28-day mortality assessed at admission between 0.74 and 0.78.[40] Reassessment 1 week later gave slightly more accurate prognoses. These models serve as helpful adjuvants in the management of patients, provided that clinicians are aware of the models' limitations. In the United States, MELD is used routinely to assess severity in many types of liver disease. A MELD score of 20 may be the simplest criterion to be used to classify a patient as having severe AH.

TREATMENT

Once a diagnosis is made, treatment should address all aspects of the disease, including alcohol cessation, correction of nutritional deficiencies, and initiation of pharmacologic therapy for severe AH (**Fig. 1**).

Nutrition

The first consideration for hospitalized patients, after evaluation and treatment of signs of alcohol withdrawal, should be nutrition and electrolyte repletion. Chlordiazepoxide (Librium) should be avoided due to its accumulation in patients with liver disease. It may induce coma and the need for intubation. Shorter-acting drugs, such as lorazepam (Ativan), should be used to treat alcohol withdrawal. The dosing interval is best determined by sequential examinations or symptom-triggered therapy rather than by a fixed schedule.

AH induces a profound catabolic state in patients who are malnourished secondary to anorexia and poor diet. Large volumes of alcohol suppress the appetite. Many admit to drinking essentially all of their calories in the form of alcohol.

Patients with long-standing alcohol abuse are known to have significant protein malnutrition. At 6 Department of Veterans Affairs Medical Centers, 363 alcoholic patients with AH were studied. The entire cohort exhibited signs of malnutrition and the severity of malnutrition correlated closely with the clinical severity of liver disease.[41] Nutritional support is key for long-term survival. In 2000, Cabré and colleagues[42] conducted a randomized trial comparing the short-term and long-term effects of total enteral nutrition with steroids in patients with AH. Patients were

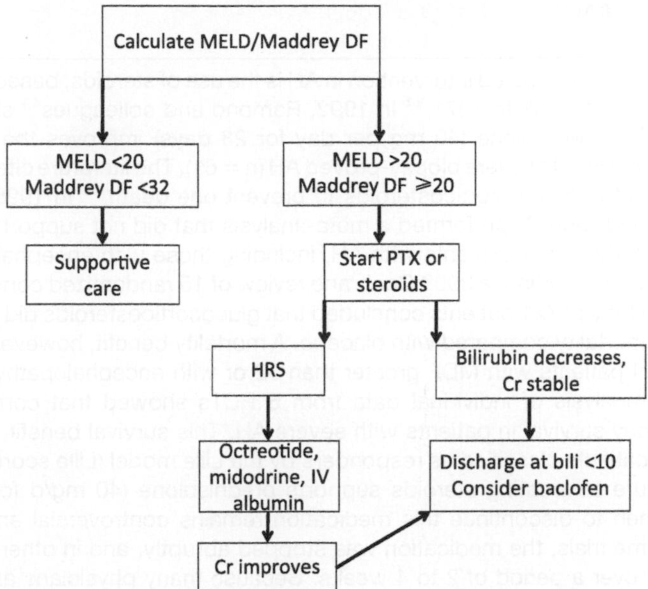

Fig. 1. Treatment algorithm for patients with acute AH. Bili, bilirubin (mg/dL); Cr, creatinine; DF, discriminant function; HRS, hepatorenal syndrome; MELD, model for end stage liver disease; PTX, pentoxifylline.

randomized to receive prednisolone (40 mg/d) or enteral tube feeding (2000 kcal/d) for 28 days, and were followed for 1 year or until death. Mortality during treatment was similar in both groups but occurred earlier with enteral feeding (median 7 vs 23 days). At 1 year's follow-up, patients treated with enteral feeding had lower mortality rates than the steroid-treated group (8% vs 37%).

Nutrition should be provided orally or via a nasojejunal tube if nausea, vomiting, or encephalopathy (with weak gag reflex and increased risk of aspiration) is a concern. The AMT Bridle Nasal Tube Retaining System is recommended for nasojejunal feeding. This bridle system reduces feeding tube pullout.[43] Finally, patients with AH also require multivitamin, folic acid, and thiamine supplementation.

Maintenance intravenous fluids should be avoided in patients with AH. These patients are frequently profoundly potassium depleted due to lack of intake of potassium-containing foods and hyperaldosteronism due to their liver disease. Replacement of potassium may be required daily until the serum potassium level is normal without supplementation. Elixirs should be avoided because they contain alcohol.

If patients with AH exhibit signs of fluid retention, and the blood urea nitrogen and creatinine are normal, spironolactone may be given, which increases urinary excretion of sodium and water and increases serum potassium. Oral furosemide may then be added, once the serum potassium normalizes without further need for potassium supplementation. If azotemia occurs, diuretics should be discontinued and patients should be evaluated for hepatorenal syndrome (HRS) (discussed later).

There may be a component of malabsorption of vitamin K due to jaundice in addition to poor synthesis of coagulation components by the diseased liver. Three daily doses of vitamin K (10 mg) intravenously or subcutaneously usually decrease the international normalized ratio (INR). Oral dosing of vitamin K is not effective because of poor absorption in the setting of deep jaundice.

PHARMACOTHERAPY

Steroids

The most extensively studied intervention in AH is the use of steroids, based on 13 clinical trials that date back to 1971.[24] In 1992, Ramond and colleagues[44] showed that treatment with prednisolone (40 mg per day for 28 days) improves the short-term survival of patients with severe biopsy-proved AH (n = 61). The literature cites a number needed to treat of 5 with corticosteroids to prevent one death.[45] In 1995, however, Christensen and Gluud[46] performed a meta-analysis that did not support the routine use of glucocorticoids in patients with AH, including those with encephalopathy. To further support this finding, a 2008 Cochrane review of 15 randomized controlled trials (RCTs) with a total of 721 patients concluded that glucocorticosteroids did not statistically reduce mortality compared with placebo. A mortality benefit, however, was seen in a subset of patients with MDF greater than 32 or with encephalopathy.[47] A more recent meta-analysis of individual data from 5 RCTs showed that corticosteroids improve 28-day survival in patients with severe AH. This survival benefit was mainly observed in patients classified as responders by the Lille model (Lille score <0.16).[48]

The literature advocating steroids supports prednisolone (40 mg/d for 28 days). How and when to discontinue this medication remains controversial and undetermined. In some trials, the medication was stopped abruptly, and in others, the dose was tapered over a period of 2 to 4 weeks. Because many physicians are reluctant to stop steroid treatment abruptly, patients may remain on unnecessarily prolonged therapy.[49] Too often these patients have no insurance and, consequently, no follow-up. Thus, prednisolone may be continued for prolonged periods of time due to reluctance on the part of the uninformed physician to discontinue it. The authors refer to this phenomenon as *steroid autopilot*, which can be disastrous. Finally, the use of steroids is associated with significant side effects, including hyperglycemia and Cushing syndrome. In the current era, many patients with AH are also obese, insulin resistant, or overtly diabetic.[10] Some also have concomitant hepatitis B or C. Steroids are problematic in these settings.

Pentoxifylline

In the past decade, PTX has emerged as a treatment of AH. PTX is an antagonist of tumor necrosis factor (TNF). The efficacy of PTX was demonstrated in an initial pilot study of 20 patients in 1991 and then in a randomized, placebo-controlled trial of 101 patients with an MDF greater than or equal to 32 in 2000.[50] Patients were given either placebo or PTX (400 mg 3 times a day for 28 days).[22] Treatment with PTX improved short-term survival in patients with severe AH. The benefit was seen in decreasing the risk of HRS.

A head-to-head study comparing PTX with prednisolone was published in 2009. The probability of dying at 3 months was higher with prednisolone compared with PTX at 35.29% versus 14.71%, respectively.[51]

In a 2009 study investigating physician preferences in treating severe AH (MDF ≥32), 25% of patients were treated with steroids, 28.7% were treated with PTX, 6.3% were treated with both steroids and PTX, and 40% were untreated (n = 254).[1]

Most recently, there was an RCT of 174 patients treated with prednisolone plus *N*-acetylcysteine or only prednisolone in severe AH.[52] Mortality was not significantly lower in the prednisolone-NAC group than the prednisolone group at 6 months. Mortality was significantly lower, however, at 1 month (8% vs 24%) but not at 3 months. Death due to HRS was less frequent in the prednisolone-NAC group (9%) than in the prednisolone-only group 22%) at 6 months.

AH is unresponsive to corticosteroid treatment in approximately 40% of patients. Nonresponders to corticosteroids do not obtain any benefit from an early switch to PTX.[53] This illustrates that AH is a morbid condition.

Anti-TNF Therapy

Two monoclonal anti-TNF agents, infliximab and etanercept, have also been studied in AH. In 2004, an RCT (n = 36) revealed treatment with infliximab (dose 10 mg/kg) plus prednisolone (vs prednisolone alone) was more harmful in patients with severe AH (MDF >32) due to a high prevalence of severe infections.[54] Similarly, a study with etanercept in patients with moderate to severe AH (DF >15) showed a significantly higher mortality rate after 6 months.[55]

The level of TNF may explain why monoclonal antibodies worsen survival. At high blood levels, TNF is toxic; however, at low levels TNF increases liver regeneration.[56] The infliximab dose in the above trial was 6 times that of the dose in the pilot study.[54] It is probable that the use of high-dose monoclonal antibodies reduces the TNF to a level unable to promote liver regeneration. In contrast, PTX reduces TNF only slightly.[22] This may explain why PTX is beneficial whereas monoclonal antibodies actually increase mortality.

Oxandrolone

In 1984, Mendenhall and colleagues[57] compared the use of oxandrolone with prednisolone with placebo for 30 days in moderate to severe AH. Although neither steroid improved short-term survival, oxandrolone was associated with a beneficial effect on long-term survival in patients with moderate disease. Among those who survived for 1 or 2 months after the start of treatment, the conditional 6-month death rate was 3.5% with oxandrolone and 19% to 20% with placebo.

A more recent review of oxandrolone use in clinical situations, including HIV-related muscle wasting, severe burn injury, neuromuscular disorders, and AH, again found clinical efficacy, notably, improvements in body composition, muscle strength and function, status of underlying disease, recovery from acute catabolic injury, and nutritional status with few side effects.[58] It has been the authors' practice to prescribe oxandrolone (40 mg orally daily for a total of 30 days) for AH patients who meet the following criterion: (1) MDF greater than 80 on admission or (2) lack of improvement in MDF or MELD after 10 to 14 days of PTX. Androgenic steroids could theoretically increase the risk of hepatocellular or prostate carcinoma; however, it seems to improve survival in patients with refractory AH.

Baclofen

Baclofen has been shown effective in reducing alcohol craving and recidivism. Addolorato and colleagues conducted a randomized, double-blind, controlled study (n = 148) of baclofen for maintenance of alcohol abstinence.[59] Patients were randomized to either oral baclofen (10 mg 3 times a day) or placebo for 12 weeks. Of 42 patients allocated to baclofen, 71% achieved and maintained abstinence compared with 29% of 42 patients assigned to the placebo group. In 2010, however, a double-blind, placebo-controlled, randomized study comparing baclofen (30 mg/d) to placebo for 12 weeks of treatment did not show that baclofen was superior to placebo in the treatment of alcohol dependence.[60] The appropriate dosing of baclofen has been criticized and debated. In 2011, Addolorato presented a secondary analysis with baclofen (60 mg orally daily).[61] Patients (all without underlying liver disease) on the higher dose of baclofen had a greater reduction in the number of drinks per day, showing a dose-effect relationship. The literature also quotes a physician who self-treated with baclofen and escalated the dose to 270 mg daily before his craving was eradicated.[62]

Baclofen is generally well tolerated and could play an important role in the treatment of individuals with AH post hospitalization. The authors start baclofen (5 mg orally 3 times a day) when the bilirubin level is declining and approaching value of 10 mg/dL. This dose is given for 3 days and then increased to 10 mg 3 times a day and prescribed indefinitely. The dose could be cautiously increased if the usual dose does not suppress craving. Patients with AH do not report the mild mental status changes that patients without AH frequently notice with this drug. Many patients notice that their alcohol craving returns when they discontinue baclofen. They usually restart it or request that it be refilled at that time. New trials are under way.

HEPATORENAL SYNDROME

HRS is often seen in AH, even on admission and in the absence of diuretics. Development of renal failure significant increases mortality. The initial evaluation for suspected HRS should begin with a careful review of potential nephrotoxic medications, urinalysis, urine electrolytes, spot urine protein, and renal ultrasound to assess for potential renal disease or obstructive nephropathy.

Diagnosis of HRS represents a difficult clinical conundrum. A retrospective review of patients with advanced liver disease and renal failure found that misdiagnosis of HRS occurred in approximately 40% of cases.[63] In response, new urinary markers are being investigated to aid in diagnosis of renal disease in cirrhosis. Neutrophil gelatinase-associated lipocalin (NGAL) has been referred to as "the troponin of the kidney." Preliminary data show that urinary excretion of NGAL is increased in parenchymal acute kidney injury (AKI) but not in functional AKI, such as prerenal azotemia. Patients with acute tubular necrosis and infection-associated renal failure have higher values of 324 and 284, respectively, whereas patients with hypovolemia-related renal failure and HRS have lower values of 30 and 74, respectively.[64] Additional data also suggest that NGAL is higher in patients with cirrhosis and HRS versus patients with cirrhosis and normal renal function.[65] Thus, advances are being made so that the old adage of HRS being a diagnosis of exclusion may no longer apply.

Diagnosis of HRS should be considered when the creatinine rises despite discontinuation of diuretics and the infusion of albumin (1 g/kg/d; 100 g maximum) for a total of 2 days. A study of octreotide and midodrine used in combination and in addition to albumin showed a significant reduction in mortality (43% vs 71%) in a cohort of 81 patients where 60 patients were treated with octreotide/midodrine compared with 21 concomitant controls.[66] Further studies support the therapeutic regimen of octreotide, midodrine, and albumin significantly improving short-term survival and renal function in both HRS type 1 and type 2.[67]

The authors recommend octreotide (50 μg/h continuous infusion rather than subcutaneously) and midodrine (7.5 mg orally every 8 hours followed by increasing the dose of midodrine by 2.5-mg increments with each dosing at each 8-hour interval unless patients becomes frankly hypertensive). It is crucial to rapidly achieve a therapeutic dose of midodrine and octreotide and to treat at least 3 days. In a randomized trial of terlipressin (not available in the United States) in the treatment of HRS, no patient with a serum creatinine greater than 5.6 mg/dL responded.[68]

Renal replacement therapy (RRT) with hemodialysis or continuous venovenous hemofiltration is not recommended in the setting of AH. Without liver transplantation as an option, many nephrologists are unwilling to provide RRT. RRT may induce cardiac arrest when first attempted and actually shorten survival in AH patients, who are usually profoundly hypotensive before RRT.

LIVER TRANSPLANT

AH is so dramatically reversible that 66% of patients who abstain from alcohol have a significant reduction in Child-Pugh score after just 3 months.[69] It is the authors' experience that many resume work and take no medications other than baclofen after 6 months. In the United States, a 6-month interval of observed abstinence from alcohol is required before patients with AH are considered for liver transplantation. Only those who are still in liver failure despite abstinence are considered for transplantation.

This 6-month interval, however, has recently been challenged in a prospective European study of liver transplantation in 26 patients with severe AH who were thought unlikely to survive 6 months. The results of transplantation were excellent, with a 6-month survival rate of 77% after transplant versus 23% without transplant. Three of 26 patients resumed drinking alcohol; of these 3, none had graft dysfunction. Further follow-up may demonstrate a reduction in graft or patient survival in the presence of alcohol.[70] These findings are not directly applicable to patients with AH in the United States, where organs are not allocated for AH.[71]

OUTPATIENT FOLLOW-UP

Once patients are clinically stable with a bilirubin of 10 mg/dL, they can be discharged. This bilirubin criterion is based on a 50-year experience at the University of Southern California Liver Unit, which had 86 beds dedicated to liver disease patients and was predominantly populated by patients with severe AH.[49] Patients released from the hospital with a bilirubin greater than 10 mg/dL often deteriorate and return by ambulance in worse condition than at the time of release. Patients are discharged with prescriptions for baclofen and other medications as needed, including diuretics and medications to treat hepatic encephalopathy. Some state Medicaid programs only pay for 6 medications per month. Thus, prescribing nonessential medications, including vitamins, may decrease compliance and deprive patients of essential medications.

In clinics, diuretics and medications for hepatic encephalopathy can usually be tapered as the liver disease improves with abstinence. PTX is continued until the bilirubin is 5 mg/dL. Baclofen is continued indefinitely given the reported recurrence of alcohol craving when discontinued. A small percentage of patients remain jaundiced and ill despite 6 months of abstinence. This subgroup should be considered for referral for liver transplantation.

REFERENCES

1. O'Shea R, Kinnard MF, Umar N, et al. Treatment of alcoholic hepatitis (AH) in clinical practice. Gastroenterology 2009;136(5):A830–1.
2. Beckett AG, Livingstone AV, Hill KR. Acute alcoholic hepatitis. Br Med J 1961; 2(5260):1113–9.
3. American Psychiatric Association. Diagnostic and statistical manual of mental disorders. 4th edition. Washington, DC: Author; 2000.
4. Kim WR, Brown RS, Terrault NA, et al. Burden of liver disease in the United States: summary of a workshop. Hepatology 2002;36(1):227–42.

5. Rehm J, Mathers C, Popova S, et al. Global burden of disease and injury and economic cost attributable to alcohol use and alcohol-use disorders. Lancet 2009;373(9682):2223–33.
6. Yoon Y. Surveillance report #88 liver cirrhosis mortality in the United States 1970–2007. Available at: http://pubs.niaaa.nih.gov/publications/surveillance88/Cirr07.htm. Accessed November 20, 2011.
7. Asrani SK, Kamath PS, Pedersen R, et al. Liver related mortality in the US is underestimated. Hepatology 2010;52(4):408A.
8. Becker U, Deis A, Sørensen TI, et al. Prediction of risk of liver disease by alcohol intake, sex, and age: a prospective population study. Hepatology 1996;23(5):1025–9.
9. Mandayam S, Jamal MM, Morgan TR. Epidemiology of alcoholic liver disease. Semin Liver Dis 2004;24(3):217–32.
10. Bellentani S, Saccoccio G, Costa G, et al. Drinking habits as cofactors of risk for alcohol induced liver damage. The Dionysos Study Group. Gut 1997;41(6): 845–50.
11. Asrani SK, Larson JJ, Benson JT, et al. Survival of patients with alcoholic hepatitis: a population-based study. Hepatology 2010;52(4):1111–2.
12. Frezza M, di Padova C, Pozzato G, et al. High blood alcohol levels in women. The role of decreased gastric alcohol dehydrogenase activity and first-pass metabolism. N Engl J Med 1990;322(2):95–9.
13. Gutierrez-Reyes G, Rosique D, Corona-Caloca LE, et al. Association of genetic polymorphisms of ADH1B, ALDH2 and CYP2E1 with alcoholism in a group of mexican mestizos. Hepatology 2011;54:522A.
14. Yoon YH, Yi HY, Thomson PC. Alcohol-related and viral hepatitis C-related cirrhosis mortality among Hispanic subgroups in the United States, 2000-2004. Alcohol Clin Exp Res 2011;35(2):240–9.
15. Singal AK. Comments on AASLD practice guidelines for alcoholic liver disease. Hepatology 2010;51(5):1860–1 [author reply: 1861].
16. Levitsky J, Mailliard ME. Diagnosis and therapy of alcoholic liver disease. Semin Liver Dis 2004;24(3):233–47.
17. Sass DA, Shaikh OS. Alcoholic hepatitis. Clin Liver Dis 2006;10(2):219–37, vii.
18. Lischner MW, Alexander JF, Galambos JT. Natural history of alcoholic hepatitis. I. The acute disease. Am J Dig Dis 1971;16(6):481–94.
19. Morales AM, Hashimoto LA, Mokhtee D. Alcoholic hepatitis with leukemoid reaction after surgery. J Gastrointest Surg 2006;10(1):83–5.
20. Mitchell RG, Michael M, Sandidge D. High mortality among patients with the leukemoid reaction and alcoholic hepatitis. South Med J 1991;84(2):281–2.
21. Juturi JV, Hopkins T, Farhangi M. Severe leukocytosis with neutrophilia (leukemoid reaction) in alcoholic steatohepatitis. Am J Gastroenterol 1998;93(6):1013.
22. Akriviadis E, Botla R, Briggs W, et al. Pentoxifylline improves short-term survival in severe acute alcoholic hepatitis: a double-blind, placebo-controlled trial. Gastroenterology 2000;119(6):1637–48.
23. Uchida T, Kao H, Quispe-Sjogren M, et al. Alcoholic foamy degeneration—a pattern of acute alcoholic injury of the liver. Gastroenterology 1983;84(4):683–92.
24. O'Shea RS, Dasarathy S, McCullough AJ. Alcoholic liver disease. Am J Gastroenterol 2010;105(1):14–32 [quiz: 33].
25. Sorbi D, Boynton J, Lindor KD. The ratio of aspartate aminotransferase to alanine aminotransferase: potential value in differentiating nonalcoholic steatohepatitis from alcoholic liver disease. Am J Gastroenterol 1999;94(4):1018–22.
26. Delanghe J, De Buyzere ML. Carbohydrate deficient transferrin and forensic medicine. Clin Chim Acta 2009;406(1–2):1–7.

27. Poynard T, Zourabichvili O, Hilpert G, et al. Prognostic value of total serum bilirubin/gamma-glutamyl transpeptidase ratio in cirrhotic patients. Hepatology 1984;4(2):324–7.
28. Milman N, Graudal N. Serum ferritin in acute viral hepatitis. Scand J Gastroenterol 1984;19(1):38–40.
29. Hoefs JC, Green G, Reynolds TB, et al. Mechanism for the abnormal liver scan in acute alcoholic liver injury. Am J Gastroenterol 1984;79(12):950–8.
30. Hoefs JC, Wang F, Kanel G. Functional measurement of nonfibrotic hepatic mass in cirrhotic patients. Am J Gastroenterol 1997;92(11):2054–8.
31. Everson GT, Shiffman ML, Hoefs JC, et al. Quantitative liver function tests improve the prediction of clinical outcomes in chronic hepatitis C: results from the HALT-C trial. Hepatology 2011 Oct 26. [Epub ahead of print]. DOI: 10.1002/hep.24752.
32. Lefkowitch JH. Morphology of alcoholic liver disease. Clin Liver Dis 2005;9(1):37–53.
33. Jensen K, Gluud C. The mallory body: morphological, clinical and experimental studies (part 1 of a literature survey). Hepatology 1994;20(4 Pt 1):1061–77.
34. Maddrey WC, Boitnott JK, Bedine MS, et al. Corticosteroid therapy of alcoholic hepatitis. Gastroenterology 1978;75(2):193–9.
35. Dunn W, Jamil LH, Brown LS, et al. MELD accurately predicts mortality in patients with alcoholic hepatitis. Hepatology 2005;41(2):353–8.
36. Forrest EH, Evans CD, Stewart S, et al. Analysis of factors predictive of mortality in alcoholic hepatitis and derivation and validation of the Glasgow alcoholic hepatitis score. Gut 2005;54(8):1174–9.
37. Srikureja W, Kyulo NL, Runyon BA, et al. MELD score is a better prognostic model than child-turcotte-pugh score or discriminant function score in patients with alcoholic hepatitis. J Hepatol 2005;42(5):700–6.
38. Forrest EH, Morris AJ, Stewart S, et al. The Glasgow alcoholic hepatitis score identifies patients who may benefit from corticosteroids. Gut 2007;56(12): 1743–6.
39. Louvet A, Naveau S, Abdelnour M, et al. The Lille model: a new tool for therapeutic strategy in patients with severe alcoholic hepatitis treated with steroids. Hepatology 2007;45(6):1348–54.
40. Sandahl TD, Jepsen P, Ott P, et al. Validation of prognostic scores for clinical use in patients with alcoholic hepatitis. Scand J Gastroenterol 2011;46(9):1127–32.
41. Mendenhall CL, Anderson S, Weesner RE, et al. Protein-calorie malnutrition associated with alcoholic hepatitis. Veterans Administration Cooperative Study Group on Alcoholic Hepatitis. Am J Med 1984;76(2):211–22.
42. Cabré E, Rodríguez-Iglesias P, Caballería J, et al. Short- and long-term outcome of severe alcohol-induced hepatitis treated with steroids or enteral nutrition: a multicenter randomized trial. Hepatology 2000;32(1):36–42.
43. Applied Medical Technology Inc. AMT Bridle Nasal Tube Retaining System. Available at: www.appliedmedical.net.
44. Ramond MJ, Poynard T, Rueff B, et al. A randomized trial of prednisolone in patients with severe alcoholic hepatitis. N Engl J Med 1992;326(8):507–12.
45. Lucey MR, Mathurin P, Morgan TR. Alcoholic hepatitis. N Engl J Med 2009; 360(26):2758–69.
46. Christensen E, Gluud C. Glucocorticoids are ineffective in alcoholic hepatitis: a meta-analysis adjusting for confounding variables. Gut 1995;37(1):113–8.
47. Rambaldi A, Saconato HH, Christensen E, et al. Systematic review: glucocorticosteroids for alcoholic hepatitis—a Cochrane Hepato-Biliary Group systematic review with meta-analyses and trial sequential analyses of randomized clinical trials. Aliment Pharmacol Ther 2008;27(12):1167–78.

48. Mathurin P, O'Grady J, Carithers RL, et al. Corticosteroids improve short-term survival in patients with severe alcoholic hepatitis: meta-analysis of individual patient data. Gut 2011;60(2):255–60.
49. Amini M, Runyon BA. Alcoholic hepatitis 2010: a clinician's guide to diagnosis and therapy. World J Gastroenterol 2010;16(39):4905–12.
50. McHutchison JG, Runyon BA, Draguesku JO, et al. Pentoxifylline may prevent renal impairment (hepatorenal-syndrome) in severe acute alcoholic hepatitis. Hepatology 1991;14(4):A96.
51. De BK, Gangopadhyay S, Dutta D, et al. Pentoxifylline versus prednisolone for severe alcoholic hepatitis: a randomized controlled trial. World J Gastroenterol 2009;15(13):1613–9.
52. Nguyen-Khac E, Thevenot T, Piquet MA, et al. Glucocorticoids plus N-acetylcysteine in severe alcoholic hepatitis. N Engl J Med 2011;365(19):1781–9.
53. Louvet A, Diaz E, Dharancy S, et al. Early switch to pentoxifylline in patients with severe alcoholic hepatitis is inefficient in non-responders to corticosteroids. J Hepatol 2008;48(3):465–70.
54. Naveau S, Chollet-Martin S, Dharancy S, et al. A double-blind randomized controlled trial of infliximab associated with prednisolone in acute alcoholic hepatitis. Hepatology 2004;39(5):1390–7.
55. Boetticher NC, Peine CJ, Kwo P, et al. A randomized, double-blinded, placebo-controlled multicenter trial of etanercept in the treatment of alcoholic hepatitis. Gastroenterology 2008;135(6):1953–60.
56. Schwabe RF, Brenner DA. Mechanisms of liver injury. I. TNF-alpha-induced liver injury: role of IKK, JNK, and ROS pathways. Am J Physiol Gastrointest Liver Physiol 2006;290(4):G583–9.
57. Mendenhall CL, Anderson S, Garcia-Pont P, et al. Short-term and long-term survival in patients with alcoholic hepatitis treated with oxandrolone and prednisolone. N Engl J Med 1984;311(23):1464–70.
58. Orr R, Fiatarone Singh M. The anabolic androgenic steroid oxandrolone in the treatment of wasting and catabolic disorders: review of efficacy and safety. Drugs 2004;64(7):725–50.
59. Addolorato G, Leggio L, Ferrulli A, et al. Effectiveness and safety of baclofen for maintenance of alcohol abstinence in alcohol-dependent patients with liver cirrhosis: randomised, double-blind controlled study. Lancet 2007;370(9603):1915–22.
60. Garbutt JC, Kampov-Polevoy AB, Gallop R, et al. Efficacy and safety of baclofen for alcohol dependence: a randomized, double-blind, placebo-controlled trial. Alcohol Clin Exp Res 2010;34(11):1849–57.
61. Addolorato G, Leggio L, Ferrulli A, et al. Dose-response effect of baclofen in reducing daily alcohol intake in alcohol dependence: secondary analysis of a randomized, double-blind, placebo-controlled trial. Alcohol Alcohol 2011;46(3):312–7.
62. Enserink M. Addiction research. Anonymous alcoholic bankrolls trial of controversial therapy. Science 2011;332(6030):653.
63. Watt K, Uhanova J, Minuk GY. Hepatorenal syndrome: diagnostic accuracy, clinical features, and outcome in a tertiary care center. Am J Gastroenterol 2002;97(8):2046–50.
64. Fagundes C, Pepin MN, Guevara M, et al. Evaluation of four different urinary biomarkers in the assessment of renal failure in cirrhosis. Role for urinary neutrophil gelatinase-associated lipocalin. Hepatology 2011;54:1234A.
65. Cavallin M, Fasolato S, Sticca A, et al. Increased urinary level of neutrophil gelatinase-associated lipocalin (NGAL) In patients with cirrhosis and type 1 HRS. Hepatology 2011;54:1254A–5A.

66. Esrailian E, Pantangco ER, Kyulo NL, et al. Octreotide/Midodrine therapy significantly improves renal function and 30-day survival in patients with type 1 hepatorenal syndrome. Dig Dis Sci 2007;52(3):742–8.
67. Skagen C, Einstein M, Lucey MR, et al. Combination treatment with octreotide, midodrine, and albumin improves survival in patients with type 1 and type 2 hepatorenal syndrome. J Clin Gastroenterol 2009;43(7):680–5.
68. Boyer TD, Sanyal AJ, Garcia-Tsao G, et al. Predictors of response to terlipressin plus albumin in hepatorenal syndrome (HRS) type 1: relationship of serum creatinine to hemodynamics. J Hepatol 2011;55(2):315–21.
69. Veldt BJ, Lainé F, Guillygomarc'h A, et al. Indication of liver transplantation in severe alcoholic liver cirrhosis: quantitative evaluation and optimal timing. J Hepatol 2002;36(1):93–8.
70. Mathurin P, Moreno C, Samuel D, et al. Early liver transplantation for severe alcoholic hepatitis. N Engl J Med 2011;365(19):1790–800.
71. Brown RS. Transplantation for alcoholic hepatitis—time to rethink the 6-month "rule". N Engl J Med 2011;365(19):1836–8.

Granulomatous Liver Disease

Steven L. Flamm, MD

KEYWORDS

- Hepatic granuloma • Sarcoidosis • Primary biliary cirrhosis
- Medication hepatotoxicity • Alkaline phosphatase • GGT
- Liver biopsy

GRANULOMATOUS LIVER DISEASE

Granulomatous liver disease is a common problem and often provides a clue to the presence of underlying systemic disease. Findings of hepatic granulomata on liver biopsy often confuse the clinician and consultant. Granulomatous liver disease may present with an abnormal liver panel but no symptoms. Patients may present with manifestations of the systemic process. Identification of the systemic process may allow proper therapy and improvement in the natural history of the underlying disease state. Careful assessment of systemic symptoms and appropriate laboratory testing frequently permits a specific diagnosis. This article reviews how to address consultation regarding a finding of hepatic granulomata on liver biopsy.

HISTOPATHOLOGY

Granulomatous liver disease is defined by the histologic findings on liver biopsy. Granulomata may be found in different tissues and represent many different disease processes.[1] A granuloma is a distinct lesion that is characterized by an accumulation of mononuclear cells, primarily macrophages, in the center. There is a surrounding rim with fibroblasts and lymphocytes. The lesion may or may not be well circumscribed, but it is separate from adjacent, uninvolved tissue (**Fig. 1**). Hepatic granulomata may be located anywhere in the hepatic lobule, but involvement of different sites may be helpful in the differential diagnoses of specific disease processes.

Granulomata develop over time as an immunologic response to exogenous and/or endogenous antigenic stimuli. The granuloma may appear as punched-out clusters of lymphocytes or histiocytes. Mononuclear cells, such as macrophages, are activated by various cytokines. These activated macrophages resemble epithelial cells and are called epithelioid cells. Macrophages may fuse to form multinucleated giant cells. Eosinophils may or may not be present.

Division of Hepatology, Northwestern University Feinberg School of Medicine, 676 North Saint Clair Street, Suite 1900, Chicago, IL 60611, USA
E-mail address: s-flamm@northwestern.edu

Clin Liver Dis 16 (2012) 387–396
doi:10.1016/j.cld.2012.03.013

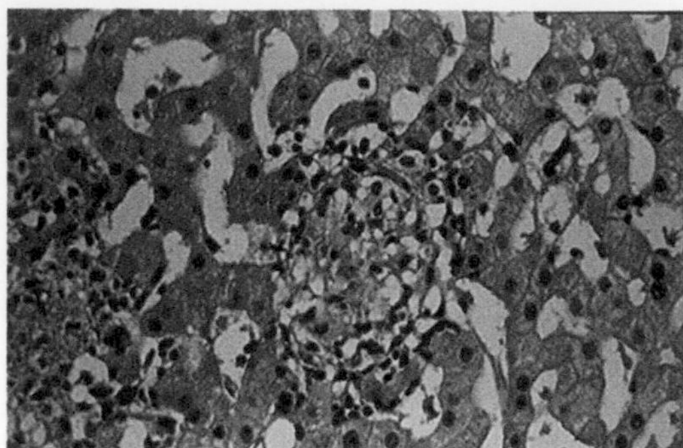

Fig. 1. Hepatic granuloma.

Four different types of hepatic granulomata have been described, and each is associated with different etiologies[2]: Caseating granulomata, characterized by central necrosis; noncaseating granulomata, do not have central necrosis; fibrin-ring granulomata, characterized by the histologic feature of a central vacuole with a fibrin-ring, surrounded by epithelioid cells; and lipogranulomas, containing a central lipid vacuole.

ASSOCIATED DISEASE STATES

Numerous disease states have been associated with hepatic granuloma. Different disease processes may be more or less common depending on the area of the world where it occurs. The presence of a single granuloma in a liver biopsy may be a spurious finding and may not indicate the presence of granulomatous liver disease.[3] In addition, hepatic granulomata may occasionally be observed in patients with known chronic liver disease and may not necessarily indicate that a second process is ongoing.[4] The presence of hepatic granulomata on diagnostic liver biopsy should spur a workup to identify the underlying cause.

Categories of disease states that may involve the liver with granulomata include the following:

1. Sarcoidosis
2. Autoimmune
3. Infectious diseases
4. Drugs
5. Cancer
6. Idiopathic.

Sarcoidosis

One of the most common causes of hepatic granulomata in the United States is sarcoidosis.[1,5] A systemic disease of unknown etiology that may or may not be autoimmune, sarcoidosis, can affect people of any age, gender, and race. However, it is more common in young African Americans.[6,7] Sarcoidosis affects many organ systems, most notably the lungs. However, involvement of the gastrointestinal system is common although frequently asymptomatic. In the liver, hepatic granulomata are often identified. Even when numerous granulomata are present, clinical evidence of chronic liver disease is rare. Occasionally, portal vein thrombosis and/or cirrhosis is observed.

The diagnosis of hepatic sarcoidosis is based on clinical presentation, biochemical profile, and characteristics of the hepatic granulomata. The patient may have a known history of sarcoidosis or may have signs and symptoms related to chronic pulmonary disease, such as cough or shortness of breath. Involvement of other organ systems, such as the eyes or skin may provide a clue to the diagnosis. Chest radiograph may reveal changes consistent with sarcoidosis. From a biochemical standpoint, patients frequently show elevated levels of serum alkaline phosphatase and γ-glutamyltransferase (GGT). Slight elevations in the level of bilirubin may be observed but are less common. In addition, the epithelioid cells of the hepatic granuloma in sarcoidosis often secrete angiotensin-converting enzyme (ACE), and ACE levels are elevated in 75% of patients.[8,9] The hepatic granuloma in sarcoidosis is usually in the portal tract and is noncaseating.

Because hepatic sarcoidosis most commonly has a benign course and there is no definitive test to confirm the diagnosis, other causes of hepatic granulomatosis must be ruled out to the satisfaction of the consultant.

Treatment of hepatic sarcoidosis is usually not recommended, despite the elevated levels of alkaline phosphatase.[10] If patients have evidence of portal hypertension and cirrhosis, a short course of corticosteroids can be considered. However, it is unclear if this is helpful, and the endpoints of therapy or outcome measures are not defined.

Autoimmune

Another common cause of hepatic granulomata in the United States is primary biliary cirrhosis (PBC).[1,5,11] A disease primarily of middle-aged women, patients may be asymptomatic or may present with progressive fatigue and/or pruritus. PBC may be associated with other autoimmune disorders such as sicca syndrome or CREST syndrome, and patients may have related symptoms such as dry eyes and/or mouth, heartburn or Raynaud syndrome.[12] The biochemical profile is similar to sarcoidosis; patients typically have elevated levels of alkaline phosphatase and GGT. Bilirubin levels are often not elevated early in the course and only modest levels of elevations are typically noted even in advanced disease.

Patients with PBC have a positive antimitochondrial antibody (AMA) in greater than 90% of cases. Elevated serum immunoglobulin (Ig) M levels also may be observed.[13] Based on histology, hepatic granulomata resemble the ones seen in sarcoidosis. However, patients with PBC may also have bile duct inflammation (cholangitis) on liver biopsy.

The diagnosis of PBC is suggested by the presence of symptoms, such as progressive fatigue and pruritus (although symptoms are frequently absent) in a middle-aged woman. A cholestatic profile is noted. AMA positivity and/or elevated IgM levels allow for a definitive diagnosis.

Treatment of PBC involves ursodeoxycholic acid (13–15 mg/kg/d in divided doses).[14] Treatment is not curative, and the condition may continue to progress and develop cirrhosis.

Other autoimmune diseases in which hepatic granulomata have been described include Crohn disease and Wegener granulomatosis (polyangiitis).[15,16]

Infectious Diseases

Many infectious diseases have been associated with hepatic granulomatosis and must be ruled out to the satisfaction of the consultant (**Box 1**).[17]

Tuberculosis

Hepatic granulomata are observed in approximately 20% of patients with pulmonary tuberculosis, approximately 75% of patients with extrapulmonary tuberculosis, and

Box 1
Infectious etiologies of granulomatous liver disease

Bacterial
- Tuberculosis
- Mycobacterium avium-intracellulare complex
- Brucellosis
- Lepromatous leprosy
- Bacille Calmette-Guérin infection
- Listeriosis
- Melioidosis
- Tularemia
- Yersiniosis
- Psittacosis
- Whipple disease
- Cat scratch fever

Viral
- Cytomegalovirus
- Epstein-Barr virus
- Hepatitis A, B, and C
- Infectious mononucleosis

Fungal
- Histoplasmosis
- Coccidioidomycosis
- Cryptococcus
- Nocardiosis
- Candidiasis
- Blastomycosis

Parasitic
- Toxoplasmosis
- Schistosomiasis
- Visceral larva migrans
- Visceral leishmaniasis

Rickettsial
- Coxiella burnetii (Q fever)
- Boutonneuse fever

Spirochetal
- Secondary syphilis

Chlamydia
- Psittacosis

more than 90% of patients with miliary tuberculosis. Systemic symptoms such as fevers, weight loss, anorexia, and night sweats may be present. The patient may or may not have known pulmonary tuberculosis. If systemic symptoms are present including fever or if the patient has pulmonary symptoms including cough and/or shortness of breath, a diagnosis of tuberculosis must be considered.[18]

The biochemical profile typically reveals an elevated level of alkaline phosphatase and GGT, bilirubin levels may be elevated but elevations are usually not prominent. Hepatic granulomata are usually in the portal tract and may or may not be caseating.

A description of the specific diagnostic strategy and treatment of tuberculosis is beyond the scope of this review. A diagnosis of tuberculosis must be considered and ruled out to the satisfaction of the consultant when hepatic granulomata are observed. Appropriate treatment should be instituted expeditiously if the diagnosis is confirmed. If the diagnosis of tuberculosis cannot be ruled out and remains of concern, antituberculous therapy should be considered before an empiric course of corticosteroids.

Mycobacterium avium-intracellulare complex

Mycobacterium avium-intracellulare complex (MAC) is associated with hepatic granulomatosis and is observed in immunocompromised patients, such as ones with HIV.[19] In patients with a cholestatic biochemical profile and fevers, a diagnosis of MAC should be considered, particularly if the patient is HIV positive and if hepatic granulomatosis has been confirmed on liver biopsy.

Fungal infections

Fungal infections should be considered in the differential diagnosis of hepatic granulomatosis.[20–24] Histoplasmosis and coccidioidomycosis are among the more common causes in the United States. Histoplasmosis should be considered in particular in patients who live or have lived in the Southern or Central United States. Coccidioidomycosis should be considered in patients from the Southwestern United States. Hepatic granulomata may also be observed in candidiasis, blastomycosis, or cryptococcosis.

A review of the diagnostic strategy and treatment of these entities is beyond the scope of this article. However, fungal infections should be considered in the differential diagnosis of patients with hepatic granulomata.

HIV-related diseases

Patients with AIDS are vulnerable to infections that are associated with hepatic granulomatosis, including tuberculosis, MAC, and fungal infections, such as histoplasmosis, toxoplasmosis, and cryptococcosis. Each infection should be ruled out in a patient with HIV and hepatic granulomatosis.

Brucellosis

Brucellosis is caused by infection with *Brucella abortus*, *Brucella suis*, *Brucella canis*, and *Brucella melitensis*.[25] *Brucella* is acquired from animals either with contact from infected cattle, goats, and swine or by ingestion of unpasteurized dairy products. The most common symptom is fever. Other symptoms may be present including decreased appetite, fatigue, weight loss, and night sweats. Symptoms may be abrupt or insidious, and can oscillate over a period of months. Many organ systems may be involved. If the liver is involved, hepatic granulomatosis may be observed. Serum agglutinins for *Brucella* are obtained as a diagnostic test.

Q fever

Q fever is caused by infection with *Coxiella burnetti*, a rickettsial organism. *Coxiella* can be acquired by inhalation, ingestion, or from tick bites. Q fever most commonly presents as pneumonia with fevers, myalgias, and headaches. If the liver is involved, hepatic granulomatosis may be involved.[26] The granuloma, known as a fibrin-ring granuloma, is characterized by a fibrinoid necrotic ring surrounded by histiocytes and lymphocytes.

Schistosomiasis

Schistosomiasis may be observed as a cause of hepatic granulomatosis.[27] Granulomata often contain abundant eosinophils.

Chronic viral hepatitis B or C

Granulomata have been observed rarely in patients with chronic hepatitis B or C viral infections. Granulomata are described as epithelioid and nonnecrotizing.[28,29]

Other infectious causes

Various other infections have been associated with hepatic granulomata. These include Lyme disease (*Borrelia burgdorferi*), toxoplasmosis, nocardiosis, actinomycosis, salmonellosis, cytomegalovirus, and Epstein-Barr virus infections.

Cancer

Hodgkin lymphoma is the most common malignancy associated with hepatic granulomatosis. Hepatic granulomata may also be observed in non–Hodgkin lymphoma and renal cell carcinoma.[30–32]

Drugs

Many commonly used medications have been associated with hepatic granulomatosis including sulfa drugs, allopurinol, isoniazid, chlorpropamide, and quinidine (**Box 2**).[5,33] Granulomata of variable size may be located anywhere in the liver. Eosinophils may be present, a clue to a drug-related etiology. A recommendation by the consultant to discontinue unnecessary medications associated with hepatic granulomatosis is in order.

Foreign Body

Granulomata typically comprises macrophages forming giant cells. Talc in intravenous drug users or suture material after surgery may be implicated.[34]

Lipogranuloma

Lipogranuloma have been associated with ingestion of mineral oil. The lipogranuloma is characterized by fat droplets surrounded by macrophages and lymphocytes. They are small and contain multinucleated giant cells. The lipogranuloma does not result in significant liver injury.[35]

Idiopathic

An exhaustive workup of the causes of hepatic granulomatosis is unremarkable.[1] Patients may have symptoms such as myalgias, arthralgias, fevers, and hepatosplenomegaly.[36] The sedimentation rate may be highly elevated. This syndrome is called idiopathic granulomatous hepatitis.

Box 2
Medications associated with granulomatous liver disease (alphabetical order)

Allopurinol
Amoxicillin-clavulanic acid
Carbamazepine
Chlorpropamide
Diltiazem
Gold
Halothane
Hydralazine
Interferon alfa
Mebendazole
Methyldopa
Nitrofurantoin
Phenylbutazone
Phenytoin
Procainamide
Quinidine
Sulfa drugs

TREATMENT

Treatment recommendations depend on the underlying diagnosis. Infectious etiologies of hepatic granulomatosis should be treated with the appropriate antibiotic, antifungal, or antimycobacterial agent. Treatment of PBC includes ursodeoxycholic acid. Medication-induced hepatic granulomatosis is treated by removal of the offending agent. Malignancy-related hepatic granulomatosis is treated by therapy of the associated malignancy.

Hepatic granulomatosis secondary to sarcoidosis is usually not treated. Concomitant pulmonary sarcoidosis may be treated with corticosteroids, but treatment of hepatic sarcoidosis alone is rarely recommended. A short course of corticosteroids can be considered if patients have portal hypertension related to hepatic sarcoidosis, but the outcome measures and length of therapy is unclear. Tuberculosis must be ruled out for the satisfaction of the consultant before commencing therapy with corticosteroids.

Idiopathic granulomatous hepatitis may also be treated with an empiric course of corticosteroids. However, as previously discussed, one must be careful to rule out tuberculosis before treatment with corticosteroids. If tuberculosis remains in the differential diagnosis, an empiric course of antituberculous therapy for 4 to 8 weeks should be considered before a therapeutic course with corticosteroids. Methotrexate can be considered if symptomatic granulomatous hepatitis remains after a course of corticosteroids.[37]

APPROACH BY THE CONSULTANT

Hepatic granulomata are not infrequently observed in diagnostic liver biopsies, and 1 or 2 granulomata do not necessarily implicate a relevant disease process. However, if hepatic granulomatosis is definitive, a thorough history, physical examination, and blood testing workup should be obtained. Regarding the history, symptoms such as fevers, weight loss, arthralgias, and myalgias should be sought. Pulmonary symptoms, such as cough and shortness of breath, may be observed in patients with sarcoidosis or infectious causes such as tuberculosis, MAC, or Q fever. A careful travel history should be obtained, with particular attention to contact with animals or ingestion of unpasteurized milk. Patients with PBC may complain of pruritus or severe fatigue, or symptoms such as dry eyes and/or mouth (sicca syndrome) or heartburn and/or Raynaud syndrome (CREST syndrome). Medication history should also be reviewed carefully. On physical examination, fevers may be a clue to underlying infection. Lymphadenopathy may be present in Hodgkin disease. Excoriations may be present in PBC.

A chest radiograph may show findings consistent with pulmonary sarcoidosis or tuberculosis. Blood testing should be obtained, including a liver panel (which usually reveals hepatic cholestasis with elevated alkaline phosphatase and GGT, AMA, serum IgM levels, and serum ACE inhibitor levels. Appropriate serologic studies should be obtained if specific infectious diseases are sought. A sedimentation rate may be elevated in several of the causes of hepatic granulomatosis. HIV testing should be considered in individuals with tuberculosis and MAC. QuantiFERON testing and/or placement of a purified protein derivative should be considered if tuberculosis remains in the differential diagnosis.

The liver biopsy results should also be reviewed with the pathologist to determine if there are any clues to the diagnosis from the appearance or location of the hepatic granulomata. Caseating granulomata are characteristic of tuberculosis. Fibrin-ring granulomata may be observed in Q fever or Hodgkin disease.

SUMMARY

Hepatic granulomatosis is a relatively common and vexing problem for which gastroenterology consultation may be sought. A careful history, physical examination, and blood testing workup can frequently identify the cause and allow design of an appropriate treatment approach.

REFERENCES

1. Drebber U, Kasper HU, Ratering J, et al. Hepatic granulomas: histological and molecular pathological approach to differential diagnosis—a study of 442 cases. Liver Int 2008;28:828.
2. Maddrey WC. Granulomas of the liver. In: Schiff ER, Sorrell MF, Maddrey WC, editors. Schiff's diseases of the liver. 8th edition. Philadelphia: Lippincott-Raven; 1989. p. 1572.
3. Klatskin G, Yesner R. Hepatic manifestations of sarcoidosis and other granulomatous diseases; a study based on histological examination of tissue obtained by needle biopsy of the liver. Yale J Biol Med 1950;23:207.
4. Tahan V, Ozaras R, Lacevic N, et al. Prevalence of hepatic granulomas in chronic hepatitis B. Dig Dis Sci 2004;49:1575.
5. Zakim D, Boyer TD. 3rd edition. Hepatology, a textbook of liver diseases, vol. 3. Philadelphia: WB Saunders; 1996. p. 1472.
6. Rybicki BA, Iannuzzi MC. Epidemiology of sarcoidosis: recent advances and future prospects. Semin Respir Crit Care Med 2007;28:22–35.
7. Ayyala US, Padilla ML. Diagnosis and treatment of hepatic sarcoidosis. Curr Treat Options Gastroenterol 2006;9:475–83.

8. Ishak KG. Granulomas of the liver. Adv Pathol Lab Med 1995;8:247.
9. Studdy PR, Bird R. Serum angiotensin converting enzyme in sarcoidosis—its value in present clinical practice. Ann Clin Biochem 1989;26(Pt 1):13.
10. Vatti R, Sharma OP. Course of asymptomatic liver involvement in sarcoidosis: role of therapy in selected cases. Sarcoidosis Vasc Diffuse Lung Dis 1997;14:73.
11. Gaya DR, Thorburn D, Oien KA, et al. Hepatic granulomas: a 10 year single centre experience. J Clin Pathol 2003;56:850–3.
12. Lindor KD, Gershwin ME, Poupon R, et al. Primary biliary cirrhosis. Hepatology 2009;50:291–308.
13. Kaplan MM, Gershwin ME. Primary biliary cirrhosis. N Engl J Med 2005;353: 1261–73.
14. Poupon RE, Poupon R, Balkau B, The UDCS-PBC Study Group. Ursodiol for the long-term treatment of primary biliary cirrhosis. N Engl J Med 1994;330:1342–7.
15. Maurer LH, Hughes RW, Folley JL, et al. Granulomatous hepatitis associated with regional enteritis. Gastroenterology 1967;53:301–5.
16. Holl-Ulrich K, Klass M. Wegener s granulomatosis with granulomatous liver involvement. Clin Exp Rheumatol 2010;28:88–9.
17. Lamps LW. Hepatic granulomas, with an emphasis on their infectious causes. Adv Anat Pathol 2008;15:309–18.
18. Alvarez SZ, Carpio R. Hepatobiliary tuberculosis. Dig Dis Sci 1983;28:193.
19. Horsburgh CR. *Mycobacterium avium* complex infection in the acquired immunodeficiency syndrome. N Engl J Med 1991;324:1332–8.
20. Lewis JH, Patel HR, Zimmerman HJ. The spectrum of hepatic candidiasis. Hepatology 1982;2:479–87.
21. Smith JW, Utz JP. Progressive disseminated histoplasmosis. A prospective study of 26 patients. Ann Intern Med 1972;103:533–8.
22. Davies SF, Khan M, Sarosi GA. Disseminated histoplasmosis in immunologically suppressed patients. Am J Med 1978;64:94–100.
23. Kovacs JA, Kovac AA, Polis M, et al. Cryptococcosis in the acquired immunodeficiency syndrome. Ann Intern Med 1985;103:533–8.
24. Deresinski SC, Stevens DA. Coccidioidomycosis in compromised hosts: experience at Stanford University Hospital. Medicine 1974;54:377–95.
25. Akritidis N, Tzivras M, Delladetsima I, et al. The liver in brucellosis. Clin Gastroenterol Hepatol 2007;5:1109.
26. Hofmann CE, Heaton JW. Q fever hepatitis. Gastroenterology 1982;83:474–9.
27. Warren KS. The pathogenesis of "clay-pipe stem cirrhosis" in mice with chronic schistomsomiasis mansoni, with a note on the longevity of the schistosomes. Am J Pathol 1966;49:477–89.
28. Emile JF, Sebagh M, Féray C, et al. The presence of epithelioid granulomas in hepatitis C virus-related cirrhosis. Hum Pathol 1993;24:1095–7.
29. Kanno A, Murakami K. A transient emergence of hepatic granulomas in a patient with chronic hepatitis B. Tohoku J Exp Med 1998;185:281–5.
30. Kadin ME, Donaldson SS, Dorfman RF. Isolated granulomas in Hodgkin's disease. N Engl J Med 1970;283:859.
31. Braylan RC, Long JC, Jaffe ES, et al. Malignant lymphoma obscured by concomitant extensive epithelioid granulomas: report of three cases with similar clinicopathologic features. Cancer 1977;39:1146.
32. Chagnac A, Gal R, Kimche D. Liver granulomas: a possible paraneoplastic manifestation of hypernephroma. Am J Gastroenterol 1985;80:989–92.
33. Ishak KG, Zimmerman HJ. Drug-induced and toxic granulomatous hepatitis. Baillieres Clin Gastroenterol 1986;2:463–80.

34. Co DO, Hogan LH, Il-Kim S, et al. T cell contributions to the different phases of granuloma formation. Immunol Lett 2004;92:135–42.
35. Boitnott JK, Margolis S. Mineral oil in human tissues. II. Oil droplets in lymph nodes of the porta hepatis. Bull Johns Hopkins Hosp 1966;118:414–22.
36. Simon HB, Wolff SM. Granulomatous hepatitis and prolonged fever of unknown origin: a study of 13 patients. Medicine (Baltimore) 1973;52:1.
37. Knox TA, Kaplan MM, Gelfand JA, et al. Methotrexate treatment of idiopathic granulomatous hepatitis. Ann Intern Med 1995;122:592.

Nonalcoholic Fatty Liver Disease

Angelo H. Paredes, MD[a], Dawn M. Torres, MD[a], Stephen A. Harrison, MD[b,*]

KEYWORDS

- Nonalcoholic fatty liver disease (NAFLD)
- Nonalcoholic steatohepatitis (NASH) • Diagnosis • Treatment

CLINICAL CASE

A 55-year-old Hispanic woman with a past medical history of obesity, type 2 diabetes, hypertension, and hyperlipidemia is referred for evaluation of asymptomatic elevation of serum aminotransferases. She was recently started on a statin for hyperlipidemia and on interval labs was noted to have a rise in her liver-associated enzymes from a baseline alkaline phosphatase (ALP) 70 IU/L → 85 IU/L, aspartate aminotransferase (AST) 60 U/L → 75 U/L, and alanine aminotransferase (ALT) 48 U/L → 85U/L. Review of her previous labs reveals a several-year history of liver enzymes 1.5 to 2.0 times normal. She is a nondrinker of alcohol or caffeine and is a nonsmoker. No risk factors for chronic hepatitis B or C identified. Current medications include metformin, lisinopril, hydrochlorothiazide, and a baby aspirin. Family history is notable for a mother with cirrhosis of unknown etiology.

Nonalcoholic fatty liver disease (NAFLD) is the most common cause of incidental elevation of liver enzymes in the Western world, as well as in rapidly developing countries.[1,2] NAFLD encompasses a spectrum of disease ranging from simple fatty liver, to inflammatory steatohepatitis with increasing levels of fibrosis and possibly cirrhosis. NAFLD is a multifactorial disease with varied clinical associations.

The prevalence of the disease is difficult to establish because of lack of effective screening tests, although NAFLD is closely linked with obesity and the metabolic syndrome. Risk factors include body mass index (BMI) of 25 kg/m^2 or greater, central obesity, and diabetes.

Disclaimer: The view(s) expressed herein are those of the author(s) and do not reflect the official policy or position of Brooke Army Medical Center, the US Army Medical Department, the US Army Office of the Surgeon General, the Department of the Army, Department of Defense or the US Government.

Grant Support: None.

[a] Division of Gastroenterology, Department of Medicine, Walter Reed National Military Medical Center, 8901 Wisconsin Avenue, Bethesda, MD 20889, USA; [b] Division of Gastroenterology and Hepatology, Department of Medicine, Brooke Army Medical Center, San Antonio Military Medical Center, 3851 Roger Brooke Drive, Fort Sam Houston, TX 78234, USA
* Corresponding author.
E-mail address: Stephen.harrison@amedd.army.mil

Clin Liver Dis 16 (2012) 397–419
doi:10.1016/j.cld.2012.03.005
1089-3261/12/$ – see front matter Published by Elsevier Inc.

Fatty liver on imaging confirms the diagnosis of NAFLD, although liver biopsy is currently required to discriminate between isolated fatty liver and those with nonalcoholic steatohepatitis (NASH). Liver biopsy is not without drawbacks, and as an invasive procedure, carries the risk of serious, albeit rare complications, and noninvasive laboratory or radiographic studies would be of tremendous benefit.

Patients with NASH are those at risk for disease progression to cirrhosis as well as hepatocellular carcinoma (HCC), so treatment efforts are primarily focused of this subset of patients. Treatment is aimed at lifestyle modification to achieve weight loss and increase cardiovascular exercise. There are no single pharmacologic agents recommended in the treatment of NAFLD, although many have been studied with generally modest benefit. Surgical weight loss procedures have also been successfully used in the treatment of NASH. Multimodality treatment approaches combining lifestyle modification with pharmacotherapy represent a newer frontier of study that has shown promise in the treatment of this growing patient population.

DEFINITIONS

NAFLD is the umbrella diagnosis that includes both isolated fatty liver (IFL) and NASH. Natural history studies have demonstrated that patients with IFL do not have increased liver-related mortality with minimal risk for disease progression. In contrast, patients who meet histopathologic criteria for NASH are at risk for progression to cirrhosis as well as HCC.

NAFLD is defined as macrovesicular fat accumulation in more than 5% of hepatocytes in those who do not consume alcohol in amounts generally considered to be harmful to the liver. Typically, this has been defined as 1 to 2 drinks per day for a women and 2–3 drinks per day for a man (average <20 g/day).[1,2] Patients are primed for NAFLD in the setting of obesity with insulin resistance (IR). The complex interplay between environmental and genetic factors that leads to the development of necroinflammation and fibrosis in certain cases is not fully understood, and the dogma of sequential progression of disease from isolated fatty liver to NASH to cirrhosis has grown out of favor. The development of steatosis is a relatively straightforward affair depending on excess free fatty acids either from lipolysis in adipocytes, dietary lipids, de novo lipogenesis, or impaired lipid disposal.[3] Ongoing research is focused on elucidating the steps that lead to steatohepatitis and fibrosis with a recent emphasis on lipotoxicity and impaired cellular repair mechanisms, including autophagy.[4] Genetic predisposition including specific alleles that have been associated with hepatic steatosis and/or advanced NASH have also added to the current understanding of NASH.[5]

Epidemiology

NAFLD is now the most common liver disease in the United States and possibly worldwide. The most common presentation is the asymptomatic, nondrinking patient with mildly elevated liver associated enzymes: alanine aminotransferase (ALT) > aspartate aminotransferase (AST). Patients will generally have associated metabolic comorbidities, such as obesity, the metabolic syndrome, diabetes, and dyslipidemia.[6] Defining criteria for the metabolic syndrome include any 3 of the following 5: laboratory and physical examination findings: increased waist circumference (men >40 in, women >35 inches), increased triglyceride levels of 150 or higher, reduced high-density lipoproteins (HDL) levels of less than 40 mg/dL in men or less than 50 mg/dL in women, increased blood pressure of greater than 130 mm Hg systolic or greater than 85 mm Hg diastolic, or increased fasting glucose levels of greater than 100 mg/dL.[7]

The prevalence in obesity in US adults has more than doubled since the 1960s, with the greatest increase occurring since 1980[8] with recent estimates suggesting an overall obesity prevalence of 33.8% and diabetes prevalence among middle-aged adults of 10.6%.[9] Concurrently, the prevalence of metabolic syndrome in US adults is estimated at 26.7% using National Health and Nutrition Examination Survey (NHANES) 1999–2000 data, an increase of 3.6% from NHANES III data (1998–1994).[10]

Although the incidence and prevalence of the NALFD and NASH is difficult to establish, autopsy studies have found evidence of hepatic steatosis in 36% of lean and 72% of obese subjects.[11] The prevalence of steatohepatitis in the same subgroup was 2.7% among lean subjects to 18.5% among markedly obese subjects. Today, it is estimated that 30% of the adult population in the United States has NAFLD,[12] with an increasing prevalence to 90% in morbidly obese populations presenting for bariatric surgery.[13] The prevalence of NASH is more difficult to determine, although a recently published prospective cohort study using ultrasound and liver biopsy determined the prevalence of NAFLD in asymptomatic middle-aged patients to be 46.0% and the prevalence of NASH to be 12.2%.[14]

Pediatric NAFLD

Childhood obesity continues to be a major focus of public health efforts in the United States and is globally recognized as a health epidemic. Population-based prevalence studies suggest that greater than 15% of children in North America, Great Britain, and western Europe are obese.[15] Similarly, a 2009 to 2010 US-based study showed the prevalence of obesity in children and adolescents was 16.9%.[16] The rise in obesity is paralleled by the rise in NAFLD, with NHANES-3 data reporting 6% of overweight adolescent and 10% of obese adolescents had abnormal ALT.[17]

Despite the prevalence of pediatric NAFLD, the condition is largely underdiagnosed. Because most children with NAFLD are asymptomatic, the diagnosis often depends on the detection of hepatomegaly on physical examination or elevated aminotransferases on screening. Autopsy studies in the United States have shown the prevalence of NAFLD to be 9.6% to 13.0% in children and adolescents, and approximately one-quarter of these cases presented with NASH.[18,19]

The risk factors for the metabolic syndrome appear to track from childhood into adulthood. A recently published retrospective longitudinal hospital-based cohort study demonstrated that the presence of NAFLD in children is associated with a significantly shorter long-term survival and a 13.8-fold higher risk of dying or requiring liver transplantation when compared with the age- and gender-matched general population.[20]

Diabetic NAFLD

Diabetic NAFLD is now recognized as a subgroup of patients with increased morbidity and mortality. The pathogenesis of both diabetes and NAFLD includes IR, and accordingly, there is a 60% to 76% prevalence of NAFLD and 22% prevalence of NASH in diabetic patients.[14,21] Patients with diabetic NAFLD have more severe inflammation and fibrosis on liver biopsy and a tendency toward more rapid fibrosis progression.[22,23] Diabetes is recognized to increase the risk of cirrhosis-related complications, as well as HCC.[24]

NAFLD and diabetes together has been shown to be associated with an increased risk of both liver-related death, as well as-all cause mortality.[25,26] Adams and colleagues[27] prospectively followed 116 diabetic subjects with NAFLD for 10.9 $\pm$ 5.2 years (range 0.1–25.0). Subjects were likely to be younger, female, and obese. The most common cause of death was malignancy (33%), liver-related complications (19%), and ischemic heart disease (19%). It is postulated that direct upregulation of fibrogenic growth factors by hyperinsulinemia and hyperglycemia, along with changes in adipo-cytokine levels that accompany diabetes, such as increased tumor necrosis factor alpha (TNF-α) and reduced adiponectin levels may play significant roles in contributing to liver damage and development of complications in patients with NAFLD who suffer from diabetes.[28,29]

Sex, age, and ethnicity

Sex, age, and ethnicity have each been identified as risk factors for NAFLD. Numerous studies have demonstrated that NAFLD and NASH are more common in men.[14,30] In women, the incidence of NAFLD increases with age, thought to be related to postmenopausal hormone changes.[31]

Hispanic individuals have been identified as the US ethnic group with the highest prevalence of NALFD and NASH. Browning and colleagues[32] reported an NAFLD prevalence of 31% using proton nuclear magnetic resonance spectroscopy (MRS) in a population with 43% obese and a mean age of 41 to 46 years. Hispanic individuals had the highest prevalence of hepatic steatosis (45%), followed by white (33%) and African American (24%) subjects. A recent cross-sectional study from Texas reported a similar NAFLD prevalence at 46%, with Hispanic individuals once again demonstrating the highest prevalence of NAFLD (58.3%) followed by white (44.4) and African American (35.1%) individuals.[14] Hispanic individuals also appear to have a higher prevalence of NASH compared with white[12] with recent study suggesting Hispanic patients with NASH are younger, less active, and have a diet higher in carbohydrates than their white counterparts.[33]

Outside the US, NAFLD has been expanding into populations previously viewed as low risk. Studies from China and Japan have demonstrated a NAFLD prevalence of 14% to 15% in accordance with their growing rates of overweight and obese.[34,35]

Clinical Presentation

Most patients with NAFLD are asymptomatic and have been referred for workup of elevated liver transaminases uncovered on routine testing. Abdominal obesity and hepatomegaly are the most common clinical findings. Fatigue, malaise, and vague right upper quadrant pain may also be endorsed, although these are not specific for NAFLD. Obstructive sleep apnea is a common diagnosis found in association with NAFLD and may contribute to reported symptoms of fatigue and malaise.[36–38] Signs of chronic liver disease are rarely present in the absence of cirrhosis.

The presence of abdominal or visceral adiposity has been strongly implicated in the development of the metabolic syndrome. The distribution of fat in other areas may also contribute to the metabolic risks associated with obesity. Increased dorsocervical lipohypertrophy was the anthropometric parameter that most correlated with the severity of inflammation, ballooning, Mallory hyaline, and fibrosis associated with severity of steatohepatitis.[39]

Laboratory Abnormalities

Aminotransferases

Levels of AST and ALT are typically modestly elevated, although the ratio of AST to ALT is typically less than 1, in contrast to alcohol-induced liver disease with a 2:1 AST-to-ALT ratio. A large retrospective study has shown the mean ALT and AST to be 83 IU/mL and 62 IU/mL, respectively.[40] Although the degree of elevation has been correlated with a higher likelihood of NASH, unfortunately serum aminotransferases are not reliably elevated in patients with NAFLD or NASH and should not be a stand-alone screening tool in clinically indicated patients.[14,41]

Elevated gamma-glutamyltransferase (GGT) has also been found in patients with NAFLD, and it has been reported to be associated with increased mortality.[42,43] Although increased GGT has been shown to be associated with advanced fibrosis in patients with NAFLD, the diagnosis of NAFLD cannot be made using only GGT. In a study of 50 patients with biopsy-proven NAFLD, increased GGT level was a risk factor for advanced fibrosis with 83% sensitivity and 69% specificity.[44] ALP has also been investigated with typically only mild elevation, but it is rarely the only liver function test abnormality.[45]

Hyperuricemia and NAFLD

NAFLD and serum uric acid (UA) levels have also been prospectively investigated.[46] UA, the final oxidation product of purine metabolism, has been found to be also associated with different cardiometabolic diseases, such as hypertension, kidney disease, metabolic syndrome, and cardiovascular disease.[47,48] UA has been shown to induce endothelial dysfunction, IR, oxidative stress, and systemic inflammation, all factors involved in NAFLD pathogenesis.[47,48] The largest study to date demonstrated that elevated UA was associated with a 1.29 hazard ratio of having NAFLD.[46] More intriguing is a possible association of elevated UA with advanced hepatic histology. In a cohort study of 166 subjects with NAFLD established by liver biopsy, 20% were found to have hyperuricemia with multivariate analysis correlating hyperuricemia with increased lobular inflammation and steatosis grade.[49] Further study is required, although an elevated UA in the absence of gout might favor early liver biopsy to assess for advanced disease.

Hyperferritinemia and NAFLD

Increased hepatic iron may also have a role in the development of NASH. Elevation in serum ferritin, an acute-phase protein as well as a marker of iron storage, has been shown in diabetes, IR, and NAFLD.[50,51] In NAFLD, increased ferritin levels are considered to be an expression of metabolic syndrome and of hepatic damage because of inflammatory cytokine activation.[52] IR is associated with increased hepatic iron levels.[53] Hyperferritinemia may also reflect increased hepatic iron deposition from chronic liver injury[54] and has been shown to correlate with the severity of fibrosis.[55] In a recent study of 628 subjects with biopsy-proven NAFLD, serum ferritin higher than 1.5 times the upper limit of normal was significantly associated with more severe histologic features, including steatosis, fibrosis, hepatocellular ballooning, and diagnosis of NASH. Elevated serum ferritin was also independently associated with higher NAFLD Activity Score (NAS).[56] In patients with radiographic evidence of NAFLD, serum ferritin may be useful in identifying those at risk for NASH and advanced fibrosis.

Vitamin D deficiency and NAFLD

Vitamin D deficiency has been notably associated with obesity and IR in recent years.[57] By corollary, NAFLD and vitamin D deficiency also appear related, with numerous studies demonstrating that patients with NAFLD have significantly lower vitamin D levels compared with matched controls.[58,59] This has been supported by animal model research demonstrating vitamin D deficiency is associated with gene expression that promotes increased hepatic inflammation and oxidative stress, leading to higher NAS in the setting of a Western high-fat/high–fructose corn syrup diet.[60]

Natural History

Patients with NAFLD with IFL on biopsy appear to have a benign prognosis and are at a low risk for the development of advanced disease, as reported by several cohort studies.[61,62] The diagnosis of NASH portends a worse clinical prognosis, with increased cardiovascular and liver-related mortality, as well as increased rates of malignancy.[63,64] In a 28-year follow-up study of patients with NAFLD in comparison to the general Swedish population, patients with NASH had an 85% increased mortality risk, with most deaths caused by cardiovascular disease, followed by extra-hepatic malignancies, and then liver-related death.

NASH with fibrosis has been shown to carry a worse prognosis than NASH without fibrosis. Fibrosis progression is associated with diabetes mellitus, severe IR, BMI, weight gain of more than 5 kg, and rising ALT and AST.[22] Progression to NASH cirrhosis has been reported at a rate of 11% over a 15-year period.[65] The progression to end-stage liver disease or HCC once advanced fibrosis or cirrhosis is present is variable. The largest study to date compared 247 patients with biopsy-confirmed NASH and cirrhosis with 264 patients with chronic hepatitis C (CHC) and cirrhosis, and followed them for a mean of 7.1 years. In comparison with patients with cirrhosis secondary to hepatitis C, patients with NASH and cirrhosis had similar rates of liver-related complications (19.4% vs 17.8%), although when accounting for confounders, such as age, sex, BMI, and diabetes, patients with CHC and cirrhosis had significantly more related liver complications, although a similar overall mortality.[66] Overall mortality was similar between the 2 groups, with 9.4% (CHC group) versus 13.4% (NAFLD group) of patients either requiring liver transplant or dying.

Diagnosis

The diagnosis of NAFLD is supported by either hepatic steatosis on imaging studies or liver biopsy, together with the exclusion of individuals who regularly consume more than 20 g ethanol per day. Computed tomography (CT), magnetic resonance (MR), and ultrasound (US) can all identify hepatic steatosis with reasonable accuracy, although the utility of US is limited in morbidly obese patients.[67] These imaging modalities are quite good in identifying patients with higher than 30% steatosis, but do not provide information on necroinflammatory activity or hepatic fibrosis.

Histology

Percutaneous liver biopsy remains the gold standard for diagnosis of NAFLD and has the additional benefit of distinguishing between NASH and simple steatosis. Liver biopsy also assesses the degree of fibrosis, providing prognostic implication and may influence the clinical management of NAFLD.[68] Liver tissue can be used to exclude other liver diseases, such as drug-induced hepatotoxicity, Wilson disease, and autoimmune hepatitis.[69] The prognosis of NAFLD is variable and depends greatly on the severity of the presenting disease on the initial liver biopsy. In a prospective repeat liver biopsy study, 31.8% of patients with NASH had worsening fibrosis occurring at a median of 4.3 years.[70]

Brunt criteria are the most commonly used to make the diagnosis of NASH. The histologic grade indicates the activity of the steatohepatitic lesions, whereas the stage reflects the degree of fibrosis. NASH is defined by a histologic pattern of hepatic injury characterized by macrovesicular steatosis, lobular inflammation, hepatocellular ballooning, and often perivenular (zone 3) fibrosis. Mallory-Denk bodies may or may not be present.[2] Microvesicular steatosis is seen in 10% of liver biopsies obtained from patients with NAFLD and has been shown to correlate with a more advanced histologic feature of NAFLD: higher grade of steatosis, ballooning cell injury, and more fibrosis.[71] It is worth mentioning that the NAS is used for the histologic assessment of NAFLD to distinguish steatosis from NASH in clinical trials.[72] NAS provides a composite score based on the degree of steatosis, lobular inflammation, and hepatocyte ballooning. The NAS does not include fibrosis and is reported separately.[73]

Liver biopsy has several disadvantages, including poor patient acceptance and potential complications, including excessive bleeding and, rarely, death. Aside from the inherently invasive nature of the procedure, other limitations of this technique include intraobserver variation and sampling variability, with features such as fibrosis often not uniformly distributed within the liver.[74,75] These risks and limitations are further increased with repeated liver biopsies, which are performed for restaging after therapeutic treatment plans have been used and to monitor progression of disease throughout a patient's lifetime. The frequency of patient refusal to undergo biopsy may exceed 50% in some centers and the frequency of physician reluctance may be as high as 30%.[76] Noninvasive testing would be of great benefit, particularly to identify NASH at an early stage with or without advanced fibrosis. Diagnostic modalities investigated to date include radiographic tests or panels that combine laboratory and clinical data.

Radiographic modalities

Many imaging modalities have been used to quantify hepatic steatosis and fibrosis. See **Table 1** for summary of the various modalities. US is the most common method for screening asymptomatic patients with suspected NAFLD. US findings include hepatomegaly, diffuse increases in the echogenicity of the liver parenchyma, and vascular blunting. Although easily performed and economical, US is operator dependent and subject to intraobserver and interobserver variability.[77] The sensitivity of US to detect steatosis decreases with a degree of fat infiltration less than 30%,[78] as well as in obese patients.[79]

Whereas standard US has been unable to assess for hepatic fibrosis, newer US-based transient elastography (TE) has become available throughout Europe, Asia,

Table 1
Radiologic studies available for the diagnosis of NAFLD

Modality	Strengths	Weaknesses
Ultrasound	• Noninvasive • Inexpensive, readily available • Good at detecting steatosis	• Operator dependent • Unable to detect fibrosis or necroinflammation
Transient elastography	• Noninvasive • Assesses fibrosis	• Operator dependent • Expense • Limited accuracy BMI >30 • Not FDA approved
CT scan	• Readily available • Good at detecting steatosis	• Unable to detect necroinflammation or mild-moderate fibrosis • Radiation exposure
MRI	• Readily available • No radiation	• Expense • Unable to detect fibrosis
MR spectroscopy	• No radiation • Sensitive steatosis measurements	• Expense • Unable to detect fibrosis • Not readily available
MR elastography	• No radiation • Sensitive fibrosis measurements	• Not readily available • Expensive • Prospective validation in NAFLD populations required

Abbreviations: BMI, body mass index; CT, computed tomography; FDA, Food and Drug Administration; MRI, magnetic resonance imaging; NAFLD, nonalcoholic fatty liver disease.

and Canada with the ability to measure liver stiffness. With progressive fibrosis, the liver begins to lose its intrinsic gross elasticity namely because of the advanced scarring. TE (FibroScan, Echosens; Paris, France) measures the velocity of a low-amplitude sheer wave that is propagated through the liver parenchyma to determine the degree of liver stiffness that is equated to hepatic fibrosis. This technology has shown benefit in numerous Asian and European studies, although the benefit is dramatically decreased in obese populations in which TE failed to provide a measurements in 20% of cases, most notably in female obese patients.[80–83] Recently, a special "XL" probe was developed to use in obese patients that has shown better accuracy, although still with significant limitations, particularly in those with a BMI greater than 30.[84] In summary, TE is a promising new technology with the benefits of good patient acceptance and ease of administration, although the drawbacks of machine expense and limited utility in obese patients must be addressed before widespread application.

MR imaging (MRI) uses the differential chemical shifts between fat and water to detect steatosis at levels down to 3%.[85] MR spectroscopy (MRS) can decompose the liver signal into its fat and water signal components and therefore assess liver fat more directly than CT or US. MRS was applied to the large Dallas Heart Study population of 2349 and showed good internal validation for detection of hepatic triglyceride.[86]

Another new MRI technology is that of MR elastography (MRE), which, similar to TE, quantitatively and noninvasively assesses liver stiffness. Multiple studies have shown that MRE accurately assesses hepatic fibrosis caused by a variety of liver diseases.[87–91] In a retrospective study involving 58 patients with NAFLD, liver stiffness had high accuracy for discriminating patients with NASH from those with simple steatosis, with a sensitivity of 94% and specificity of 73%.[92] Although application of this technology is currently limited by availability, prospective study validating these results may increase the utility of MRE.

CT is another cross-sectional imaging modality that has been able to detect hepatic steatosis with reasonable accuracy.[93] Noncontrast CT scanning is more useful for detecting steatosis than contrast-enhanced scans; however, the application of CT scan to the general population is limited given the radiation exposure with each examination.[94,95] In addition, CT scan is unable to accurately gauge fibrosis, except in cases of cirrhosis with additional findings suggestive of portal hypertension, such as collateral formation (varices) or splenomegaly.

Biomarkers

Accurate laboratory tests or a panel of tests that would identify those at high risk for NASH and fibrosis to allow for more discreet selection of biopsy candidates would be valuable. Serum aminotransferases do not correlate with advanced disease but have been used as part of clinical scoring systems.[96] Biomarkers studied to date include collagen or extracellular matrix enzymes, cytokines, such as TNF-α, proteomic markers, and most recently genetic markers shown to be associated with NASH.[97] See **Table 2** for a summary of these tests.

Clinical scoring systems

Several clinical scoring systems based on readily available clinical and laboratory indices have been developed to identify advanced fibrosis in patients with NAFLD. The AST-to-platelet ratio index (APRI) is a promising tool with limited expense and widespread availability. APRI has been studied in CHC and NAFLD cohorts and has been shown to reliably predict advanced fibrosis.[98]

The BMI, AST/ALT ratio, Diabetes (BARD) score is another clinical scoring system that is easy to use during an office visit and requires little additional testing. The

Table 2
Clinical and biomarker scoring systems for the diagnosis of advanced fibrosis in NAFLD

Test	Strengths	Weaknesses
AST: platelet (APRI)	• Easy to obtain • Inexpensive • Accurately predicts advanced fibrosis	• Less accurate with little to moderate fibrosis
BARD score: BMI, AST/ALT, diabetes	• Easy to obtain • Inexpensive	• Best used as negative predictor for advanced fibrosis
NAFLD fibrosis score: age, hyperglycemia, BMI, platelets, albumin, AST/ALT ratio	• Easy to obtain • Inexpensive • Accurately predicts advanced fibrosis • Most validated	• Requires mathematical calculation • Less accurate with little to moderate fibrosis
Enhanced Liver Fibrosis Panel : hyaluronic acid, tissue inhibitor of metalloproteinase 1, aminoterminal peptide of procollagen III	• Commercially available • Accurately predicts advanced fibrosis	• Expensive • Less accurate with little to moderate fibrosis • Lacks adequate validation in NAFLD populations
FibroTest-FibroSURE (Biopredictive): α2-macroglobulin, apolipoprotein A1, haptoglobin, total bilirubin, γ-glutamyltransferase levels	• Commercially available • Accurately predicts advanced fibrosis	• Expensive • Less accurate with little to moderate fibrosis • Lacks adequate validation in NAFLD populations
FibroSpect II: hyaluronic acid, tissue inhibitor of metalloproteinase-1, α2-macroglobulin	• Commercially available • Accurately predicts advanced fibrosis	• Expensive • Less accurate with little to moderate fibrosis • Lacks adequate validation in NAFLD populations
Cytokeratin-18	• Accurately predicts moderate and advanced fibrosis • Good predictor of NASH • May parallel changes in histology over time (early study)	• Not commercially available

Abbreviations: ALT, alanine aminotransferase; AST, aspartate aminotransferase; BMI, body mass index; NAFLD, nonalcoholic fatty liver disease; NASH, nonalcoholic steatohepatitis.

BARD score reliably predicts significant fibrosis by combining BMI of 28 kg/m^2 or higher (1 point), AST/ALT ratio of 0.8 or higher (1 point), and diabetes (2 points). A score of 2 to 4 was associated with an odds ratio for advanced fibrosis of 17 (confidence interval 9.2–31.9) and a negative predictive value of 96%.[40]

Similarly, the NAFLD fibrosis score uses routinely measured data, including age, hyperglycemia, BMI, platelet count, albumin, and AST/ALT ratio. Although this score requires more complex mathematical calculation, an online calculator has become readily available. The NAFLD fibrosis score shows good positive predictive value between 82% and 90% in identifying the presence of advanced fibrosis and similar negative predictive value to the BARD score.[99,100]

Biomarker panels

To augment a clinical approach to noninvasive testing of patients with NAFLD, there are several commercially available testing panels that highlight cellular matrix turnover as a marker of fibrosis. These tests are relatively expensive and are limited by the inability to identify mild to moderate disease. The Enhanced Liver Fibrosis Panel (ELF) is a panel of automated immunoassays to detect 3 markers: hyaluronic acid, tissue inhibitor of metalloproteinase 1, and aminoterminal peptide of procollagen III (P3NP). The ELF panel had an area under the curve of 0.90 for distinguishing severe fibrosis, 0.82 for moderate fibrosis, and 0.76 for no fibrosis.[101]

The FibroTest-FibroSURE (Biopredictive, Paris, France) is based on α2-macroglobulin, apolipoprotein A1, haptoglobin, total bilirubin, and γ-glutamyltransferase levels.[102] In a cohort of 170 patients with NAFLD, the FibroTest-FibroSURE was noted to have a 90% negative predictive value and 70% positive predictive value for advanced fibrosis with a receiver operating curve of 0.92 (F3-F4). Accuracy was diminished in settings of more modest fibrosis (F1-F2).

FibroSpect II (Prometheus, San Diego, CA, USA), a biochemical index using 3 biomarkers (hyaluronic acid, tissue inhibitor of metalloproteinase-1, and α2-macroglobulin) has been extensively investigated in CHC. In a cohort of 696 patients with CHC, FibroSPECT II was shown to have an 80.6% sensitivity and 71.4% specificity in predicting advanced fibrosis.[103] In a smaller cohort of 129 morbidly obese patients with awaiting Roux-en-Y gastric bypass, FibroSPECT II had a negative predictive value of 100%, positive predictive value of 15%, sensitivity of 100%, and specificity of 42% to predict stage 2 fibrosis or higher.[104] FibroSPECT II requires further validation in larger cohorts of patients with biopsy-proven NAFLD.

Although these commercially available tests provide additional information in terms of likelihood of advanced fibrosis, they do not appear markedly better than the clinical staging systems, such as the NAFLD fibrosis score. Other biomarkers, such as cytokeratin-18 (CK-18), have shown early promise in pilot trials, although is not commercially available.[105] A recent study with CK-18 suggests that change in this biomarker over time parallels change in hepatic histology.[106] Prospective large-scale trials are required to validate this exciting potential application of CK-18.

CLINICAL CASE, CONTINUED

Our female Hispanic patient underwent a full serologic workup that was negative for other causes of chronic liver disease. Her laboratories were notable for a hemoglobin A1C of 7.6. Right upper quadrant US showed hepatic steatosis and mild hepatomegaly but was otherwise unremarkable. Her BARD and NAFLD fibrosis score were calculated on her follow-up visit and predicted advanced disease. At this time, she elected to proceed with a liver biopsy. Biopsy demonstrated grade 2, stage 3 NASH. She returns now to the clinic to discuss treatment options.

Management

Lifestyle modification

Obesity and IR are closely associated with NAFLD, and therefore targeted weight loss and increased physical activity should be the first line of treatment. Lifestyle modification has been shown to improve IR and serum aminotransferases, as well as reduce hepatic steatosis, necroinflammation, and fibrosis.[107–109] In a study of 23 patients with NASH, a 1-year dietary program aimed at reducing IR and promoting weight loss resulted in improved histology in 60% of patients who successfully completed the program.[110] Weight loss should not exceed more than 1 kg per week, because rapid weight loss can exacerbate steatosis with 5% to 10% total body weight loss over a 6-month period recommended.[111–113] Patients who are able to lose between 5% and 10% of their baseline body weight improve not only insulin resistance and serum aminotransferases, but also hepatic histopathologic changes.[114]

The optimal weight loss program has not been established, and further investigation regarding the clinical and histologic efficacy of the various popular diets on NASH is required. These diet programs include Weight Watchers, carbohydrate restriction without fat restriction (Atkins diet), macronutrient and glycemic load modification (Zone diet), and fat restriction (Ornish diet). In obese patients with BMI greater than 35 kg/m^2, no significant difference in weight loss was seen with any of the dietary approaches. When comparing these diets head-to-head, weight loss correlated with a reduction in cardiovascular risk factors regardless of the dietary composition.[115] At this point, counseling on a specific dietary program is less important than tailoring a diet to a patient's lifestyle to achieve in maintaining long-term weight loss.

Adjunct weight loss pharmacotherapy

Despite a substantial need, the options for efficacious and safe weight-loss medications are currently quite limited. In fact, orlistat, a reversible inhibitor of gastric and pancreatic lipase that blocks the absorption of 30% of dietary triglycerides, is the only long-term weight loss medication available approved by the Food and Drug Administration (FDA) that has been studied in populations with NAFLD. Orlistat in combination with diet has shown efficacy in increased weight loss in obese adults after 1 year of therapy.[116] In a study of 50 overweight patients with biopsy-proven NASH, Harrison and colleagues[116] randomized patients to orlistat/diet/vitamin E or diet/vitamin E. Orlistat did not enhance weight loss or improve liver enzymes, measures of insulin resistance, and histopathology; however, patients who lost 5% or more of body weight over 9 months improved insulin resistance and steatosis, and those subjects who lost 5% or more or body weight also achieved hepatic histologic changes. This study emphasizes that weight loss, however achieved, is the underlying impetus for improvements in serum aminotransferases and IR, as well as hepatic steatosis, ballooning, and lobular inflammation.

Surgical therapy for weight loss

Surgical therapies for weight loss are viable alternative in select patient populations. Newer surgical techniques, such as the adjustable gastric banding and Roux-en-Y gastric bypass, are overall better tolerated and have shown to improve metabolic syndrome, IR, and hepatic histology. Independent of the type of bariatric surgery, most studies show a decrease in ALT and GGT levels after 10 to 41 months of follow-up.[117–119] More clinically relevant is the improvement in the metabolic risk factor profile along with a decrease in grade of steatosis, inflammation, and stage of fibrosis after bariatric surgery.[120–122] Given the potential complications and expense of bariatric surgery, the decision for referral should be limited to morbidly obese patients with other medical conditions that warrant the risks of surgical intervention.

Other NAFLD pharmacotherapy

Several medications have been used in an attempt to treat NASH with the largest amount of data involving the thiazolidinediones (TZDs), such as pioglitazone and antioxidants, specifically vitamin E. Other diabetic medications, cytoprotective agents, and antifibrotic medications have also been studied.

Antioxidants

The depletion of antioxidants within hepatocytes, resulting in impaired reactive oxygen species inactivation is the basis for antioxidant supplementation as a potential treatment for NASH. In a study of 247 patients with NASH without diabetes, subjects were randomized to pioglitazone at a dosage of 30 mg/d, vitamin E at a dosage of 800 IU/d, or placebo. Only vitamin E therapy showed significantly higher rates of reductions in hepatic steatosis and lobular inflammation.[123] Both agents were associated with reductions in hepatic steatosis, but not with improvement in fibrosis scores after 96 weeks of treatment. Other smaller trials have shown modest fibrosis improvement when used in combination with vitamin C.[124] Unfortunately, vitamin E does not appear beneficial in pediatric patient populations where a randomized controlled trial (RCT) found vitamin E to be no better than placebo in the treatment of NASH.[125]

The combination of vitamin E and ursodeoxycholic acid (UDCA), a cytoprotective agent, in patients with NASH has also been investigated and shown improvement of aminotransaminases. In a study group of 101 patients all given vitamin E and UDCA, 10 underwent repeat liver biopsy during follow-up, with 7 patients showing improvement in NAS score and 1 patient showing worsening NAS.[126] Clearly, further study in a prospective randomized placebo-controlled trial is required, particularly because vitamin E has been associated with increased risk for hemorrhagic stroke and all-cause mortality when used in higher doses than recommended for NAFLD.[127]

Another antioxidant that has been studied on a smaller scale in populations with NAFLD is betaine. In animal models, betaine has been shown to decrease hepatic steatosis, which was confirmed in the only RCT that exists.[128,129] Unfortunately, other parameters of hepatic histology were unchanged. Additional data are required before betaine can be recommended for the treatment of NASH.

Cytoprotective agents

UDCA as a cytoprotective agent has been studied independently of vitamin E in the treatment of NASH. Unfortunately, an early large RCT comparing UDCA with placebo showed a similar improvement in both groups.[130] This study was notable for an unexpectedly high improvement rate in the placebo group and has considerably tempered enthusiasm for UDCA in NASH. A recent RCT of 126 patients with biopsy-proven NASH given high-dose UDCA or placebo for 12 months showed notable improvement in serum aminotransferases, metabolic parameters, and FibroTest serum fibrosis markers with ursodiol treatment.[131] Future study with UDCA with histologic endpoints is required to determine UDCA's true utility in NASH.

Pentoxifylline (PTX) is another cytoprotective agent that has been shown to improve steatosis in NASH.[132] In the largest placebo-controlled trial using PTX to date (n = 55), Zein and colleagues[133] reported a 50% decrease of 2 or more points in NAS score in the PTX cohort versus 15.4% on placebo ($P = .01$). PTX also showed a trend toward improvement in fibrosis over placebo (35% vs 15%). PTX was well tolerated, although larger studies are necessary before this can be recommended as first-line therapy.

Diabetic medications

TZDs are potent insulin sensitizers that act as peroxisome proliferator-activated receptor-γ agonists to improve insulin resistance in skeletal muscle, adipose tissue, and the liver. The 2 major drugs of this class, pioglitazone and rosiglitazone, have generally been effective in improving NASH histology.[123,134–136] The major drawback of TZD therapy is weight gain on the order of 2 to 3 kg per year of treatment. Other side effects include exacerbation of congestive heart failure and increased risk of osteopenia and fractures.[137] The benefits of therapy appear to reverse after stopping treatment.[138] Recent evidence linking rosiglitazone to increased rates of myocardial infarction and heart failure have essentially removed this agent as a treatment choice, but pioglitazone remains available and can be considered as a potential treatment for patients with NASH, particularly those with diabetes.[139,140]

Metformin is a diabetic medication that improves insulin sensitivity and promotes weight loss. Unfortunately, recent RCTs have not shown histologic benefit of metformin therapy in either adult or pediatric populations with NASH.[141,142] Low-dose metformin in combination with rosiglitazone in a study comparing the efficacy of rosiglitazone alone versus rosiglitazone and metformin or rosiglitazone and losartan failed to produce any additional histologic benefit above monotherapy and did not significantly ameliorate the weight gain side effect of TZD therapy.[143] Metformin use is limited in patients with NASH to those with diabetes with the understanding that it does not provide significant hepatic histologic benefit, although it may improve metabolic profiles.

A new and promising class of medications currently approved for the treatment of diabetes are incretin mimetics including exenatide. Incretin mimetics promote insulin secretion, suppress inappropriate glucagon secretion, and slow gastric emptying, leading to metabolic improvements and modest weight loss. Both animal models and pilot study in humans have shown promising results, although large-scale study is required.[144–146]

Other agents

The use of angiotensin-receptor blockers (ARBs) has shown promise in the treatment of NASH. ARBs have shown to inhibit stellate cell activity in obese mice, leading to decreased hepatic fibrosis,[147] and in recent human studies with telmisartan, improve insulin sensitivity.[148] ARBs should be considered in patients with NASH with hypertension and not as first-line therapy for NASH.

Statins[149–151] and ezetimibe,[152,153] lipid-lowering agents, have shown some early promise in the treatment of NASH in animal models and small pilot studies but have yet to be proven as first-line therapies. Nevertheless, these agents can safely be used in patients with NAFLD to improve their metabolic profile.

Omega 3 fatty acid supplementation

Observational studies in patients with NAFLD suggest that omega 3 fatty acid consumption is diminished[154] and studies in murine models suggest that omega 3 fatty acid depletion is associated with hepatic steatosis mediated via upregulation of sterol regulatory binding protein-1c.[155] Histopathologic studies assessing the benefits of omega 3 fatty acid supplementation in humans with NAFLD are lacking, but a recent meta-analysis suggests improvement in hepatic steatosis without concomitant weight loss.[156] Cardiovascular benefits also exist for omega 3 fatty acid supplementation,[157] and given that this is the number one cause for mortality in this patient population, consideration should be given to its use while prospective, randomized clinical trials evaluating a possible histopathologic benefit on NASH are anxiously awaited.

Coffee consumption

The beneficial effects of coffee consumption in patients with chronic liver disease is becoming more evident. First described 20 years ago, coffee consumption was linked to decreased risk of alcoholic liver disease.[158] More recently, data suggest a fibrosis benefit in patients with chronic hepatitis C who consume 2 to 3 cups of coffee daily.[159,160] These data have recently been extended to patients with NASH, where an inverse association was found between regular coffee caffeine consumption and fibrosis.[161]

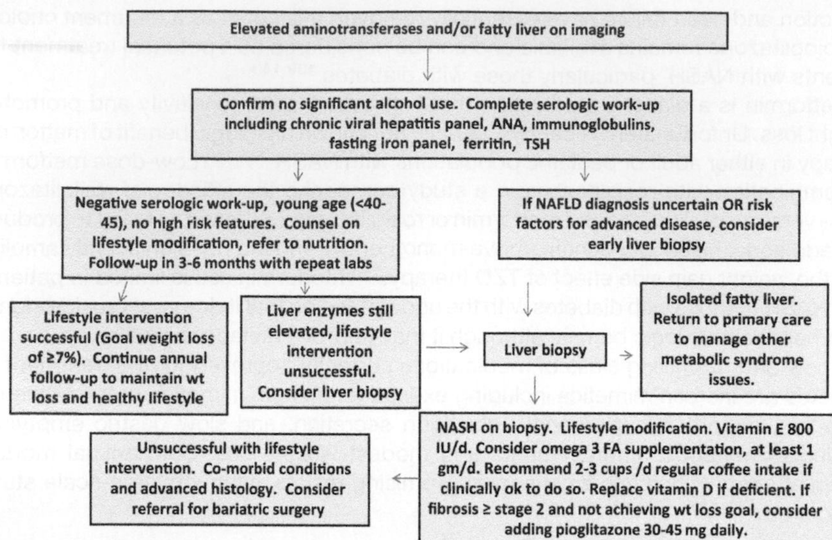

Fig. 1. NAFLD diagnosis and treatment algorithm.

CLINICAL CASE, CONTINUED

We referred our patient to a nutritionist for dietary counseling and recommended increasing physical activity with the goal of burning 400 kCal/ 5 times per week. She was started on vitamin E 800 IU/day. With regard to her poorly controlled diabetes, she was started on actos 15 mg, which was increased to 30 mg after 1 month. She was also noted to have vitamin D deficiency and was replaced with 12 weeks of 50,000 IU weekly and then placed on a daily maintenance regimen of 2000 IU. Her lipid panel was notable for an LDL of 164 mg/dL and she was started on atorvastatin. Furthermore, it was recommend that she take omega 3 fatty acid supplementation at a dosage of 1 g daily. Given that she had no significant health issues related to caffeine ingestion, it was also recommended that she start drinking 2 to 3 cups of regular coffee daily. She will continue to be followed every 3 to 6 months.

SUMMARY

As the hepatic manifestation of the metabolic syndrome, NAFLD has become the most common cause of asymptomatic liver enzyme elevations in Western nations. Although it is easy to diagnose NAFLD, a liver biopsy is currently required to diagnosis NASH. Patients with NASH are those at greatest risk of progression to cirrhosis and, thus, treatment efforts are targeted at these individuals. Although currently there are no FDA-approved treatments for NASH, a multidisciplinary approach that addresses comorbid conditions and promotes modest weight loss comprises the backbone of therapy (**Fig. 1**).

REFERENCES

1. Neuschwander-Tetri BA, Caldwell SH. Nonalcoholic steatohepatitis: summary of an AASLD Single Topic Conference. Hepatology 2003;37:1202–19.

2. Brunt EM, Janney CG, Di Bisceglie AM, et al. Nonalcoholic steatohepatitis: a proposal for grading and staging the histological lesions. Am J Gastroenterol 1999;94:2467–74.
3. Cohen JC, Horton JD, Hobbs HH. Human fatty liver disease: old questions and new insights. Science 2011;332:1519–23.
4. Syn WK, Jung Y, Omenetti A, et al. Hedgehog-mediated epithelial-to-mesenchymal transition and fibrogenic repair in nonalcoholic fatty liver disease. Gastroenterology 2009;137:1478–88.
5. Romeo S, Kozlintina J, Xing C, et al. Genetic variation in PNPLA3 confers susceptibility to nonalcoholic fatty liver disease. Nat Genet 2008;40:1461–5.
6. Clark JM, Brancati FL, Diehl AM. The prevalence and etiology of elevated aminotransferase levels in the United States. Am J Gastroenterol 2003;98:960–7.
7. Grundy SM, Cleeman JL, Daniels SR, et al. Diagnosis and management of the metabolic syndrome. Circulation 2005;112:2735–52.
8. Klein S, Wadden T, Sugerman HJ. AGA technical review on obesity. Gastroenterology 2002;123:882–932.
9. Flegal KM, Carroll MD, Ogden CL, et al. Prevalence and trends in obesity among US adults, 1999–2008. JAMA 2010;303:235–41.
10. Ogden CL, Carroll MD, Curtin LR, et al. Prevalence of overweight and obesity in the United States, 1999–2004. JAMA 2006;295:1549–55.
11. Wanless IR, Lentz JS. Fatty liver hepatitis (steatohepatitis) and obesity: an autopsy study with analysis of risk factors. Hepatology 1990;12:1106–10.
12. Lazo M, Clark JM. The epidemiology of nonalcoholic fatty liver disease: a global perspective. Semin Liver Dis 2008;28:339–50.
13. Machado M, Marques-Vidal P, Cortez-Pinto H. Hepatic histology in obese patients undergoing bariatric surgery. J Hepatol 2006;45:600–6.
14. Williams CD, Stengel J, Asike MI, et al. Prevalence of nonalcoholic fatty liver disease and nonalcoholic steatohepatitis among a largely middle-aged population utilizing ultrasound and liver biopsy: a prospective study. Gastroenterology 2011;140:124–31.
15. Janssen I, Katzmarzyk PT, Boyce WF, et al. Comparison of overweight and obesity prevalence in school-aged youth from 34 countries and their relationships with physical activity and dietary patterns. Obes Rev 2005;6:123–32.
16. Ogden CL, Carrol MD, Curtin LR, et al. Prevalence of high body mass index in US children and adolescents, 2007–2008. JAMA 2010;303:242–9.
17. Strauss RS, Barlow SE, Dietz WH. Prevalence of abnormal serum aminotransferase values in overweight and obese adolescents. J Pediatr 2000;136:727–33.
18. Schwimmer JB, Deutsch R, Kahen T, et al. Prevalence of fatty liver in children and adolescents. Pediatrics 2006;118:1388–93.
19. Riley MR, Bass NM, Rosenthal P, et al. Under diagnosis of pediatric obesity and under screening for fatty liver disease and metabolic syndrome by pediatricians and pediatric subspecialists. J Pediatr 2005;147:839–42.
20. Feldstein AE, Charatcharoenwitthaya P, Treeprasertsuk S, et al. The natural history of non-alcoholic fatty liver disease in children: a follow-up study for up to 20 years. Gut 2009;58:1538–44.
21. Targher G, Bertolini L, Padovani R, et al. Prevalence of nonalcoholic fatty liver disease and its association with cardiovascular disease in type 2 diabetic patients. Diabetes Care 2007;30:1212–8.
22. Adams LA, Sanderson S, Lindor KD, et al. The histological course of nonalcoholic fatty liver disease: a longitudinal study of 103 patients with sequential liver biopsies. J Hepatol 2005;42:132–8.

23. Angulo P, Keach JC, Batts KP, et al. Independent predictors of liver fibrosis in patients with nonalcoholic steatohepatitis. Hepatology 1999;30:1356–62.
24. Tolman KG, Fonseca V, Tan MH, et al. Narrative review: hepatobiliary disease in type 2 diabetes mellitus. Ann Intern Med 2004;141:946–56.
25. Younossi ZM, Gramlich T, Matteoni CA, et al. Nonalcoholic fatty liver disease in patients with type 2 diabetes. Clin Gastroenterol Hepatol 2004;2:262–5.
26. Adams LA, Lymp JF, St Sauver J, et al. The natural history of nonalcoholic fatty liver disease: a population-based cohort study. Gastroenterology 2005;129: 113–21.
27. Adams LA, Harmsen S, St Sauver JL, et al. Nonalcoholic fatty liver disease increases risk of death among patients with diabetes: a community-based cohort study. Am J Gastroenterol 2010;105:1567–73.
28. Paradis V, Perlemuter G, Bonvoust F, et al. High glucose and hyperinsulinemia stimulate connective tissue growth factor expression: a potential mechanism involved in progression to fibrosis in nonalcoholic steatohepatitis. Hepatology 2001;34:738–44.
29. Hui JM, Hodge A, Farrell GC, et al. Beyond insulin resistance in NASH: TNF-alpha or adiponectin? Hepatology 2004;40:46–54.
30. Caballeria L, Pera G, Auladell MA, et al. Prevalence and factors associated with the presence of nonalcoholic fatty liver disease in an adult population in Spain. Eur J Gastroenterol Hepatol 2010;21:24–32.
31. Ruhl CE, Everhart JE. Epidemiology of nonalcoholic fatty liver. Clin Liver Dis 2004;8:501–19.
32. Browning JD, Szczepaniak LS, Dobbins R, et al. Prevalence of hepatic steatosis in an urban population in the United States: impact of ethnicity. Hepatology 2004;40:1387–95.
33. Bambha K, Belt P, Abraham M, et al. Ethnicity and nonalcoholic fatty liver disease. Hepatology 2012;55(3):769–80.
34. Fan JG, Farrell GC. Epidemiology of non-alcoholic fatty liver disease in China. J Hepatol 2009;50:204–10.
35. Zhang H, He SM, Sun J, et al. Prevalence and etiology of abnormal liver function tests in adult population in Jilin, China. Int J Med Sci 2011;8(3):254–62.
36. Minoguchi K, Yokoe T, Tanaka A, et al. Association between lipid peroxidation and inflammation in obstructive sleep apnoea. Eur Respir J 2006;28:378–85.
37. Botros N, Concato J, Mohsenin V, et al. Obstructive sleep apnea as a risk factor for type 2 diabetes. Am J Med 2009;122:1122–7.
38. Chin K, Nakamura T, Takahashi K, et al. Effects of obstructive sleep apnea syndrome on serum aminotransferase levels in obese patients. Am J Med 2003;114:370–6.
39. Cheung O, Kapoor A, Puri P, et al. The impact of fat distribution on the severity of nonalcoholic fatty liver disease and metabolic syndrome. Hepatology 2007;46: 1091–100.
40. Harrison SA, Oliver D, Arnold HL, et al. Development and validation of a simple NAFLD clinical scoring system for identifying patients without advanced disease. Gut 2008;57:1414–7, 1441–47.
41. Fracanzani AL, Valenti L, Bugianesi E, et al. Risk of severe liver disease in nonalcoholic fatty liver disease with normal aminotransferase levels: a role for insulin resistance and diabetes. Hepatology 2008;48:792–8.
42. Haring R, Wallaschofski H, Nauck H, et al. Ultrasonographic hepatic steatosis increases prediction of mortality risk from elevated serum gamma-glutamyl transpeptidase levels. Hepatology 2009;50:1403–11.

43. Ruhl CE, Everhart JE. Elevated serum alanine aminotransferase and gamma glutamyltransferase and mortality in the United States population. Gastroenterology 2009;136:477–85.
44. Tahan V, Canbakan B, Balci H, et al. Serum gammaglutamyltranspeptidase distinguishes non-alcoholic fatty liver disease at high risk. Hepatogastroenterology 2008;55:1433–8.
45. Pantsari MW, Harrison SA. Nonalcoholic fatty liver disease presenting with an isolated elevated alkaline phosphatase. J Clin Gastroenterol 2006;40:633–5.
46. Li Y, Xu C, Yu C, et al. Association of serum uric acid level with non-alcoholic fatty liver disease: a cross-sectional study. J Hepatol 2009;50:1029–34.
47. Edwards NL. The role of hyperuricemia in vascular disorders. Curr Opin Rheumatol 2009;21:132–7.
48. Feig DI, Kang DH, Johnson RJ. Uric acid and cardiovascular risk. N Engl J Med 2008;359:1811–21.
49. Petta S, Camma C, Cabibi D, et al. Hyperuricemia is associated with histological liver damage in patients with non-alcoholic fatty liver disease. Aliment Pharmacol Ther 2011;34:757–66.
50. Ford ES, Cogswell ME. Diabetes and serum ferritin concentration among U.S. adults. Diabetes Care 1999;22:1978–83.
51. Manousou P, Kalambokis G, Grillo F, et al. Serum ferritin is a discriminant marker for both fibrosis and inflammation in histologically proven non-alcoholic fatty liver disease patients. Liver Int 2011;31:730–9.
52. Jehn M, Clark JM, Guallar E. Serum ferritin and risk of the metabolic syndrome in U.S. adults. Diabetes Care 2004;27:2422–8.
53. Mendler MH, Turlin B, Moirand R, et al. Insulin resistance associated hepatic iron overload. Gastroenterology 1999;117:1155–63.
54. Ferrara F, Ventura P, Vegetti A, et al. Serum ferritin as a predictor of treatment outcome in patients with chronic hepatitis C. Am J Gastroenterol 2009;104: 605–16.
55. George DK, Goldwurm S, MacDonald GA, et al. Increased hepatic iron concentration in nonalcoholic steatohepatitis is associated with increased fibrosis. Gastroenterology 1998;114:311–8.
56. Kowdley KV, Belt P, Wilson LA, et al. Serum ferritin is an independent predictor of histologic severity and advanced fibrosis in patients with nonalcoholic fatty liver disease. Hepatology 2012;55:77–85.
57. Holick MF. Vitamin D deficiency. N Engl J Med 2007;257:266–81.
58. Barchetta I, Angelico F, Del Ben M, et al. Strong association between nonalcoholic fatty liver disease (NAFLD) and low 25(OH)vitamin D levels in an adult population with normal liver enzymes. BMC Med 2011;9:85.
59. Nseir W, Taha H, Khateeb J. Fatty liver is associated with recurrent bacterial infections independent of metabolic syndrome. Dig Dis Sci 2011;56(11):3328–34.
60. Roth CL, Elfers CT, Figlewicz DP, et al. Vitamin D deficiency in obese rats exacerbates NAFLD and increases hepatic resistin and toll-like receptor activation. Hepatology 2012. [Epub ahead of print].
61. Teli MR, James OF, Burt AD, et al. The natural history of nonalcoholic fatty liver: a follow-up study. Hepatology 1995;22:1714–9.
62. Dam-Larsen S, Becker U, Franzmann MG, et al. Final results of a long-term, clinical follow-up in fatty liver patients. Scand J Gastroenterol 2009;44:1236–43.
63. Soderberg C, Stal P, Askling J, et al. Decreased survival of subjects with elevated liver function tests during a 28-year follow-up period. Hepatology 2010;51:595–602.

64. Ekstedt M, Franzen LE, Mathiesen UL, et al. Long-term follow-up of patients with NAFLD and elevated liver enzymes. Hepatology 2006;44:865–73.
65. Angulo P. Diagnosing steatohepatitis and predicting liver-related mortality in patients with NAFLD: two distinct concepts. Hepatology 2011;53:1792–4.
66. Bhala N, Angulo P, Van der Poorten D, et al. The natural history of nonalcoholic fatty liver disease with advanced fibrosis or cirrhosis: an international collaborative study. Hepatology 2011;54:1208–16.
67. Palmentieri B, de Sio I, La Mura V, et al. The role of bright liver echo pattern on ultrasound B-mod examination in the diagnosis of liver steatosis. Dig Liver Dis 2006;38:485–9.
68. Adams LA, Angulo P. Role of liver biopsy and serum markers of liver fibrosis in non-alcoholic fatty liver disease. Clin Liver Dis 2007;11:25–35.
69. Van Ness MM, Diehl AM. Is liver biopsy useful in the evaluation of patients with chronically elevated liver enzymes? Ann Intern Med 1989;111:473–8.
70. Fassio E, Alvarez E, Dominguez N, et al. Natural history of nonalcoholic steatohepatitis: a longitudinal study of repeat liver biopsies. Hepatology 2004;40: 820–6.
71. Tandra S, Yeh MM, Brunt EM, et al. Presence and significance of microvesicular steatosis in nonalcoholic fatty liver disease. J Hepatol 2011;55:654–9.
72. Kleiner DE, Brunt EM, Van Natta M, et al. Design and validation of a histological scoring system for nonalcoholic fatty liver disease. Hepatology 2005;41: 1313–21.
73. Brunt EM, Kleiner DE, Wilson LA, et al. Nonalcoholic fatty liver disease (NAFLD) activity score and the histopathologic diagnosis in NAFLD: distinct clinicopathologic meanings. Hepatology 2011;53:810–20.
74. Ratziu V, Charlotte F, Heurtier A, et al. Sampling variability of liver biopsy in nonalcoholic fatty liver disease. Gastroenterology 2005;128:1898–906.
75. Janiec DJ, Jacobson ER, Freeth A, et al. Histologic variation of grade and stage of non-alcoholic fatty liver disease in liver biopsies. Obes Surg 2005;15: 497–501.
76. Sporea I, Popescu A, Sirli R. Why, who and how should perform liver biopsy in chronic liver diseases. World J Gastroenterol 2008;14:3396–402.
77. Strauss S, Gavish E, Gottlieb P, et al. Interobserver and intraobserver variability in the sonographic assessment of fatty liver. Am J Roentgenol 2007;189:32–3.
78. Ryan CK, Johnson LA, Germin BI, et al. One hundred consecutive hepatic biopsies in the workup of living donors for right lobe liver transplantation. Liver Transpl 2002;8:1114–22.
79. Mottin CC, Moretto M, Padoin AV, et al. The role of ultrasound in the diagnosis of hepatic steatosis in morbidly obese patients. Obes Surg 2004;14:635–7.
80. Yoneda M, Mawatari H, Fujita K, et al. Non-invasive assessment of liver fibrosis by measurements of stiffness in patients with nonalcoholic fatty liver disease. Dig Liver Dis 2008;40:371–8.
81. Nobili V, Vizzutti F, Arena U, et al. Accuracy and reproducibility of transient elastography for the diagnosis of fibrosis in pediatric nonalcoholic steatohepatitis. Hepatology 2008;48:442–8.
82. Wong VW, Vergniol J, Wong GL, et al. Diagnosis of fibrosis and cirrhosis using liver stiffness measurement in nonalcoholic fatty liver disease. Hepatology 2010; 51:454–62.
83. Myers RP, Elkashab M, Ma M, et al. Transient elastography for the noninvasive assessment of liver fibrosis: a multicentre Canadian study. Can J Gastroenterol 2010;24:661–70.

84. De Ledinghen V, Wong WV, Vergniol J, et al. Diagnosis of liver fibrosis and cirrhosis using liver stiffness measurement: comparison between M and XL probe of FibroScan. J Hepatol 2011;56:833–9.
85. Fishbein M, Castro F, Cheruku S, et al. Hepatic MRI for fat quantitation: its relationship to fat morphology, diagnosis, and ultrasound. J Clin Gastroenterol 2005; 39:619–25.
86. Szczepaniak LS, Nurenberg P, Leonard D, et al. Magnetic resonance spectroscopy to measure hepatic triglyceride content: prevalence of hepatic steatosis in the general population. Am J Physiol Endocrinol Metab 2005;288: E462–8.
87. Talwalkar JA, Yin M, Fidler JL, et al. Magnetic resonance imaging of hepatic fibrosis: emerging clinical applications. Hepatology 2008;47:332–42.
88. Huwart L, Sempoux C, Vicaut E, et al. Magnetic resonance elastography for the noninvasive staging of liver fibrosis. Gastroenterology 2008;135:32–40.
89. Asbach P, Klatt D, Hamhaber U, et al. Assessment of liver viscoelasticity using multifrequency MR elastography. Magn Reson Med 2008;60:373–9.
90. Yin M, Talwalkar JA, Glaser KJ, et al. Assessment of hepatic fibrosis with magnetic resonance elastography. Clin Gastroenterol Hepatol 2007;5:1207–13.
91. Lee VS, Miller FH, Omary RA, et al. Magnetic resonance elastography and biomarkers to assess fibrosis from recurrent hepatitis C in liver transplant recipients. Transplantation 2011;92:581–6.
92. Chen J, Talwalkar JA, Yin M, et al. Early detection of nonalcoholic steatohepatitis in patients with nonalcoholic fatty liver disease by using MR elastography. Radiology 2011;259:749–56.
93. Jacobs JE, Birnbaum BA, Shapiro MA, et al. Diagnostic criteria for fatty infiltration of the liver on contrast-enhanced helical CT. Am J Roentgenol 1998;171: 659–64.
94. Kodama Y, Ng CS, Wu TT, et al. Comparison of CT methods for determining the fat content of the liver. Am J Roentgenol 2007;188:1307–12.
95. Park SH, Kim PN, Kim KW, et al. Macrovesicular hepatic steatosis in living liver donors: use of CT for quantitative and qualitative assessment. Radiology 2006; 239:105–12.
96. Sorrentino P, Tarantino G, Conca P, et al. Silent nonalcoholic fatty liver disease—a clinical histological study. J Hepatol 2004;41:751–7.
97. Adams LA. Biomakers of Liver Fibrosis. J Gastroenterol Hepatol 2011;26: 802–9.
98. Shaheen AA, Myers RP. Diagnostic accuracy of the aspartate aminotransferase-to-platelet ratio index for the prediction of hepatitis C-related fibrosis: a systematic review. Hepatology 2007;46:912–21.
99. Angulo P, Hui JM, Marchesini G, et al. The NAFLD fibrosis score: a noninvasive system that identifies liver fibrosis in patients with NAFLD. Hepatology 2007;45: 846–54.
100. McPherson S, Stewart SF, Henderson E, et al. Simple non-invasive fibrosis scoring systems can reliably exclude advanced fibrosis in patients with non-alcoholic fatty liver disease. Gut 2010;59:1265–9.
101. Guha IN, Parkes J, Roderick P, et al. Noninvasive markers of fibrosis in nonalcoholic fatty liver disease: validating the European Liver Fibrosis Panel and exploring simple markers. Hepatology 2008;47:455–60.
102. Ratziu V, Massard J, Charlotte F, et al. Diagnostic value of biochemical markers (FibroTest-FibroSURE) for the prediction of liver fibrosis in patients with non-alcoholic fatty liver disease. BMC Gastroenterol 2006;6:6.

103. Patel K, Gordon SC, Jacobson I, et al. Evaluation of a panel of non-invasive serum markers to differentiate mild from moderate-to-advanced liver fibrosis in chronic hepatitis C patients. J Hepatol 2004;41:935–42.
104. Carlson JJ, Kowdley KV, Sullivan SD, et al. An evaluation of the potential cost-effectiveness of non-invasive testing strategies in the diagnosis of significant liver fibrosis. J Gastroenterol Hepatol 2009;24:786–91.
105. Wieckowska A, Zein NN, Yerian LM, et al. In vivo assessment of liver cell apoptosis as a novel biomarker of disease severity in nonalcoholic fatty liver disease. Hepatology 2006;44:27–33.
106. Wong VW, Wong GL, Choi PC, et al. Disease progression of non-alcoholic fatty liver disease: a prospective study with paired liver biopsies at 3 years. Gut 2010; 59(7):969–74.
107. Dixon JB, Bhathal PS, Hughes NR, et al. Nonalcoholic fatty liver disease: improvement in liver histological analysis with weight loss. Hepatology 2004; 39:1647–54.
108. Eriksson S, Eriksson KF, Bondesson L. Nonalcoholic steatohepatitis in obesity: a reversible condition. Acta Med Scand 1986;220:83–8.
109. Shah K, Stufflebam A, Hilton TN, et al. Diet and exercise interventions reduce intrahepatic fat content and improve insulin sensitivity in obese older adults. Obesity (Silver Spring) 2009;17:2162–8.
110. Huang MA, Greenson JK, Chao C, et al. One-year intense nutritional counseling results in histological improvement in patients with non-alcoholic steatohepatitis: a pilot study. Am J Gastroenterol 2005;100:1072–81.
111. Angulo P. Current best treatment for nonalcoholic fatty liver disease. Expert Opin Pharmacother 2003;4:611–23.
112. Kugelmas M, Hill DB, Vivian B, et al. Cytokines and NASH: a pilot study of the effects of lifestyle modification and vitamin E. Hepatology 2003;38:413–9.
113. Harrison SA, Brunt EM, Neuschwander-Tetri BA. Orlistat for overweight subjects with nonalcoholic steatohepatitis: a randomized, prospective trial. Hepatology 2009;49:80–6.
114. Harrison SA, Day CP. Benefits of lifestyle modification in NAFLD. Gut 2007;56: 1760–9.
115. Dansinger M, Gleason J, Griggith J, et al. Comparison of the Atkins, Ornish, Weight Watchers, and Zone diets for weight loss and heart disease risk reduction. JAMA 2005;93:43–53.
116. Davidson MH, Hauptman J, DiGirolamo M, et al. Weight control and risk factor reduction in obese subjects treated for 2 years with orlistat: a randomized controlled trial. JAMA 1999;281:235–42.
117. Barker KB, Palekar NA, Bowers SP, et al. Non-alcoholic steatohepatitis: effect of Roux-en-Y gastric bypass surgery. Am J Gastroenterol 2006;101:368–73.
118. Stratopoulos C, Papakonstantinou A, Terzis I, et al. Changes in liver histology accompanying massive weight loss after gastroplasty for morbid obesity. Obes Surg 2005;15:1154–60.
119. Keshishian A, Zahriya K, Willes EB. Duodenal switch has no detrimental effects on hepatic function and improves hepatic steatohepatitis after 6 months. Obes Surg 2005;15:1418–23.
120. Tai CM, Huang CK, Hwang JC, et al. Improvement of nonalcoholic fatty liver disease after bariatric surgery in morbidly obese Chinese patients. Obes Surg 2011. [Epub ahead of print].
121. Moretto M, Kupski C, da Silva VD, et al. Effect of bariatric surgery on liver fibrosis. Obes Surg 2011. [Epub ahead of print].

122. Clark JM, Alkhuraishi AR, Solga SF, et al. Roux-en-Y gastric bypass improves liver histology in patients with non-alcoholic fatty liver disease. Obes Res 2005;13:1180–6.
123. Sanyal AJ, Chalasani N, Kowdley KV, et al. Pioglitazone, vitamin E, or placebo for nonalcoholic steatohepatitis. N Engl J Med 2010;362:1675–85.
124. Harrison SA, Torgerson S, Hayashi P, et al. Vitamin E and C treatment improves fibrosis in patients with nonalcoholic steatohepatitis. Am J Gastroenterol 2003; 98:2485–90.
125. Wong VW, Wong GL, Choi PC, et al. Disease progression of non-alcoholic fatty liver disease: a prospective study with paired liver biopsies at 3 years. JAMA 2010;59(7):969–74.
126. Pietu F, Guillaud O, Walter T, et al. Ursodeoxycholic acid with vitamin E in patients with nonalcoholic steatohepatitis: long-term results. Clin Res Hepatol Gastroenterol 2012;36:146–55.
127. Sesso HD, Buring JE, Christen WG, et al. Vitamins E and C in the prevention of cardiovascular disease in men: the Physicians' Health Study II randomized controlled trial. JAMA 2008;300:2123–33.
128. Song Z, Deaciuc I, Zhou Z, et al. Involvement of AMP-activated protein kinase in beneficial effect of betain on high sucrose diet-induced hepatic steatosis. Am J Physiol Gastrointest Liver Physiol 2007;293:G894–902.
129. Abdelmalek MF, Sanderson SO, Angulo P, et al. Betaine for nonalcoholic steatohepatitis, results of a randomized placebo-controlled trial. Hepatology 2009;50: 1818–26.
130. Lindor KD, Kowdley KV, Heathcote EJ, et al. Ursodeoxycholic acid for treatment of nonalcoholic steatohepatitis: results of a randomized trial. Hepatology 2004; 39:770–8.
131. Ratziu V, de Ledinghen V, Obert F, et al. A randomized controlled trial of high-dose ursodesoxycholic acid for nonalcoholic steatohepatitis. J Hepatol 2011; 54(5):1011–9.
132. Van Wagner LB, Koppe SW, Brunt EM, et al. Pentoxifylline for the treatment of non-alcoholic steatohepatitis: a randomized controlled trial. Ann Hepatol 2011; 10:277–86.
133. Zein CO, Yerian LM, Gogate P, et al. Pentoxifylline improves nonalcoholic steatohepatitis: a randomized placebo-controlled trial. Hepatology 2011;54: 1610–9.
134. Mahady SE, Webster AC, Walker S, et al. The role of thiazolidinediones in non-alcoholic steatohepatitis—a systematic review and meta analysis. J Hepatol 2011;55:1383–90.
135. Belfort R, Harrison SA, Brown K, et al. A placebo-controlled trial of pioglitazone in subjects with nonalcoholic steatohepatitis. N Engl J Med 2006;355: 2297–307.
136. Ratziu V, Charlotte F, Bernhardt C, et al. Long term efficacy of rosiglitazone in nonalcoholic steatohepatitis, results of the fatty liver improvement by rosiglitazone (FLIRT 2) extension trial. Hepatology 2010;51:445–53.
137. Murphy CE, Rodgers PT. Effect of thiazolidinediones on bone loss and fracture. Ann Pharmacother 2007;41:2014–8.
138. Lutchman G, Modi A, Kleiner DE, et al. The effects of discontinuing pioglitazone in patients with nonalcoholic steatohepatitis. Hepatology 2007;46:424–9.
139. Nissen SE, Wolski K. Effect of rosiglitazone on the risk of myocardial infarction and death from cardiovascular causes. N Engl J Med 2007;356: 2457–71.

140. Singh S, Loke Y, Furberg C. Long-term risk of cardiovascular events with rosiglitazone. A meta-analysis. JAMA 2007;98:1189–95.
141. Haukeland JW, Konopski Z, Eggesbo HB, et al. Metformin in patients with non-alcoholic fatty liver disease: a randomized, controlled trial. Scand J Gastroenterol 2009;44:853–60.
142. Lavine JE, Schwimmer JB, Van Natta ML, et al. Effect of vitamin E or metformin for treatment of nonalcoholic fatty liver disease in children and adolescents: the TONIC randomized controlled trial. JAMA 2011;305:1659–68.
143. Torres DM, Frances FJ, Shaw JC, et al. Rosiglitazone versus rosiglitazone and metformin versus rosiglitazone and losartan in the treatment of nonalcoholic steatohepatitis in humans: a 12-month randomized, prospective, open-label trial. Hepatology 2011;54:1631–9.
144. Ding X, Saxena NK, Lin S, et al. Exendin-4, a glucagon-like protein-1 (GLP-1) receptor agonist reverse hepatic steatosis in ob/ob mice. Hepatology 2006; 43:173–81.
145. Tushuizen ME, Bunck MC, Pouwels PJ, et al. Incretin mimetics as a novel therapeutic option for hepatic steatosis. Liver Int 2006;26:1015–7.
146. Kenny PR, Brady DE, Torres DM, et al. Exendatide in the treatment of diabetic patients with nonalcoholic fatty steatohepatitis: a case-series. Am J Gastroenterol 2010;105:2707–9.
147. Hirose A, Ono M, Saibara T, et al. Angiotensin II type 1 receptor blocker inhibits fibrosis in rat nonalcoholic steatohepatitis. Hepatology 2007;45:1375–81.
148. Ichikawa Y. Comparative effects of telmisartan and valsartan on insulin resistance in hypertensive patients with metabolic syndrome. Intern Med 2007;46: 1331–6.
149. Hyogo H, Ikegami T, Tokushige K, et al. Efficacy of pitavastatin for the treatment of non-alcoholic steatohepatitis with dyslipidemia: an open-lab, pilot study. Hepatol Res 2011;41:1057–65.
150. Foster T, Budoff MJ, Saab S, et al. Atorvastatin and antioxidants for the treatment of nonalcoholic fatty liver disease: the St. Francis Heart Study randomized clinical trial. Am J Gastroenterol 2011;106:71–7.
151. Athyros VG, Tziomalos K, Gossios TD, et al. Safety and efficacy of long-term statin treatment for cardiovascular events in patients with coronary heart disease and abnormal liver function tests in the GREACE study: a post-hoc analysis. Lancet 2010;376:1916–22.
152. Nozaki Y, Fujita K, Yoneda M, et al. Long-term combination therapy of ezetimibe and acarbose for non-alcoholic fatty liver disease. J Hepatol 2009;51: 548–56.
153. Park H, Shima T, Yamaguchi K, et al. Efficacy of long-term ezetimibe therapy in patients with nonalcoholic fatty liver disease. J Gastroenterol 2001;46:101–7.
154. Zelber-Sagi S, Ratziu V, Oren R. Nutritional and physical activity in NAFLD: an overview of the epidemiological evidence. World J Gastroenterol 2011;17: 3377–89.
155. Pachikian BD, Essaghir A, Demoulin JB, et al. Hepatic n-3 polyunsaturated fatty acid depletion promotes steatosis and insulin resistance in mice: genomic analysis of cellular targets. PLoS One 2011;6(8):e23365.
156. Parker HM, Johnson NA, Burdon CA, et al. Omega-3 supplementation and non-alcoholic fatty liver disease: a systemic review and meta-analysis. J Hepatol 2012;56:944–51.
157. Marik PE, Varon J. Omega-3 dietary supplements and the risk of cardiovascular events: a systematic review. Clin Cardiol 2009;32:365–72.

158. Klatsky AL, Armstrong MA. Alcohol, smoking, coffee, and cirrhosis. Am J Epidemiol 1992;136:1248–57.
159. Freedman ND, Everhart JE, Lindsay KL, et al. Coffee intake is associated with lower rates of liver disease progression in chronic hepatitis C. Hepatology 2009;50:1360–9.
160. Modi AA, Feld JJ, Park Y, et al. Increased caffeine consumption is associated with reduced hepatic fibrosis. Hepatology 2010;51:201–9.
161. Molloy JW, Calcagno CJ, Williams CD, et al. Association of coffee and caffeine consumption with fatty liver disease, nonalcoholic steatohepatitis, and degree of hepatic fibrosis. Hepatology 2012;55:429–36.

Surgical Clearance for the Patient with Chronic Liver Disease

Andrew J. Muir, MD, MHS

KEYWORDS

- End-stage liver disease • Hepatocellular carcinoma
- Liver cirrhosis • Portal hypertension
- Postoperative complications

Although any surgical procedure carries risks, these risks have historically been greater among certain groups of patients with liver disease.[1] For the patient requiring emergent surgery in a life-threatening situation, the role of the gastroenterologist or hepatologist may be to guide the surgeon and anesthesiologist regarding the strategies to avoid potential complications. Most consults regarding surgical risk concern patients requiring elective or urgent procedures with the time to make an assessment and potentially optimize the patient before the surgical procedure. The medical literature provides greatest insight into the risks for patients with cirrhosis, and the risks vary with the degree of hepatic insufficiency and the type of surgery. Although hepatotoxicity has long been associated with halothane, current medications are generally safe, and the different approaches to anesthesia (general, spinal, epidural) seem to carry similar risks.[2,3] This review discusses the approach to the consult for surgical clearance in a patient with chronic liver disease through discussion of several typical consults.

THE APPROACH TO THE CONSULT FOR SURGICAL CLEARANCE IN A PATIENT WITH CHRONIC LIVER DISEASE

History and Physical Examination

The consult for surgical clearance in a patient with chronic liver disease begins with a history and physical examination, and there are several key issues that deserve focus (**Box 1**). Although different surgical procedures carry different risks, the degree of liver disease is a critical factor to be evaluated. This article focuses on chronic liver

Disclosures: The author has no relationships with any commercial companies that have a direct financial interest in the subject matter or materials discussed in the article, or with any companies making competing products.

Division of Gastroenterology, Duke Clinical Research Institute, Duke University School of Medicine, PO Box 17969, Durham, NC 27715, USA
E-mail address: andrew.muir@duke.edu

Clin Liver Dis 16 (2012) 421–433
doi:10.1016/j.cld.2012.03.008 liver.theclinics.com
1089-3261/12/$ – see front matter

Box 1
Key items in the history and physical examination of a consult for surgical clearance

- Presence of acute liver failure
- History of alcohol use and possible presence of alcoholic hepatitis
- Prior liver biopsy: cirrhosis present?
- Features of portal hypertension
  - Ascites
  - Esophageal or gastric varices
  - Hepatic encephalopathy
  - TIPS placement
    - Recent assessment of TIPS patency?
- Renal function
- Calculation of the Child-Pugh score
- Calculation of the MELD score
- Evaluated for liver transplantation?

disease, but alcoholic hepatitis and acute liver failure have generally been considered contraindications to elective surgery.[4–9] Although one study of patients undergoing emergent portacaval shunt surgery reported no increased risk of mortality among patients with alcoholic hepatitis, other studies of patients with alcoholic hepatitis have reported mortality rates ranging from 55% to 100%.[5–9] These older studies have not been repeated in the modern era and therefore do not consider advances in surgery and anesthesia, but general recommendations have been to delay elective surgery to achieve resolution of the alcoholic hepatitis. As a result, the history of alcohol use is an important part of the history, followed by consideration of the diagnosis of alcoholic hepatitis. Involvement of other organs with liver diseases should be considered, such as the potential for cardiomyopathy or diabetes in a patient with hemochromatosis or lung disease in a patient with α1-antitrypsin deficiency.

The literature on the surgical risk among patients with liver disease highlights the increased risk among patients with cirrhosis and portal hypertension. If the patient has previously had a liver biopsy, the results should be sought to understand the degree of fibrosis and possible presence of cirrhosis. The history should include possible complications of portal hypertension such as ascites, spontaneous bacterial peritonitis, hepatic encephalopathy, and esophageal or gastric varices, with clarification as to whether these have bled and have required endoscopic therapy or transjugular intrahepatic portosystemic shunt (TIPS). If a TIPS is present, the indication for the TIPS should be clarified whether for refractory ascites or variceal bleeding. If placed for ascites, the lack of ascites gives confidence that the TIPS remains patent. If the TIPS has been placed for esophageal variceal bleeding, assessment of TIPS patency should be performed in the preoperative setting unless performed recently.

Child-Pugh Versus MELD

Recent studies of surgical risk have continued to evaluate the role of the Child-Pugh classification system but have also used the Model for End-Stage Liver Disease (MELD). The MELD score is a logarithmic calculation using the prothrombin time international normalized ratio (PT-INR), total serum bilirubin, and serum creatinine.[10,11] The MELD score was originally developed to predict mortality following TIPS and later became the basis for organ transplantation in the United States in 2002. For purposes of illustration, a patient with compensated cirrhosis, and therefore no ascites or encephalopathy and serum creatinine 1 mg/dL, total bilirubin 1 mg/dL, and PT-INR 1.0, would have a MELD score of 6. In an analysis of patients listed for transplantation in the United States between 2003 and 2007, patients with MELD scores less than 15 had a survival benefit in the analysis by not undergoing transplantation related to the perioperative risks of transplantation.[12]

With the transition from a Child-Pugh–based liver transplant allocation system to a system based on the MELD score, the role of the MELD score in the prediction of postoperative mortality has also been raised. A large retrospective study from the Mayo Clinic evaluated the role of the MELD score in 772 patients with cirrhosis who underwent digestive, orthopedic, or cardiovascular surgeries in cohorts from 1980 to 1990 and from 1994 to 2004.[13] Although both the MELD score and the Child-Pugh score were predictors of postoperative mortality in the univariate analysis, the multivariable analysis revealed that MELD score was an independent predictor, but not the Child-Pugh score. Age and American Society of Anesthesiologists (ASA) score were also independent predictors of postoperative mortality. Age appeared to be predictive at the extremes with no mortality among patients younger than 30 years, whereas patients older than 70 years had increased mortality. ASA class 5 (a moribund patient who is not expected to survive 24 hours with or without operation) was the strongest predictor of 7-day mortality, and MELD was the strongest predictor of mortality at time points of 30 days and beyond. Based on these results, these investigators have developed a calculator using these predictors to help determine the postoperative mortality at 7 days, 30 days, 90 days, 1 year, and 5 years (http://www.mayoclinic.org/meld/mayomodel9.html).

Several other studies have evaluated the role of the MELD score in predicting postoperative mortality, with somewhat variable results.[14–18] These generally small studies have evaluated heterogeneous populations, and based on the literature to date no clear recommendation can be made to use the MELD score instead of the Child-Pugh classification. Studies in patients receiving cardiac surgery have suggested that Child-Pugh may be more appropriate than MELD for these patients.[19–21] The heterogeneous nature of the literature makes it challenging to refer to one study with confidence for a particular patient. At the author's center, the Child-Pugh class and the MELD score are calculated to allow consideration of several studies, to guide surgeons and their patients regarding the range of risks reported in the literature.

Liver Transplantation Status

In the preoperative assessment of patients with cirrhosis, their status in terms of liver transplantation should be evaluated. If the patient is listed for liver transplantation and experiences decompensation in the postoperative setting, liver transplantation might be an option. Although evaluation for liver transplantation can be done in emergent settings, the preferred approach would be for evaluation to be done before any surgical procedure, when the patient and family can go through the experience in the outpatient setting without the urgency and stress of the critical care setting. If a patient has been evaluated previously without being offered listing for transplantation, the patient would need to take this into consideration when considering the risks versus benefits of the surgical procedure under consideration. If a patient is listed and transplantation is scheduled in the near future, the patient may be advised to defer elective procedures until after transplantation. In their study of 772 patients undergoing surgery at the Mayo Clinic, Teh and colleagues[13] recommend postponing elective procedures if the MELD score is greater than 20, and making sure that liver-transplant evaluation has been completed in patients with cirrhosis and a MELD score ranging from 12 to 19.

Medical Management in the Perioperative Period

Once the gastroenterologist/hepatologist has offered an opinion on surgical risk, the consult should also include recommendations for management in the perioperative period. If the patient has prolonged prothrombin time, vitamin K should be given for 3 days in the event of deficiency. The patient may also require fresh frozen plasma or platelets preoperatively. Thrombopoietin agonists have been approved by the US Food and Drug Administration for the treatment of idiopathic thrombocytopenic purpura, but a study of eltrombopag for patients with thrombocytopenia before an elective invasive procedure was halted for safety concerns. In this study of 292 patients, 6 patients in the eltrombopag arm developed thrombotic events compared with 2 patients in the placebo group (odds ratio [95% confidence interval] 2.827 [0.695–11.501]).[21] Thrombopoietin agonists, therefore, cannot be recommended in this setting. Patients with cirrhosis are also in a fibrinolytic state, and therefore cryoprecipitate should be available for the procedure as well.

The complications of portal hypertension should be evaluated and addressed. Patients with cirrhosis or any clinical concern for cirrhosis should have upper endoscopy to rule out varices.[22] If varices are present, primary prophylaxis with nonselective β-blocker or band ligation should be considered. If the patient has history of variceal hemorrhage, upper endoscopy should be repeated with band ligation before the surgical procedure. If the patient has ascites, efforts should be made to reduce the ascites before surgery through the use of a low-sodium diet, diuretics, and large-volume paracentesis. If not already on prophylaxis to prevent spontaneous bacterial peritonitis, prophylaxis with norfloxacin or trimethoprim/sulfamethoxazole should be considered in the patient with persistent ascites.[23] For patients with refractory ascites with an elective surgical procedure planned, TIPS can be considered.[24] All patients should be assessed for the presence of hepatic encephalopathy with appropriate medical management if needed. The surgeon and anesthesiologist should be alerted to the likelihood of encephalopathy in the postoperative setting, with the need for early identification and treatment.

Patients with liver disease are also at risk for renal insufficiency. If the patient has renal insufficiency, he or she should be evaluated for hepatorenal syndrome, which would be a sign of significant liver disease with poor prognosis that might affect decisions regarding the risk/benefit analysis for surgical procedures.[25] Patients with liver disease may develop acute kidney injury from excessive diuresis, and diuretic management may require adjustment. Electrolytes should also be evaluated, with efforts to maintain the potassium level greater than 4.0 mmol/L.

Medications for the treatment of liver disease should be addressed as part of the consultation. Current therapy for hepatitis C with peginterferon-α, ribavirin, and a protease inhibitor (boceprevir or telaprevir) results in anemia, leukopenia, and thrombocytopenia, and may lead to the suggestion that a patient has portal hypertension related, for example, to the thrombocytopenia.[26,27] Interruptions in these medications can lead to viral breakthrough, therefore elective procedures should be delayed until therapy for hepatitis C has been completed. If the patient requires emergent therapy, minimizing the duration of the interruption of treatment is important if the patient is to continue therapy for hepatitis C postoperatively. In addition, the anesthesiologist should be aware of the drug-drug interactions with the protease inhibitors and in particular with the increased risk of toxicity with benzodiazepines. The antiviral medications for hepatitis B pose little risk but may get interrupted during the perioperative period until oral medications are resumed, and the risk of viral breakthrough with prolonged interruption should be considered. For the patient with autoimmune hepatitis currently receiving steroids, stress doses of steroids may be required perioperatively.

Patients with liver disease require close monitoring postoperatively to evaluate for any signs of hepatic decompensation and to prevent complications, and admission to a critical care bed or intermediate care bed should be considered. Prolongation of the prothrombin time is a good marker of synthetic function, and elevated bilirubin and ongoing difficulties with ascites management would also be signs of concern. For pain management and anxiolysis in the perioperative period, patients with cirrhosis may be at risk for excessive sedation and the precipitation of hepatic encephalopathy because of the prolonged half-life of narcotics and benzodiazepines. The author recommends the use of short-acting agents in the perioperative period with close monitoring and treatment if there are any signs of hepatic encephalopathy. Patients with cirrhosis are often malnourished and may benefit from nutrition consultation preoperatively.

ILLUSTRATIVE CASES OF SURGICAL RISK IN PATIENTS WITH CHRONIC LIVER DISEASE

Case 1: Abdominal Surgery in a Patient with Cirrhosis

The patient is a 57-year-old woman with primary biliary cirrhosis being evaluated for cholecystectomy for symptomatic cholelithiasis. The patient was diagnosed with primary biliary cirrhosis 2 years earlier when she presented with esophageal variceal bleeding. She continues in a variceal banding protocol, and most recent upper endoscopy 16 months previously revealed no varices. She has moderate ascites despite diuretics and no history of hepatic encephalopathy. Her laboratory data include PT-INR 1.2, albumin 3.0 g/dL, total bilirubin 2.5 mg/dL, and creatinine 1.1 mg/dL. Child-Pugh score was 8 (grade B) and the MELD score was 13. The patient had not been evaluated previously for liver transplantation.

Although several factors have been found to predict the outcome of patients with cirrhosis undergoing abdominal surgery, the Child-Pugh classification has consistently performed well in this regard (**Table 1**).[17,18,24,28,29] The studies have generally shown a stepwise increase in risk of perioperative mortality with each Child-Pugh class and especially with Child-Pugh class C. A retrospective review from Louisville General Hospital and the Veterans Affairs Medical Center in Louisville, Kentucky included 100 patients with cirrhosis undergoing abdominal surgery between 1975 and 1982.[28] Cholecystectomy was the most common procedure in 29 patients. Thirty patients died, and the most common cause of death was sepsis with multisystem organ failure. The postoperative mortality rates were 10% for Child-Pugh class A, 31% for Child-Pugh class B, and 76% for Child-Pugh class C. A similar retrospective study from Loyola University Medical Center in Chicago, Illinois included 92 patients from 1984

Table 1
Risk of mortality with abdominal surgery according to Child-Pugh class

Child-Pugh Class	Garrison et al[28] (N = 100) (%)	Mansour et al[29] (N = 92) (%)	Neeff et al[18] (N = 138) (%)	Telem et al[17] (N = 100) (%)
A	10	10	10	2
B	31	30	17	2
C	76	82	63	12

through 1996 with a wide variety of abdominal surgical procedures including 17 cholecystectomies plus a mixture of both emergent and elective cases.[29] The postoperative mortality rates were 10%, 30%, and 82% in patients with Child-Pugh class A, B, and C, respectively. The mortality rate was 50% among patients requiring emergent surgery compared with 18% for elective cases.

A retrospective study from the University of Freiburg in Germany evaluated 138 patients undergoing intra-abdominal or abdominal wall surgery.[18] Postoperative mortality increased with the Child-Pugh score with 10% for Child-Pugh class A, 17% for Child-Pugh class B, and 63% for Child-Pugh class C. A similar analysis with the MELD score found postoperative mortality rates were 9% for MELD score less than 10, 19% for MELD score with a range of 10 to 15, and 54% if the MELD was greater than 15. In their multivariate analysis examining elective procedures, only the preoperative serum creatinine predicted perioperative mortality. When considering emergent procedures only, predictors of postoperative mortality were Child-Pugh class, requirement for blood transfusions, and lower sodium level. The MELD score did not predict postoperative mortality.

Another recent retrospective study conducted in 2010 evaluated 100 patients with cirrhosis undergoing abdominal surgery from 2002 through 2008 at Mount Sinai Hospital in New York, and reported more encouraging results.[17] Mortality rates were 2%, 12%, and 12% for Child-Pugh class A, B, and C, respectively. Among the 26 cholecystectomies that were all done laparoscopically, there was one death in a Child-Pugh class B patient. The investigators describe their approach to the management of cirrhotic patients perioperatively, including the restriction of crystalloid intraoperatively and postoperatively with the use of an albumin drip until an oral diet is tolerated. The diet is designed for cirrhotic patients with low sodium, low fat, and adequate protein balance. The patients may receive lactulose as early as hospital day 1 to prevent encephalopathy, and the general surgical procedures are generally performed by the liver-transplant surgeons with postoperative care provided by the multidisciplinary liver service. The morbidity results highlight the challenge of taking care of patients with cirrhosis undergoing surgical procedures, with wound complications in 12, liver decompensation in 12, postoperative ileus or obstruction in 4, respiratory failure in 10 of whom 4 required tracheostomy, sepsis in 7, postoperative variceal bleed in 3, and anastomotic leak in 1. The significant morbidity but lower mortality overall supports the recommendation for these procedures to be performed by experienced surgeons with postoperative care being the responsibility of a multidisciplinary team.

One important aspect of this case was the presence of ascites, which has often been associated with the risk of postoperative morbidity and mortality. Optimal management of ascites before surgery should be a goal. If refractory to low-sodium diet and diuretics, placement of a TIPS before an elective surgery has been considered as a management strategy.[24] In an early report of TIPS in 7 patients (3 for refractory ascites), the placement of the TIPS delayed surgery from 1 to 5 months. The investigators commented that only 2 patients received transfusions during surgery and only 1 patient died 36 days after colon resection.

In considering the patient in the case presented in this section, the last upper endoscopy for the banding protocol was 16 months ago. If the TIPS is placed to manage the ascites, this would also alleviate concerns about variceal bleeding. If the TIPS is not placed, the patient should have an upper endoscopy for possible esophageal band ligation to reduce the risk of variceal bleeding in the perioperative setting. In addition, this patient was not listed for transplantation at the time of the evaluation for transplantation. The author recommends immediate evaluation for liver transplantation before the surgical procedure so that the patient and her surgeon would know if transplantation was an option in the event of decompensation in the postoperative period.

Case 2: Resection of Hepatocellular Carcinoma in a Patient with Cirrhosis

The patient is a 64-year-old man with history of alcohol abuse who presented with a recent diagnosis of hepatocellular carcinoma (HCC). He had history of daily alcohol use for many years and quit all alcohol during a presentation with alcoholic hepatitis 6 months ago. His recent ultrasonogram for HCC surveillance revealed a 3.2-cm mass in the right lobe, and this was confirmed by magnetic resonance imaging. The patient has no history of ascites or hepatic encephalopathy. Upper endoscopy 2 months ago revealed no varices. His laboratory data include PT-INR 1.0, albumin 4.1 g/dL, total bilirubin 0.9 mg/dL, and creatinine 0.9 mg/dL. Child-Pugh score was 5 (grade A) and the MELD score was 6. The patient was believed to have compensated cirrhosis and had not been evaluated previously for liver transplantation.

Patients with early identification of HCC should be evaluated for curative therapies including hepatic resection and liver transplantation. Early experience with hepatic resection in patients was a concerning variable, with significant risk of morbidity and mortality related to liver decompensation.[30,31] More recent series have reported improved outcomes through improvements in surgical techniques and appropriate patient selection, and resection is the treatment of choice for patients who develop HCC without cirrhosis.[32–36] For patients with cirrhosis, the current guideline from the American Association for the Study of Liver Diseases recommends consideration of resection only in patients with lack of portal hypertension.[32] In a classic study by Bruix and colleagues[35] published in 1996, 29 patients with Child-Pugh class A cirrhosis underwent resection for HCC. All patients had an extensive assessment before surgery including measurement of the hepatic venous pressure gradient. Seventeen patients experienced decompensation with ascites in 16, jaundice in 2, and encephalopathy in 2. Eleven of these patients experienced decompensation that was unresolved by 3 months after surgery, and only the hepatic venous pressure gradient was a predictor of this unresolved decompensation in a multivariate analysis with an odds ratio of 1.90 (95% confidence interval 1.12–3.22). The preoperative gradient was 13.9 mm Hg in the unresolved decompensation group compared with 7.4 mm Hg (*P*<.001) among patients without unresolved decompensation. A threshold of 10 mm Hg for a gradient appeared to be a threshold in the analysis. No unresolved decompensation occurred in patients with a gradient less than 10 mm Hg, and 11 of 15 patients with a gradient greater than 10 mm Hg experienced unresolved decompensation. A follow-up study by Llovet and colleagues[36] reported the experience of the University of Barcelona with 1265 patients with HCC between 1989 and 1997. Comparisons between the 77 patients undergoing hepatic resection and the 87 patients receiving liver transplantation demonstrated similar survival outcomes at 1, 3, and 5 years. This study was not a randomized controlled trial, and the patients undergoing resection were less likely to have portal hypertension and more likely to be Child-Pugh class A. Among all patients in this analysis, the best outcomes were achieved by patients with a hepatic venous pressure gradient less than 10 mm Hg and serum bilirubin less than 1 mg/dL with 1-, 3-, and 5-year survival rates of 91%, 87%, and 74%. These studies have demonstrated that resection is the treatment of choice for patients without portal hypertension.

In evaluating the patient considering resection of HCC, the main goal of the consultant will be to evaluate for any features of portal hypertension. If there are no obvious signs of portal hypertension such as varices, ascites, or encephalopathy, measurement of the hepatic venous pressure gradient can confirm that the patient is a potential candidate for resection if the gradient is less than 10 mm Hg.

Case 3. Gastric Bypass in a Patient with Cirrhosis Secondary to Nonalcoholic Fatty Liver Disease

The patient is a 42-year-old woman presenting for evaluation of bariatric surgery. She has been obese since childhood. She has had history of mild elevations in alanine aminotransferase (ALT), and an ultrasonogram 3 years earlier had revealed hepatic steatosis. Her medical history includes hypertension and diabetes mellitus. Her body mass index is 43 kg/m^2. Her physical examination revealed no obvious stigmata of portal hypertension. Her laboratory data include aspartate aminotransferase 37 U/L, ALT 68 U/L, alkaline phosphatase 102 U/L, total bilirubin 1.2 mg/dL, albumin 4.2 g/dL, PT-INR 1.0, and platelet count 94 $\times$ 10^9/L.

The increase in bariatric surgery in the last decade has heightened awareness of the risk of nonalcoholic fatty liver disease in this population. Obesity and hepatic steatosis are known to be associated with increased risk of surgical complications from resection, but bariatric surgery offers the potential to improve liver histology.[37,38] The first knowledge of significant liver disease may come during preoperative evaluation for bariatric surgery or at the time of bariatric surgery. A review of 12 observational studies that included 1620 morbidly obese patients undergoing bariatric surgery found that the prevalence of steatosis was 91% (range 85%–98%) with steatohepatitis present in 37% (range 24%–98%).[39] Cirrhosis was present in 1.7% (range 1%–7%). Limited data are available on the risk of bariatric surgery in patients with cirrhosis. A 2004 retrospective review evaluated 30 patients with cirrhosis who underwent laparoscopic Roux-en-Y gastric bypass at the University of Pittsburgh.[40] The diagnosis was made intraoperatively in 90% of patients. There were no cases of hepatic decompensation or deaths. In 1998, surgeons at the University of Medicine and Dentistry of New Jersey published a survey of 126 bariatric surgeons regarding an unexpected finding of cirrhosis at the time of bariatric surgery.[41] Of the 126 respondents, 49 (39%) reported their experience, with 125 patients having an unexpected finding of cirrhosis. In 91 (73%) of the cases, the planned procedure was performed, but 17 (14%) of the cases were closed when cirrhosis was discovered. Of the 91 patients undergoing bariatric surgery with cirrhosis, 8 (8.8%) died of hepatic failure with 2 within the first 30 days and 6 beyond 30 days. In addition, 2 more patients with cirrhosis died of sepsis within the first 30 days. Of the 126 surgeons surveyed about cases with an unexpected finding of cirrhosis, 60% reported they would proceed with the operation while 40% reported they would biopsy the patient and close the abdomen.

Although there are no formal recommendations to biopsy all patients with nonalcoholic fatty liver disease before bariatric surgery, an evaluation for the presence of cirrhosis in advance of surgery might affect the decision of some surgeons to offer the procedure. For those willing to proceed, awareness of the presence of cirrhosis would allow the surgical and anesthesia teams to be better prepared. Preoperative biopsy should be considered in patients with stigmata of portal hypertension. Normal aminotransferases cannot rule out cirrhosis, and factors associated with advanced fibrosis in nonalcoholic fatty liver disease, including age over 45 years and diabetes mellitus, might also prompt consideration of a preoperative biopsy.[42] The patient in this case has the history of diabetes mellitus and although there are no obvious features of portal hypertension, the low platelet count would warrant further evaluation to exclude cirrhosis. Bariatric surgical programs should consider a plan proactively for patients with an unexpected finding of cirrhosis at the time of surgery.

Case 4: Coronary Artery Bypass Grafting in a Patient with Cirrhosis

The patient is a 57-year-old man with history of hepatitis C virus cirrhosis who presented for liver-transplant evaluation because of refractory ascites. He developed acute kidney injury with diuretics and required weekly paracentesis. He has no history of hepatic encephalopathy or variceal hemorrhage, and upper endoscopy 1 month ago revealed grade-2 varices. His laboratory data include PT-INR 1.4, albumin 3.1 g/dL, total bilirubin 2.8 mg/dL, and creatinine 1.3 mg/dL. Child-Pugh score was 9 (grade B) and the MELD score was 17. As part of his transplant evaluation, stress echocardiogram was concerning for ischemia. Cardiac catheterization revealed preserved left ventricular function but diffuse 3-vessel disease that was not amenable to percutaneous coronary intervention. Coronary artery bypass graft (CABG) surgery was recommended. The cardiac surgeon asks for consultation regarding operative risk.

Several series have evaluated the risks associated with cardiac surgery in patients with cirrhosis (**Table 2**).[19,20,43] Some series did not include patients with Child-Pugh class C cirrhosis, reflecting decisions by many clinicians to not offer cardiac surgery to the patients with more advanced cirrhosis. Some of these studies have also assessed the predictive value of the Child-Pugh score compared with MELD, with the Child-Pugh score generally performing better in predicting postoperative mortality.[20,43] The previously described large study from the Mayo Clinic included 79 patients undergoing cardiovascular surgery, and their Web site using the MELD score is available for patients undergoing cardiac surgery. Their multivariable regression analysis of prediction of postoperative mortality found that MELD and not Child-Pugh score was a predictor, but the analysis did not specifically break out the cardiac surgery patients.[17] At the author's center the approach with abdominal surgeries is followed, both Child-Pugh and MELD are considered in evaluating these patients.

A retrospective review from the New York Hospital/Cornell University Medical Center was performed to determine the outcome after cardiac operations from 1990 through 1996 in patients with cirrhosis.[43] Thirteen patients were identified with 8 Child-Pugh class A, 5 class B, and no class C patients. The investigators commented that chest-tube output and transfusion requirements were considerably higher than average for patients at their institution undergoing cardiac surgery. Four (80%) of Child-Pugh B and 1 class A patient returned to the operating room for concerns about excessive mediastinal bleeding. Four of the 5 Child-Pugh class B patients suffered perioperative mortality compared with no deaths in the class A patients. Causes of death were gastrointestinal and septic complications, with no deaths related to cardiovascular failure. From this small series, these investigators concluded that patients with Child-Pugh class B cirrhosis should not be offered cardiac surgery.

The Cleveland Clinic reported their experience from 1992 through 2002 with 44 cirrhosis patients undergoing cardiac surgery using cardiopulmonary bypass, including CABG (16), valve surgeries (16), simultaneous CABG and valve surgery (10), and

Table 2
Risk of mortality with cardiac surgery according to Child-Pugh class

Child-Pugh Class	Klemperer et al[43] (N = 13)	Suman et al[19] (N = 44)	Filsoufi et al[20] (N = 27)
A	0/8 (0%)	1/31 (3%)	1/10 (10%)
B	4/5 (80%)	5/12 (42%)	2/11 (18%)
C	No data	1/1 (100%)	4/6 (67%)

pericardiectomy.[19] Only 1 Child-Pugh class C patient received cardiac surgery and died. Child-Pugh class B patients had worse outcomes than class A patients in terms of both hepatic decompensation (8/12 vs 3/31, respectively) and mortality (5/12, 42% vs 1/31, 3%). A Child-Pugh score of greater than 7 predicted mortality, with sensitivity of 86% and specificity of 92%. The investigators commented that a similar predictive value could not be determined for MELD. It was concluded that cardiac surgery with cardiopulmonary bypass could be performed safely in patients with a Child-Pugh score less than or equal to 7 but that patients with a score greater than or equal to 8 had significant mortality risk.

The Mount Sinai Hospital performed a retrospective review of cardiac surgery between 1998 and 2004 in 27 patients with cirrhosis.[20] Outcomes were worse for Child-Pugh class C patients, with mortality in 4 of 6 (67%) and major postoperative complications in all 6 patients. Operative mortality was lower for Child-Pugh class A (1/10, 10%) and class B (2/11, 18%) patients, and major postoperative complications occurred in 22% of class A patients compared with 56% of class B patients. No mortality occurred in the 5 patients who had revascularization without the use of cardiopulmonary bypass, highlighting the need for alternative options with less risk for these patients. In anticipating risks, the Child-Pugh classification did predict mortality, but the MELD scores were not associated with hospital mortality.

These series highlight the risks associated with cardiac surgery in patients with cirrhosis. When possible, less invasive options including percutaneous coronary intervention and valvuloplasty should be considered. If surgery is necessary, significant risk of morbidity is present for all patients with cirrhosis, but the risk of mortality generally appears to be lower for Child-Pugh class A patients. Patients with Child-Pugh B and C cirrhosis, and their surgeons and anesthesiologists, must be aware of the significant risk of morbidity and mortality. Any patient with cirrhosis should be evaluated for candidacy for liver transplantation so that they are aware if transplantation is available to them in the event of decompensation in the postoperative setting. Case reports of cardiac surgery at the time of liver transplantation have been reported with variable outcomes, and the general aim for patients considering liver transplantation would be to achieve effective revascularization before transplantation.[44,45]

SUMMARY

Patients with chronic liver disease face greater risk of perioperative morbidity and mortality, and the evidence demonstrates that the risk is greater among patients with cirrhosis. The Child-Pugh score has consistently performed well in estimating relative risk or mortality, with the best outcomes among Child-Pugh class A patients and poor outcomes for patients with Child-Pugh class C cirrhosis. Variable results have been reported on the ability of the MELD score to predict surgical outcomes, but the combination of the Child-Pugh score and the MELD score provides access to more studies to guide patients and their surgeons regarding operative risks. When considering the risk for the individual patient, other factors to consider include other comorbidities, age, and ASA grade. For patients considering elective surgery, the procedure should be delayed to allow for a complete evaluation of the severity of liver disease and optimization of complications such as varices, ascites, and encephalopathy. Elective surgery should not be offered to patients with acute liver failure and alcoholic hepatitis. For patients with cirrhosis, the patient's candidacy for liver transplantation should be considered before the procedure in the event of postoperative decompensation.

REFERENCES

1. Friedman LS, Maddrey WC. Surgery in the patient with liver disease. Med Clin North Am 1987;71:453–76.
2. Walton B, Simpson BR, Strunin L, et al. Unexplained hepatitis following halothane. Br Med J 1976;1(6019):1171–6.
3. Nishiyama T, Fujimoto T, Hanaoka K. A comparison of liver function after hepatectomy in cirrhotic patients between sevoflurane and isoflurane in anesthesia with nitrous oxide and epidural block. Anesth Analg 2004;98(4):990–3.
4. Harville DD, Summerskill WH. Surgery in acute hepatitis. Causes and effects. JAMA 1963;184:257–61.
5. Greenwood SM, Leffler CT, Minkowitz S. The increased mortality rate of open liver biopsy in alcoholic hepatitis. Surg Gynecol Obstet 1972;134:600–4.
6. Bell RH Jr, Miyai K, Orloff MJ. Outcome in cirrhotic patients with acute alcoholic hepatitis after emergency portacaval shunt for bleeding esophageal varices. Am J Surg 1984;147:78–84.
7. Mikkelsen WP, Kern WH. The influence of acute hyaline necrosis on survival after emergency and elective portacaval shunt. Major Probl Clin Surg 1974;14:233–42.
8. Mikkelsen WP, Turrill FL, Kern WH. Acute hyaline necrosis of the liver. A surgical trap. Am J Surg 1968;116:266–72.
9. Powell-Jackson P, Greenway B, Williams R. Adverse effects of exploratory laparotomy in patients with unsuspected liver disease. Br J Surg 1982;69:449–51.
10. Kamath PS, Wiesner RH, Malinchoc M, et al. A model to predict survival in patients with end-stage liver disease. Hepatology 2001;33(2):464–70.
11. Wiesner R, Edwards E, Freeman R, et al. Model for end-stage liver disease (MELD) and allocation of donor livers. Gastroenterology 2003;124(1):91–6.
12. Perkins JS, Halldorson JB, Bakthavatsalam R, et al. Should liver transplantation in patients with model for end-stage liver disease scores < or = 14 be avoided? A decision analysis approach. Liver Transpl 2009;15(2):242–54.
13. Teh SH, Nagorney DM, Stevens SR, et al. Risk factors for mortality after surgery in patients with cirrhosis. Gastroenterology 2007;132:1261–9.
14. Farnsworth N, Fagan SP, Berger DH, et al. Child-Turcotte-Pugh versus MELD score as a predictor of outcome after elective and emergent surgery in cirrhotic patients. Am J Surg 2004;188:580–3.
15. Perkins L, Jeffries M, Patel T. Utility of preoperative scores for predicting morbidity after cholecystectomy in patients with cirrhosis. Clin Gastroenterol Hepatol 2004;2: 1123–8.
16. Befeler AS, Palmer DE, Hoffman M, et al. The safety of intra-abdominal surgery in patients with cirrhosis: model for end-stage liver disease score is superior to Child-Turcotte-Pugh classification in predicting outcome. Arch Surg 2005;140:650–4.
17. Telem DA, Schiano T, Goldstone R, et al. Factors that predict outcome of abdominal operations in patients with advanced cirrhosis. Clin Gastroenterol Hepatol 2010;8:451–7.
18. Neeff H, Mariaskin D, Spangenberg HC, et al. Perioperative mortality after non-hepatic general surgery in patients with liver cirrhosis: an analysis of 138 operations in the 2000s using Child and MELD scores. J Gastrointest Surg 2011;15:1–11.
19. Suman A, Barnes DS, Zein NN, et al. Predicting outcome after cardiac surgery in patients with cirrhosis: a comparison of Child-Pugh and MELD scores. Clin Gastroenterol Hepatol 2004;2:719–23.
20. Filsoufi F, Salzberg SP, Rahmanian PB, et al. Early and late outcome of cardiac surgery in patients with liver cirrhosis. Liver Transpl 2007;13(7):990–5.

21. Afdhal N, Giannini E, Tayyab GN, et al. Eltrombopag in chronic liver disease patients with thrombocytopenia undergoing elective invasive procedure: results from ELEVATE, a randomized clinical trial. J Hepatol 2010;52:S460.
22. Garcia-Tsao G, Sanyal AJ, Grace ND, et al. Prevention and management of gastroesophageal varices and variceal hemorrhage in cirrhosis. Hepatology 2007;46:922–38.
23. Runyon BA. Management of adult patients with ascites due to cirrhosis: an update. Hepatology 2009;49:2087–107.
24. Azoulay D, Buabse F, Damiano I, et al. Neoadjuvant transjugular intrahepatic portosystemic shunt: a solution for extrahepatic abdominal operation in cirrhotic patients with severe portal hypertension. J Am Coll Surg 2001;193:46–51.
25. Cárdenas A, Ginès P. Management of patients with cirrhosis awaiting liver transplantation. Gut 2011;60(3):412–21.
26. Ghany MG, Strader DB, Thomas DL, et al. Diagnosis, management, and treatment of hepatitis C: an update. Hepatology 2009;49(4):1335–74. No abstract available.
27. Ghany MG, Nelson DR, Strader DB, et al. An update on treatment of genotype 1 chronic hepatitis C virus infection: 2011 practice guideline by the American Association for the Study of Liver Diseases. Hepatology 2011;54(4):1433–44.
28. Garrison RN, Cryer HM, Howard DA, et al. Clarification of risk factors for abdominal operations in patients with hepatic cirrhosis. Ann Surg 1984;199:648–55.
29. Mansour A, Watson W, Shayani V, et al. Abdominal operations in patients with cirrhosis: still a major surgical challenge. Surgery 1997;122:730–5.
30. Clavien PA, Petrowsky H, DeOliveira ML, et al. Strategies for safer liver surgery and partial liver transplantation. N Engl J Med 2007;356:1545–59.
31. Bruix J. Treatment of hepatocellular carcinoma. Hepatology 1997;25:259–62.
32. Bruix J, Sherman M. Management of hepatocellular carcinoma: an update. Hepatology 2011;53(3):1020–2.
33. Mor E, Tur-Kaspa R, Sheiner P, et al. Treatment of hepatocellular carcinoma associated with cirrhosis in the era of liver transplantation. Ann Intern Med 1998;129:643–53.
34. Grazi GL, Ercolani G, Pierangeli F, et al. Improved results of liver resection for hepatocellular carcinoma on cirrhosis give the procedure added value. Ann Surg 2001;234:71–8.
35. Bruix J, Castells A, Bosch J, et al. Surgical resection of hepatocellular carcinoma in cirrhotic patients: prognostic value of preoperative portal pressure. Gastroenterology 1996;111:1018–22.
36. Llovet JM, Fuster J, Bruix J. Intention-to-treat analysis of surgical treatment for early hepatocellular carcinoma: resection versus transplantation. Hepatology 1999;30:1434–40.
37. Behrns KE, Tsiotos GG, DeSouza NF, et al. Hepatic steatosis as a potential risk factor for major hepatic resection. J Gastrointest Surg 1998;2(3):292–8.
38. Furuya CK Jr, de Oliveira CP, de Mello ES, et al. Effects of bariatric surgery on nonalcoholic fatty liver disease: preliminary findings after 2 years. J Gastroenterol Hepatol 2007;22(4):510–4.
39. Machado M, Marques-Vidal P, Cortez-Pinto H. Hepatic histology in obese patients undergoing bariatric surgery. J Hepatol 2006;45(4):600–6.
40. Dallal RM, Mattar SG, Lord JL, et al. Results of laparoscopic gastric bypass in patients with cirrhosis. Obes Surg 2004;14(1):47–53.
41. Brolin RE, Bradley LJ, Taliwal RV. Unsuspected cirrhosis discovered during elective obesity operations. Arch Surg 1998;133(1):84–8.

42. Angulo P, Keach JC, Batts KP, et al. Independent predictors of liver fibrosis in patients with nonalcoholic steatohepatitis. Hepatology 1999;30(6):1356–62.
43. Klemperer JD, Ko W, Krieger KH, et al. Cardiac operations in patients with cirrhosis. Ann Thorac Surg 1998;65:85–7.
44. Morris JJ, Hellman CL, Gawey BJ, et al. Case 3—1995. Three patients requiring both coronary artery bypass surgery and orthotopic liver transplantation. J Cardiothorac Vasc Anesth 1995;9:322–32.
45. Eckhoff DE, Frenette L, Sellers MT, et al. Combined cardiac surgery and liver transplantation. Liver Transpl 2001;7:60–1.

Is the Patient a Candidate for Liver Transplantation?

Alyson N. Fox, MD, MSCE[a,b,*], Robert S. Brown Jr, MD, MPH[a,c]

KEYWORDS

- Liver failure • Transplantation • Hepatic decompensation
- Liver disease • Transplant evaluation

Liver transplantation provides a lifesaving alternative to medical therapy for patients with a variety of liver diseases. The goal of liver transplantation is to prolong both the length and quality of life in a recipient. The major indications for liver transplantation include acute and irreversible liver failure, hepatic decompensation caused by chronic liver disease, primary hepatic malignancy, and metabolic disorders. Both the number of patients listed for liver transplantation and the number of liver transplants performed in the United States continues to grow annually. In 2010, approximately 11,350 patients were added to the national liver transplant waiting list and approximately 6000 were removed because of receipt of a deceased or living-donor transplant.[1] Despite growing numbers of patients listed for liver transplantation and the ability to successfully perform liver transplants, the availability of donor organs remains limited. Consideration for liver transplant involves a rigorous evaluation process that is time consuming, expensive, and potentially dangerous when it includes invasive testing. With donor organs remaining a scarce resource and the process of transplant evaluation being so complex, it is critical to distinguish the patients who will most benefit from transplantation.

HISTORICAL PERSPECTIVE

In the last 50 years, liver transplantation has emerged as a life-prolonging technique for patients suffering from end-stage liver disease. The first liver transplant was performed in 1963, but it was not until the 1980s that liver transplantation became a common procedure. Advances in surgical technique, immunosuppressive medications, and prevention of postoperative infections allowed liver transplantation to

[a] Center for Liver Disease and Transplantation, New York Presbyterian Hospital, New York, NY, USA; [b] Weill Cornell Medical Center, 1305 York Avenue New York, NY 10021, USA; [c] Columbia University College of Physicians and Surgeons, 622 West 168th Street, New York, NY 10032, USA
* Corresponding author. Weill Cornell Medical Center, 1305 York Avenue New York, NY 10021, USA.
E-mail address: alf9011@med.cornell.edu

Clin Liver Dis 16 (2012) 435–448
doi:10.1016/j.cld.2012.03.014

become a life-sustaining possibility.[2] During the past 20 years, the expertise with transplant surgery and transplant medicine has evolved to the point at which there are currently more than 6000 liver transplants performed annually in the United States.

DETERMINING THE SEVERITY OF ILLNESS AND ORGAN ALLOCATION: FROM CHILD-TURCOTTE-PUGH TO THE MODEL FOR END-STAGE LIVER DISEASE SCORE

A key concept in deciding whether a patient is an appropriate candidate for transplantation is determining the severity of illness as it relates to prognosis. In those under consideration for transplantation because of chronic liver diseases, the Child-Turcotte-Pugh (CTP) score and the Model for End-Stage Liver Disease (MELD) score have been instrumental in helping clinicians gauge mortality risk and necessity of transplantation.

The CTP score takes into account the presence of hepatic encephalopathy, ascites, the serum bilirubin, albumin, and increase in prothrombin time to more than the control values.[3] Between 1 and 3 points are assigned for each degree of variation among these 5 parameters and, based on the total number of points assigned, an individual is classified as class A (5–6), B (7–9), or C (10–15). Child class A represents compensated disease with better prognosis and class C represents severely decompensated disease with poor prognosis. Before 2002, the CTP score was used to grade severity of illness and prioritization for the liver transplant waiting list. Under this system, patients were listed for liver transplantation using a status code (1, 2a, 2b, 3) based on their CTP class and whether they were at home, in the hospital, or in the intensive care unit. Priority was given to the patients with longer waiting time within each status. Because each status was broad, there were many patients in each group and thus waiting time was a significant driver of transplant priority. Thus, under this system, it was common for available organs to go to people whose liver disease was less decompensated (eg, a Child-Pugh score of 11 vs 14) if they had been on the waiting list longer. A more severity-based system was clearly needed. In addition, because the CTP score incorporates subjective data into its calculation (ie, ascites and encephalopathy), a more objective disease severity index was sought to make the system more reproducible between centers.

The MELD score is a mathematically derived score based on measurement of the serum bilirubin, International Normalization Ratio, and creatinine. Because its calculation is based on biochemical parameters that are increased in the presence of liver disease, the MELD score increases concomitantly with increasing severity of liver disease. The MELD scoring system was initially developed to predict survival after elective transjugular intrahepatic shunt placement in patients with end-stage liver disease.[4] It was later validated to predict survival in those with advanced liver disease, including those on the transplant waiting list, and in February 2002 was adopted by the United Network for Organ Sharing (UNOS) as the preferred scoring system for organ allocation.[5] In this system, waiting time is deemphasized because it is not carried forward as the MELD increases and is only used to break ties at a given MELD score. The cornerstone of MELD-based allocation ensures that those with the highest scores (the sickest patients) receive organs first despite competing factors such as cause of liver disease or list waiting time. After the introduction of the MELD allocation system, analyses of list dynamics revealed a decreased waiting time, decreased list size (6% reduction), decreased list registration (12% reduction between February 2002 and February 2003), and increased rates of transplantation (6% increase).[6,7] It also reduced waiting list mortality without adversely affecting posttransplant survival, thus increasing the survival benefit of transplantation. Based on these results, the implementation of the MELD system has objectively improved the state of liver transplantation in the United States.

WHO BENEFITS FROM LIVER TRANSPLANTATION?

Simply stated, a patient needs to be sick enough to derive a benefit from transplantation, but well enough to survive a complex surgical procedure. During its advanced stages, cirrhosis is associated with a high rate of morbidity and mortality. After experiencing a first decompensation event (**Box 1**), prognosis is poor.[8] Thus, expectant medical management of those with cirrhosis in an attempt to prevent complications is paramount. A higher MELD score connotes more severe illness, and the MELD score is known to accurately predict 3-month mortality in those awaiting transplantation.[9] It is therefore reasonable that those whose mortality without a transplant exceeds mortality with a transplant are the ideal candidates for transplantation. A pivotal study by Merion and colleagues[10] helped to better define the survival benefit of liver transplantation. By comparing the mortality between those listed and those transplanted, the investigators were able to show that, at low MELD scores, undergoing transplantation is associated with a significant risk of death. A MELD score of 15 to 17 represented a transition point beyond which there was a survival benefit at 1 year observed with transplantation. With a longer time horizon (3–5 years), all but those with a MELD score less than 10 benefit from transplantation.

MINIMAL LISTING CRITERIA

Before the implementation of the MELD score as the method of liver allocation, the liver transplant community held a meeting in 1997 to compose minimal listing criteria for transplantation. It was determined that listed patients should have a predicted 1-year survival rate without transplantation of 90% or less. Based on the published data at the time, the patient cohort meeting these criteria were those patients with Child-Pugh scores of 7 or greater.[11] In December of 2003, another meeting was held to analyze the patterns in organ allocation after the first 18 months of MELD-based allocation.[12] Among the topics discussed was the issue of minimum listing criteria. With the practice of minimum listing as CTP score greater than or equal to 7, a considerable percentage of patients meeting the criteria had low MELD scores. At that time, Organ Procurement and Transplantation Network (OPTN) data indicated that approximately 17% of transplants were occurring in those with MELD scores of 7 to 15 at the time of removal from the list. However, there was great variability based on

Box 1
Complications of liver disease warranting transplant evaluation

Refractory ascites

Hepatic encephalopathy

Portal hypertensive bleeding

Hepatocellular malignancy

Pruritus

Recurrent cholangitis

Hepatopulmonary syndrome

Portopulmonary hypertension

region. Although the group recognized that the 18-month data suggested that there were likely sufficient data to support the establishment of a minimal listing MELD score, no such criteria were established.

Despite the lack of national guidelines on this issue, many centers have established a MELD cut point, at less than which they consider patients too early for transplant consideration. However the MELD score may not accurately portray an individual patient's severity of illness because the MELD score lacks subjective information that can strongly affect quality of life, particularly complications of portal hypertension. In cases in which the calculated MELD is low but the patient has severe encephalopathy, uncontrolled ascites, or frequent gastrointestinal bleeding, consideration is typically given to listing despite a low MELD score. The American Association for the Study of Liver Diseases (AASLD) guidelines recommend that patients with cirrhosis should be referred for transplant evaluation when they develop a decompensation or when they reach a CTP score of greater than or equal to 7 or MELD score greater than or equal to 10.[13]

THE EVALUATION PROCESS

The evaluation process for liver transplantation seeks to define the patients who will obtain the most benefit from transplantation, have the best chance for postoperative recovery and survival, and who will be good stewards for the limited resource (the organ graft) they receive.[14] The process involves intense medical, psychiatric, social, and financial screening to identify those who might have contraindications to solid organ transplantation (**Table 1**). Once the screening is completed, a committee, usually composed of hepatologists, transplants surgeons, transplant coordinators, psychiatrists, and social workers, convenes to determine who is most appropriate for listing based on both objective and subjective measures. When a person is deemed suitable for transplantation, they are placed on the national UNOS waiting list.

INDICATIONS FOR LIVER TRANSPLANTATION AND SPECIAL CONSIDERATIONS BY DIAGNOSIS

Hepatitis C

Cirrhosis caused by chronic hepatitis C infection remains the leading indication for liver transplantation in the United States (**Fig. 1**, **Table 2**). Without curative treatment before transplantation, nearly all grafts become reinfected immediately after transplantation.[15] In the posttransplant setting, hepatitis C virus (HCV) infection seems to be accelerated, such that those transplanted for HCV experience high rates of graft dysfunction and loss with decreased survival compared with those transplanted for other indications.[16,17] To prevent graft compromise, consideration should be given to treating those with compensated disease who are awaiting transplantation with modified interferon and ribavirin dosing, especially if the genotype is favorable.[18] This strategy may be helpful to prevent graft infection; however, treatment in this setting may be poorly tolerated. Once transplantation has occurred, consideration should be given to antiviral therapy, although it is associated with its own set of unique challenges in the posttransplantation setting.

Hepatitis B

Before the use of hepatitis B immune globulin (HBIG) as immunoprophylaxis after transplantation for chronic hepatitis B, recurrence of hepatitis B virus (HBV) in the liver allograft occurred in up to 80%, and was usually complicated by graft dysfunction and death. Because of these outcomes, HBV was initially viewed as a contraindication to

Table 1
Components of evaluation for liver transplantation

Component	Details
Medical evaluation	Review of medical records History and physical examination by transplant hepatologist and transplant surgeon
Laboratory evaluation	Electrolytes, liver function tests, complete blood count, coagulation studies, hepatitis serologies, markers for autoimmune, inherited and metabolic liver diseases, blood typing with antibody screen, RPR, EBV, CMV, HIV testing, thyroid function studies
Radiology	Abdominal sonogram with Doppler evaluation Contrast-enhanced abdominal imaging Bone density scan CT scan of the chest (if HCC)
Cardiac evaluation	Electrocardiogram Echocardiogram (with agitated saline injection) Nuclear stress test (if age >45 y or cardiac risk factors are present) Coronary catheterization (if stress test is abnormal or high risk for cardiac disease) Right heart catheterization (if increased pulmonary pressures on noninvasive studies) Cardiology consultation
Pulmonary evaluation	PPD testing Chest radiograph Pulmonary function testing Room air arterial blood gas Shunt fraction study if evidence of intrapulmonary shunt Pulmonary consultation
Neurologic evaluation	Carotid Doppler if age >60 y Neuroimaging and neurology consultation if history of neurologic disorder
Age-appropriate cancer screening	PAP smear Mammogram Colonoscopy PSA
Psychosocial evaluation	Psychiatry consultation Social work consultation Financial counselor consultation Nutritionist consultation

Abbreviations: CMV, cytomegalovirus; CT, computed tomography; EBV, Epstein-Barr virus; HCC, hepatocellular carcinoma; HIV, human immunodeficiency virus; PAP, Papanicolaou; PPD, purified protein derivative; PSA, prostate-specific antigen; RPR, rapid plasma reagin.

transplantation. Control of the virus before transplantation is critical in preventing graft reinfection. With the availability of antiviral medications with a high genetic barrier to resistance, suppression of the virus before transplantation is feasible. The combination of HBIG with oral antivirals has allowed HBV-infected patients to go from having the poorest posttransplantation outcomes to having survival rates among the best of all transplant recipients.[19] With the use of HBIG and oral nucleos(t)ide therapy, the 5-year graft survival for those transplanted for HBV is 85% and retransplantation for recurrent HBV cirrhosis is rare.

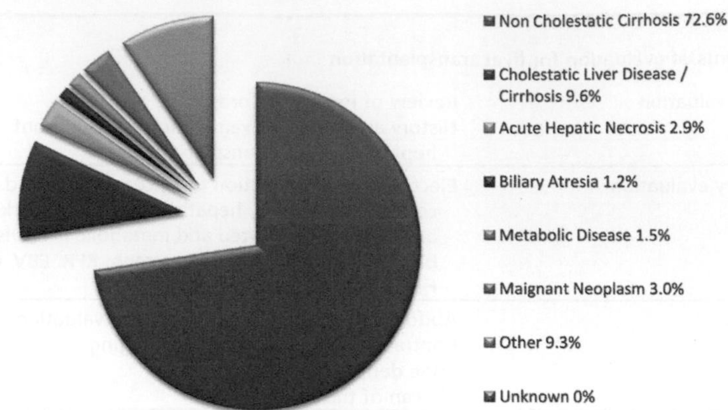

Fig. 1. Distribution of Diagnoses US Waitlist Characteristics, 2008. (*Courtesy of* the US Department of Health and Human Services. Available at: http://optn.transplant.hrsa.gov.)

Alcohol-related Liver Disease

Alcohol-related liver disease is the most common cause of cirrhosis in the United States. Despite this, it is not the leading indication for transplantation, because active alcohol use represents an absolute contraindication to transplantation, and because, in those with decompensation caused by alcohol-related liver disease, abstinence can reverse the severity of illness such that transplantation may be avoided. In those with a history of excessive alcohol use, most centers require a period of documented abstinence before consideration of transplantation. Typically, many centers require this period to be at least 6 months in duration.[20] Although a time frame of 6 months is not based on rigorous well-controlled data, it is known that longer abstinence periods predict lower rates of alcohol recidivism. In addition, the rationale behind a 6-month sobriety period is that 6 months may be adequate time to allow for hepatic recovery if the alcoholic injury is reversible with abstinence, which could prevent an unnecessary transplant in a patient who will recover without the need for transplantation. This period also allows those at risk for return to drinking to be identified and allows intensive therapy and counseling. In those who can achieve the period of abstinence, a transplant team may rely heavily on a social worker, counselor, or psychiatry consultant and a structured rehabilitation program to maximize the likelihood of a successful intervention. Although recidivism after transplantation is common (~30%), problem drinking is rare, and recurrent alcohol use rarely causes significant graft dysfunction and is not associated with decreased survival.[21]

Cholestatic Liver Disease

Primary biliary cirrhosis (PBC) and primary sclerosing cholangitis (PSC) are the 2 adult-onset cholestatic disorders that commonly lead to end-stage liver disease requiring transplantation. PBC is associated with all of the complications typical of cirrhosis and, in addition, patients may suffer from xanthelasma, metabolic bone disease, and intractable pruritus. The pruritus that accompanies PBC can be so detrimental to quality of life that additional MELD exception points can be assigned when the native MELD score is low. The Mayo Risk Score is a model developed in the late 1980s that incorporates patient age, total bilirubin, serum albumin, prothrombin time, and severity of edema to predict survival in patients with PBC.[22] Although this

Table 2 Medical conditions for which liver transplantation is indicated	
Viral	Hepatitis C Hepatitis B
Autoimmune liver disease	—
Alcohol-related liver disease	—
Inherited/metabolic liver diseases	Hereditary hemochromatosis α-1-Antitrypsin deficiency Wilson disease Nonalcoholic fatty liver disease Tyrosinemia Type IV glycogen storage disease Neonatal hemochromatosis Amyloidosis Hyperoxaluria Urea cycle defects Amino acid defects
Cholestatic liver disease	Primary biliary cirrhosis Primary sclerosing cholangitis Biliary atresia Alagille syndrome Progressive familial intrahepatic cholestasis Cystic fibrosis Bile duct loss
Malignancy	Hepatocellular carcinoma Cholangiocarcinoma Fibrolamellar carcinoma Epithelioid hemangioendothelioma Hepatoblastoma Metastatic neuroendocrine tumor
Polycystic liver disease	—
Vascular disorder	Budd-Chiari syndrome
Fulminant hepatic failure	—
Retransplantation	—

risk score is not used as an allocation tool for transplantation, it can be helpful to predict which patients should be considered for transplant evaluation. Based on the minimal listing criteria mentioned earlier, it has been suggested that patients with a Mayo Risk Score that denotes greater than 10% 1-year mortality risk should be sent for transplant evaluation.[11] Outcomes of transplantation for PBC are good, with survival rates at 1 year, 5 years, and 10 years of 83%, 78%, and 67% respectively.[23] Compared with those not undergoing transplantation, the survival benefit of transplantation for PBC is clear. PBC is a condition that can recur after transplantation, but it is unclear whether or not this affects survival.[23]

Severity of illness from PSC has also been modeled with a Mayo Risk Score by using age, bilirubin, albumin, aspartate aminotransferase, and history of variceal bleeding to determine survival.[24] Patients with PSC are another group who may be at a disadvantage for transplantation with MELD-based allocation. PSC can be associated with recurrent bouts of cholangitis and those episodes can be used to petition for MELD exception points as a way to augment the native MELD score. Because up to 90% of those with PSC may be affected by inflammatory bowel disease (IBD) and the risk of developing colorectal neoplasia in those with PSC is even greater than with IBD alone, it is critical that these patients undergo routine endoscopy before and after transplantation to detect gastrointestinal malignancy.[25]

Inherited/Metabolic Liver Disease

α-1-Antitrypsin deficiency, hereditary hemochromatosis, Wilson disease, and nonalcoholic fatty liver disease (NAFLD) are all causes of cirrhosis and can lead to end-stage liver disease. This cluster of diseases is marked by systemic involvement that can occasionally preclude safe liver transplantation. α-1-Antitrypsin deficiency is a cause of panlobular pulmonary emphysema and liver disease in those with the PiZZ phenotype. Both acute and chronic liver disease can develop in childhood or adulthood. In adults, liver disease typically does not present until the fifth decade. Because of the coexistent lung disease seen in this condition, a thorough pulmonary evaluation should be mandated during transplant evaluation. Both adult and pediatric patients undergoing liver transplantation for α-1-antitrypsin deficiency have excellent outcomes with 1-year, 3-year, and 5-year survival reported at 89%, 85%, and 83% respectively for adults and 92%, 90%, and 90% in children.[26]

Hereditary hemochromatosis (HH) is a disorder of iron overload that results in hepatic damage and cirrhosis. Survival after transplantation for HH is low compared with other causes, with 1-year, 3-year, and 5-year survival rates of 64%, 48%, and 34%.[27] These low survival rates may be attributed to increased rates of infectious and cardiac complications seen in this population.[28,29] It is therefore critical that patients with HH undergo a rigorous cardiac assessment before transplantation to identify potential problems.

Wilson disease is a rare disorder that results in abnormal copper accumulation in the liver, brain, and eye. Patients with this disorder can present with either chronic liver disease or an acute fulminant disease. Liver transplantation in the fulminant setting universally requires transplantation, because most patients do not recover hepatic function. Survival after transplantation is excellent, with one series showing 1-year, 3-year, and 5-year survival at 89.1%, 82.9%, and 75.6%, respectively.[30] Because neuropsychiatric symptoms are found in one-third of patients with Wilson disease, it is important to have both a comprehensive neurologic and psychiatric assessment before transplantation, because patients with neuropsychiatric symptoms can have decreased survival after transplantation.[30]

A diagnosis of NAFLD accounted for 1.2% of liver transplants in 2001 and has risen steadily such that, in 2009, it accounted for 9.7% of all transplants.[31] Survival after transplantation is comparable with survival for other indications. Because NAFLD is associated with the metabolic syndrome, it is crucial to carefully screen patients for conditions such as cardiovascular disease, renal disease, insulin resistance, and hyperlipidemia during the transplant evaluation, because these conditions are associated with an independent risk of mortality.

Autoimmune Liver Disease

Autoimmune hepatitis that is unrecognized or unresponsive to treatment can develop into progressive liver disease resulting in cirrhosis and decompensation. Liver transplant outcomes for autoimmune liver disease are favorable; however, age at transplantation greater than 50 years has been associated with impaired survival.[32] After surgery, episodes of acute cellular rejection are more common in those with autoimmune liver disease.[33] Because autoantibodies persist after transplantation, recurrent disease is known to occur and, although usually treatable with augmentation of immunosuppression, can lead to progressive graft dysfunction and affect survival.[34,35]

Vascular Disorders of the Liver

Disorders such as Budd-Chiari syndrome or sinusoidal obstruction syndrome (formerly known as veno-occlusive disease) can result in liver failure when they occur rapidly. Although shunt procedures can be temporizing, many patents have progressive liver disease and require transplantation. Because most patients with Budd-Chiari syndrome have underlying hematologic disorders, they can be at risk for recurrent thrombosis despite transplantation and usually require lifelong anticoagulation. Transplant survival outcomes vary, with some groups reporting 5-year survival of 65% and some reporting better rates at 88%.[36,37] Aggressive anticoagulation therapy after transplantation may decrease thrombotic complications and enhance survival.

Fulminant Hepatic Failure

Fulminant hepatic failure (FHF) is the rapid development of encephalopathy, coagulopathy, and jaundice in someone without known preexisting liver disease. Acetaminophen toxicity accounts for approximately half of all causes of FHF in the United States.[38] Patients can rapidly progress to a state of critical illness. Patients with this condition from any cause should be referred for liver transplant evaluation emergently, because these cases are best managed at a transplant center with expertise in dealing with the complications of FHF. Although some patents recover hepatic function, some causes of FHF are uniformly fatal if transplantation does not occur. There are several tools to help predict which patients will recover and which will ultimately require transplantation, such as the Kings College Criteria, Clichy Criteria, and, more recently, the MELD score.[39–42] Patients with FHF are given a special UNOS status 1, which gives them priority over all forms of chronic liver disease. This status allows rapid transplantation before developing cerebral edema. Although these prognostic models can be helpful, clinical judgment should take precedence. Transplant outcomes for FHF are excellent, and exceed outcomes for those transplanted for chronic liver diseases.[43] Transplants for FHF account for less than 10% of all transplants done annually in the United States.

Hepatocellular Carcinoma

Hepatocellular carcinoma (HCC) has become an increasingly important indication for liver transplantation. A landmark study by Mazzaferro and colleagues[44] showed that the 4-year survival after transplantation was 75% and the recurrence-free survival was 83% if the intrahepatic tumors were of a certain size and quantity, termed the Milan Criteria (1 lesion ≤5 cm, or 2–3 lesions each ≤3 cm). Patients diagnosed with HCC who are within the Milan Criteria are automatically assigned a MELD priority score of 22. This score increases every 3 months until the patient is either offered a liver, suffers a complication, or until they progress beyond the Milan Criteria. Frequently, these patients have low calculated MELD scores and exception points afford them the chance to be competitive for liver allocation before their malignancy worsens, which would preclude them from transplantation. When patients listed with HCC exception scores of 22 or higher are compared with the cohort of patients with calculated MELD scores in the same range, the patients with HCC have higher rates of transplantation, lower rates of dropout, and receive livers more rapidly once listed.[45]

All patients with HCC confined to the liver should be evaluated for transplantation, because there are increasing options for those with tumors that exceed the Milan Criteria. It has been shown that extending the size limits beyond the Milan Criteria may be possible without sacrificing survival outcome.[46] However, these patients are not given additional MELD priority and it can be difficult to access a deceased donor graft. Likewise, tumors beyond the Milan Criteria may be eligible for downstaging with the ultimate goal of transplantation.[47] Patients successfully downstaged to within the Milan Criteria can petition for MELD exception points.

Cholangiocarcinoma

Early experience with liver transplantation for cholangiocarcinoma (CCA) was associated with high recurrence rates and poor survival.[48] Only recently, under a specific protocol requiring neoadjuvant chemotherapy and radiation (either external beam or brachytherapy), have patients with stage I and II hilar CCAs achieved 1-year, 3-year, and 5-year survival rates of 92%, 82%, and 82%.[49] Currently, only select US centers offer transplantation for CCA under these highly specialized protocols with high rates of dropout on the waiting list. However, early referral to one of those centers for transplant consideration is warranted in those with limited stage disease.

CONTRAINDICATIONS TO LIVER TRANSPLANTATION

The contraindications for liver transplantation are divided into those that are absolute and those that represent relative contraindications (**Table 3**). In general, contraindications are factors that either make the surgical risk prohibitive or the likelihood of long-term survival or quality of life after transplantation low.

Absolute Contraindications

Because the goal of liver transplantation is to prolong survival, it is critical to select recipients who have an acceptable chance of survival during and after transplantation. On its own, end-stage liver disease can be debilitating and can cause severe systemic illness. It is therefore crucial to exclude those who have a high mortality resulting from conditions other than liver disease. Severe cardiopulmonary disease or other severe comorbidities pose a risk that is independent of liver disease. Patients with such conditions are at high risk from operative and postoperative death. Transplantation is contraindicated in those with uncontrolled hepatocellular carcinoma, because rates of recurrence are high. For those with extrahepatic malignancies, most centers require low projected 5-year rates of recurrence, and some a period of recurrence-free survival, before transplantation. Once on immunosuppression after transplantation, patients are at a higher risk for developing de novo malignancy and may be at increased risk for recurrent malignancy.[50]

Table 3
Contraindications to liver transplantation

Absolute Contraindications to Transplant	Relative Contraindications to Transplant
Severe cardiopulmonary disease	Advanced age
Other outstanding comorbidity	Obesity
Hepatic malignancy with vascular invasion or beyond transplantable criterion	Psychiatric disease
Extrahepatic malignancy	HIV infection
Active infection	Surgical challenges: prior extensive intra-abdominal surgeries, extensive vascular thrombosis
Active substance abuse	
Poor psychosocial support	
Poor compliance	

Active, uncontrolled infection, particularly with resistant bacteria or fungi, at the time of transplantation is associated with poor survival.

Psychosocial contraindications to transplantation are as important as medical contraindications. Patients being considered for transplantation need to have an adequate psychosocial support system, because the medical illness and transplantation process can be stressful. In addition, a care partner other than the medical team is necessary to provide care and support during the postoperative period. Because many patients with liver disease have a history of significant substance abuse, strict abstinence from addictive drugs and alcohol is of paramount importance. Abuse of any substance, even legal prescription drugs, is prohibited. Some centers require abstinence from smoking cigarettes as well. In addition, poor compliance with medical advice and instructions represents a contraindication to transplantation. Because organs represent a scarce resource, it is critical that recipients adhere to immunosuppression regimens and, most often, pretransplant behaviors portend posttransplant behaviors.

Relative Contraindications

Relative contraindications to transplantation are often not based on data and can vary widely from center to center. Relative contraindications can sometimes be corrected. The evaluation of patients with advanced age is commonly faced by most transplant centers. As the population ages, many older individuals present with indications for transplantation. Although no firm age cutoff exists, there is heightened concern to transplanting patients older than 70 years, because mortality and risk for malignancy are higher. More important perhaps than chronologic age is physiologic age, which is relevant when examining patients' overall risk and benefit from transplant. Obesity is a growing epidemic and many patients seen for liver transplant evaluation are overweight or obese by body mass index (BMI) classification. Analysis has shown that the 1-year and 2-year mortality after transplantation are significantly higher in those with morbid obesity, and 5-year mortality was significantly higher both in those defined as severely obese and morbidly obese, owing to increased adverse cardiovascular events.[51] Based on these data, many centers have established BMI criteria for listing. A history of psychiatric disease is not a firm contraindication for transplantation, but those with preexisting psychiatric illness need to be under the care of a mental health professional and have their disease well controlled before being considered for transplantation.

Human immunodeficiency virus (HIV) infection was previously considered an absolute contraindication to transplantation, because there was great concern about the tolerability of combined effect of viral and medication-induced immune suppression. With the advent of highly active antiretroviral (HAART) medications, liver transplantation in the HIV population has become an acceptable procedure. In the last decade, transplantation of HIV-positive patients has become increasingly prevalent, although total numbers still remain low (0.3% of total liver transplants in the United States between 1999 and 2008).[52] Although cutoff values for CD4 count targets may vary between centers, it is generally accepted that the HIV viral load should be fully suppressed. Disease-specific issues such as multidrug-resistant disease, opportunistic infection, and HIV-associated malignancies or wasting still represent contraindications to transplantation. Patients with HIV should be referred to a transplant center with expertise in managing the specific issues related to the management of HIV infection both before and after transplantation.

In addition, complicated surgical anatomy can represent a relative contraindication to transplantation. Those with prior abdominal surgeries and with extensive portal/

mesenteric vascular thromboses can present a considerable surgical challenge. Contrast-enhanced cross-sectional imaging studies can be valuable in providing a road map and may facilitate anticipation of using vascular grafts or alternative techniques. Close evaluation by the transplanting surgeon is advised.

Delisting

Despite extensive work-up before transplantation, those affected by complications related to cirrhosis or end-stage liver disease often have a complicated course. Once listed for transplantation, patients should be regularly evaluated by the transplant team to assess for changes in their medical and psychosocial circumstances. As with fulminant liver failure, many potential recipients improve and do not require transplantation. In some, the condition worsens to the point at which the risk of transplantation outweighs the benefit. In the latter group, consideration should be given to temporary or permanent delisting.

SUMMARY

Identifying whether someone is a good candidate for liver transplantation is a complex process that requires a team approach. There are several medical and psychosocial considerations involved, each of which is thoroughly explored during the evaluation process. Both the indications and contraindications to transplant can change over time, reflecting advances in understanding of and ability to treat certain disease processes. Ultimately, the goal of liver transplantation remains to provide a survival benefit to those with acute or chronic liver diseases.

REFERENCES

1. Based on OPTN data as of October 7. Available at: http://optn.transplant.hrsa.gov. Accessed October 7, 2011.
2. Ahmed A, Keeffe EB. Current indications and contraindications for liver transplantation. Clin Liver Dis 2007;11(2):227–47.
3. Pugh RN, Murray-Lyon IM, Dawson JL, et al. Transection of the oesophagus for bleeding oesophageal varices. Br J Surg 1973;60(8):646–9.
4. Malinchoc M, Kamath PS, Gordon FD, et al. A model to predict poor survival in patients undergoing transjugular intrahepatic portosystemic shunts. Hepatology 2000;31(4):864–71.
5. Kamath PS, Wiesner RH, Malinchoc M, et al. A model to predict survival in patients with end-stage liver disease. Hepatology 2001;33(2):464–70.
6. Hanto DW, Fishbein TM, Pinson CW, et al. Liver and intestine transplantation: summary analysis, 1994-2003. Am J Transplant 2005;5(4 Pt 2):916–33.
7. Martin AP, Bartels M, Hauss J, et al. Overview of the MELD score and the UNOS adult liver allocation system. Transplant Proc 2007;39(10):3169–74.
8. D'Amico G, Garcia-Tsao G, Pagliaro L. Natural history and prognostic indicators of survival in cirrhosis: a systematic review of 118 studies. J Hepatol 2006;44(1): 217–31.
9. Wiesner R, Edwards E, Freeman R, et al. Model for End-Stage Liver Disease (MELD) and allocation of donor livers. Gastroenterology 2003;124(1):91–6.
10. Merion RM, Schaubel DE, Dykstra DM, et al. The survival benefit of liver transplantation. Am J Transplant 2005;5(2):307–13.
11. Lucey MR, Brown KA, Everson GT, et al. Minimal criteria for placement of adults on the liver transplant waiting list: a report of a national conference organized by

the American Society of Transplant Physicians and the American Association for the Study of Liver Diseases. Liver Transpl Surg 1997;3(6):628–37.
12. Olthoff KM, Brown RS Jr, Delmonico FL, et al. Summary report of a national conference: evolving concepts in liver allocation in the MELD and PELD era. December 8, 2003, Washington, DC, USA. Liver Transpl 2004;10(10 Suppl 2):A6–22.
13. Murray KF, Carithers RL Jr. AASLD practice guidelines: evaluation of the patient for liver transplantation. Hepatology 2005;41(6):1407–32.
14. O'Leary JG, Lepe R, Davis GL. Indications for liver transplantation. Gastroenterology 2008;134:1764–76.
15. Garcia-Retortillo M, Forns X, Feliu A, et al. Hepatitis C virus kinetics during and immediately after liver transplantation. Hepatology 2002;35(3):680–7.
16. Forman LM, Lewis JD, Berlin JA, et al. The association between hepatitis C infection and survival after orthotopic liver transplantation. Gastroenterology 2002; 122(4):889–96.
17. Berenguer M, Ferrell L, Watson J, et al. HCV-related fibrosis progression following liver transplantation: increase in recent years. J Hepatol 2000;32(4):673–84.
18. Everson GT, Trotter J, Forman L, et al. Treatment of advanced hepatitis C with a low accelerating dosage regimen of antiviral therapy. Hepatology 2005;42(2):255–62.
19. Kim WR, Poterucha JJ, Kremers WK, et al. Outcome of liver transplantation for hepatitis B in the United States. Liver Transpl 2004;10(8):968–74.
20. Everhart JE, Beresford TP. Liver transplantation for alcoholic liver disease: a survey of transplantation programs in the United States. Liver Transpl Surg 1997;3(3):220–6.
21. Lim JK, Keeffe EB. Liver transplantation for alcoholic liver disease: current concepts and length of sobriety. Liver Transpl 2004;10(10 Suppl 2):S31–8.
22. Dickson ER, Grambsch PM, Fleming TR, et al. Prognosis in primary biliary cirrhosis: model for decision making. Hepatology 1989;10(1):1–7.
23. Liermann Garcia RF, Evangelista Garcia C, McMaster P, et al. Transplantation for primary biliary cirrhosis: retrospective analysis of 400 patients in a single center. Hepatology 2001;33(1):22–7.
24. Kim WR, Therneau TM, Wiesner RH, et al. A revised natural history model for primary sclerosing cholangitis. Mayo Clin Proc 2000;75(7):688–94.
25. Soetikno RM, Lin OS, Heidenreich PA, et al. Increased risk of colorectal neoplasia in patients with primary sclerosing cholangitis and ulcerative colitis: a meta-analysis. Gastrointest Endosc 2002;56(1):48–54.
26. Kemmer N, Kaiser T, Zacharias V, et al. Alpha-1-antitrypsin deficiency: outcomes after liver transplantation. Transplant Proc 2008;40(5):1492–4.
27. Kowdley KV, Brandhagen DJ, Gish RG, et al. Survival after liver transplantation in patients with hepatic iron overload: the national hemochromatosis transplant registry. Gastroenterology 2005;129(2):494–503.
28. Brandhagen DJ, Alvarez W, Therneau TM, et al. Iron overload in cirrhosis-HFE genotypes and outcome after liver transplantation. Hepatology 2000;31(2):456–60.
29. Tung BY, Farrell FJ, McCashland TM, et al. Long-term follow-up after liver transplantation in patients with hepatic iron overload. Liver Transpl Surg 1999;5(5):369–74.
30. Medici V, Mirante VG, Fassati LR, et al. Liver transplantation for Wilson's disease: the burden of neurological and psychiatric disorders. Liver Transpl 2005;11(9):1056–63.
31. Charlton MR, Burns JM, Pedersen RA, et al. Frequency and outcomes of liver transplantation for nonalcoholic steatohepatitis in the United States. Gastroenterology 2011;141(4):1249–53.
32. Schramm C, Bubenheim M, Adam R, et al. Primary liver transplantation for autoimmune hepatitis: a comparative analysis of the European Liver Transplant Registry. Liver Transpl 2010;16(4):461–9.

33. Vogel A, Heinrich E, Bahr MJ, et al. Long-term outcome of liver transplantation for autoimmune hepatitis. Clin Transplant 2004;18(1):62–9.
34. Prados E, Cuervas-Mons V, de la Mata M, et al. Outcome of autoimmune hepatitis after liver transplantation. Transplantation 1998;66(12):1645–50.
35. Ratziu V, Samuel D, Sebagh M, et al. Long-term follow-up after liver transplantation for autoimmune hepatitis: evidence of recurrence of primary disease. J Hepatol 1999;30(1):131–41.
36. Cruz E, Ascher NL, Roberts JP, et al. High incidence of recurrence and hematologic events following liver transplantation for Budd-Chiari syndrome. Clin Transplant 2005;19(4):501–6.
37. Chinnakotla S, Klintmalm GB, Kim P, et al. Long-term follow-up of liver transplantation for Budd-Chiari syndrome with antithrombotic therapy based on the etiology. Transplantation 2011;92(3):341–5.
38. Larson AM, Polson J, Fontana RJ, et al. Acetaminophen-induced acute liver failure: results of a United States multicenter, prospective study. Hepatology 2005;42(6):1364–72.
39. O'Grady JG, Alexander GJ, Hayllar KM, et al. Early indicators of prognosis in fulminant hepatic failure. Gastroenterology 1989;97(2):439–45.
40. Katoonizadeh A, Decaestecker J, Wilmer A, et al. MELD score to predict outcome in adult patients with non-acetaminophen-induced acute liver failure. Liver Int 2007;27(3):329–34.
41. Schmidt LE, Larsen FS. MELD score as a predictor of liver failure and death in patients with acetaminophen-induced liver injury. Hepatology 2007;45(3):789–96.
42. Bernuau J, Goudeau A, Poynard T, et al. Multivariate analysis of prognostic factors in fulminant hepatitis B. Hepatology 1986;6(4):648–51.
43. Ascher NL, Lake JR, Emond JC, et al. Liver transplantation for fulminant hepatic failure. Arch Surg 1993;128(6):677–82.
44. Mazzaferro V, Regalia E, Doci R, et al. Liver transplantation for the treatment of small hepatocellular carcinomas in patients with cirrhosis. N Engl J Med 1996; 334(11):693–9.
45. Freeman RB Jr, Steffick DE, Guidinger MK, et al. Liver and intestine transplantation in the United States, 1997-2006. Am J Transplant 2008;8(4 Pt 2):958–76.
46. Yao FY, Ferrell L, Bass NM, et al. Liver transplantation for hepatocellular carcinoma: expansion of the tumor size limits does not adversely impact survival. Hepatology 2001;33(6):1394–403.
47. Yao FY, Hirose R, LaBerge JM, et al. A prospective study on downstaging of hepatocellular carcinoma prior to liver transplantation. Liver Transpl 2005;11(12):1505–14.
48. Goldstein RM, Stone M, Tillery GW, et al. Is liver transplantation indicated for cholangiocarcinoma? Am J Surg 1993;166(6):768–71 [discussion: 71–2].
49. Rea DJ, Heimbach JK, Rosen CB, et al. Liver transplantation with neoadjuvant chemoradiation is more effective than resection for hilar cholangiocarcinoma. Ann Surg 2005;242(3):451–8 [discussion: 8–61].
50. Watt KD, Pedersen RA, Kremers WK, et al. Long-term probability of and mortality from de novo malignancy after liver transplantation. Gastroenterology 2009; 137(6):2010–7.
51. Nair S, Verma S, Thuluvath PJ. Obesity and its effect on survival in patients undergoing orthotopic liver transplantation in the United States. Hepatology 2002; 35(1):105–9.
52. Kemmer NM, Sherman KE. Liver transplantation trends in the HIV population. Dig Dis Sci 2011;56(11):3393–8.

Index

Note: Page numbers of article titles are in **boldface** type.

Clin Liver Dis 16 (2012) 449–466
doi:10.1016/S1089-3261(12)00043-8
liver.theclinics.com
1089-3261/12/$ – see front matter

D

I

J

L

M

T

U

V

W

Moving?

Make sure your subscription moves with you!

To notify us of your new address, find your **Clinics Account Number** (located on your mailing label above your name), and contact customer service at:

Email: journalscustomerservice-usa@elsevier.com

800-654-2452 (subscribers in the U.S. & Canada)
314-447-8871 (subscribers outside of the U.S. & Canada)

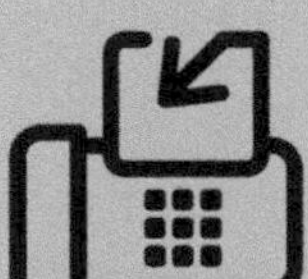

Fax number: 314-447-8029

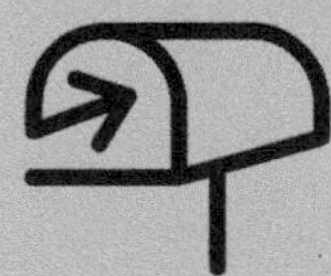

Elsevier Health Sciences Division
Subscription Customer Service
3251 Riverport Lane
Maryland Heights, MO 63043

*To ensure uninterrupted delivery of your subscription, please notify us at least 4 weeks in advance of move.

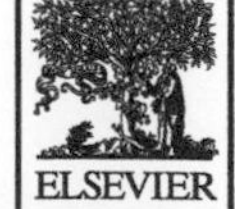

Printed and bound by CPI Group (UK) Ltd, Croydon, CR0 4YY

03/10/2024

01040454-0008